Managing Money, Measurement and Marketing in the Allied Health Professions

T0133884

Edited by

Robert Jones

and

Fiona Jenkins

Series Foreword by
Penny Humphris

Foreword by
Karen Middleton

Radcliffe Publishing
Oxford • New York

Radcliffe Publishing Ltd
18 Marcham Road
Abingdon
Oxon OX14 1AA
United Kingdom

www.radcliffepublishing.com
Electronic catalogue and worldwide online ordering facility.

British Library Cataloguing in Publication Data

A catalogue record for this book is available from the British Library.

ISBN-13: 978 1 84619 198 5

The paper used for the text pages of this book is FSC certified. FSC (The Forest Stewardship Council) is an international network to promote responsible management of the world's forests.

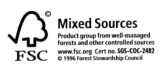

Mixed Sources
Product group from well-managed forests and other controlled sources
www.fsc.org Cert no. SGS-COC-2482
© 1996 Forest Stewardship Council

FSC

Typeset by Phoenix Photosetting, Chatham, Kent
Printed and bound by TJI Digital, Padstow, Cornwall

Contents

List of figures

List of tables

List of boxes

Series foreword

The NHS, the biggest organisation in the UK and reputedly the third largest in the world, is undergoing massive transformation. We know that effective leadership is essential if the health service is to achieve continuous improvement in the services it offers. It needs people from all types of backgrounds – clinical and managerial – to step up and take on leadership roles to shape the future of health improvement and healthcare delivery.

Leaders are needed at every level of the health service. The concept of leadership only coming from the top and being defined by position and title is now out of date. It is much more about ways of thinking and behaving and individuals seeing themselves as having the potential to make a real difference for patients. Effective leadership is about working in partnerships and teams to develop a vision for the future, set the direction, influence those whose input is needed and deliver results – a high quality, safe, timely and accessible health service for all.

Allied health professionals operate in every setting in which healthcare is delivered. You have unparalleled opportunities to help patients to lead their own care and to see how services to patients, clients and carers can be improved across entire patient pathways, crossing traditional professional and organisational boundaries to improve patients' experiences. You have the potential to make a difference by leading improvement and managing services and resources well.

There are already many outstanding leaders in the NHS in the allied health professions making a real difference to services. Two of them had the vision for this series of books and have worked with formidable energy and commitment to make them a reality. Robert and Fiona have both made a considerable investment in their own professional and personal development and delivered substantial improvements in the services for which they are responsible. They have increased their awareness, skills and knowledge and taken on leadership roles, putting into practice many of their ideas and learning. They have worked tirelessly to spread their learning and skilfully persuaded a great many academics and practitioners to contribute to these books to provide a rich collection of theories, tools, techniques and insights to help you.

This series of books has been written to encourage and support many more of you to embark on or to continue your development, to enhance your leadership and management skills, knowledge and experience and to give you confidence to take on new roles and responsibilities. I am sure that many of you, who have not previously considered yourselves as leaders will, when you have read these books, reconsider your roles and potential and take the next steps on your journeys.

Penny Humphris
Former Director of the NHS Leadership Centre
June 2010

Foreword

As we look to train and develop clinicians as practitioners, partners, managers and leaders in order to drive up the quality of healthcare, we must make sure that continuing professional development balances these aspects of any clinical professional role.

For the Allied Health Professions, pre-registration and continuing professional development have largely focused on the skills and competencies required of practitioners and partners, but the training required to develop managers and leaders has been rather ad hoc and pretty much left to individual clinicians who may be interested. We must take a more comprehensive approach in the future across the health and care system to developing the talent of clinicians as managers and leaders.

Traditionally, clinicians, as practitioners, have been the champions for the quality of clinical care and general managers have been the champions for corporate governance, in particular, finance. This 'splitting' of responsibilities is simply not sustainable in a world where every clinical decision has a resource implication and where disregarding the quality of clinical care for the sake of the 'bottom line' can have very serious consequences.

In order for clinicians to develop as leaders of their profession, of services across a care group, of organisations, regionally, nationally and internationally, it is crucial that we educate ourselves in the art and science of management. Not all managers are leaders, but all leaders must have sound generic management skills – these are what this book in the Essential Guides Series can help with.

Whilst health policy changes and varies in different countries, there are some basic concepts that clinicians must get to grips with if they are to ensure the sustainability of their services for the public and patients; this book together with the first three books in this series takes you through these concepts and their practical application.

Clinicians will have to apply even greater rigour to the measurement of their clinical practice in terms of patient safety, clinical outcomes and patient experience. They will need to take full advantage of digital technology in order to ensure the efficiency of their services. Clinicians simply *must* develop an understanding of the financial implications of the decisions they make, how to manage budgets and contracts and how to use the information they have to market their services. Being a professional clinician means understanding more than simply clinical practice!

I believe allied health professionals have a unique contribution to make in the transformation of the health and care system and ensuring it is fit for purpose now and in the future. I believe, however, that that contribution is under-valued at present and our services to patients and the public could be in jeopardy as a result – the difference we can make to people's lives could be lost. In order to change the situation, we must change ourselves and improve our development as clinicians. The prestigious authors in this book certainly facilitate this.

Fiona Jenkins and Robert Jones are two people who model exactly what can be achieved by taking control of one's own development outside of one's comfort zone and I am delighted that they are collaborating with others to share their expertise and experience.

Karen Middleton BSc(Hons)
Chief Health Professions Officer (England)
June 2010

Preface

In order to provide and facilitate effective management and leadership in the Allied Health Professions in the ever changing and dynamic environment of healthcare provision, AHP managers and leaders must be business 'savvy' as well as being clinical heads of clinical services. We need the knowledge, skills, experience, expertise and ability to ensure our services are responsive to patients' needs and expectations, that services are up to date, proactive rather than reactive and grounded in robust evidence. This evidence-base and solid foundation of expertise and knowledge is equally important in management and leadership as is the evidence base and expertise in clinical work. An environment in which we develop a motivated workforce with wide-ranging expertise, providing a quality experience for users of services is dependent not only on the commitment of staff to provide the best possible care, but also on management quality.

The main focus of this book is money, measurement and marketing – essential components – in the context of our management quality and leadership framework.

As the authors and editors of *Managing Money, Measurement and Marketing in the Allied Health Professions* we are privileged and excited to have brought together 18 nationally and internationally acknowledged and recognised experts from around the world as chapter contributors with great expertise and stature; all experts in their fields. As managers and leaders of healthcare services we can only provide what we have planned and worked out carefully, based on our knowledge, expertise, skills and abilities and we believe that this book is an important contribution towards supporting AHPs in the healthcare business management and leadership environment.

We need, for example, to understand how the finances of healthcare work, particularly in a cash-strapped environment so as to maximise the use of all resources. Nobody benefits from 'bean counting' for the sake of it, but everyone benefits from accountability and service provision based on quality evidence. Information and its management in the broadest sense is integral to almost everything we do and we need a thorough understanding of what it is about and how to use it. If you can't measure it, you can't manage it; that's equally true whether in relation to activity, performance management, clinical outcomes, risk, business planning or purchasing services – all of which are discussed in this book. Marketing our services – in the broadest sense – based on a robust foundation of business planning and business-case development, project management, service level agreements and specification are presented together with information and guidance about marketing as essential aspects of what we need to know and do. In order to market our services successfully, it is necessary to write clear, concise reports and hone our presentation skills; all of this – and much more – is set out and included within this book.

We present our own AHP toolkit for Benchmarking, Activity Sampling and Management Quality Matrix based on fourteen standards which we have developed over many years to help managers, leaders and their teams to both benchmark and assess management quality in their services; the Matrix can be used as a whole or in sections – Standard by Standard – as an on-going evaluation methodology. In common with our 'Assessment Tool' for the evaluation of management and leadership structures and organisation presented in the first book in our Allied Health Profession series – *Managing and Leading in the Allied Health Professions* – we have developed the Benchmarking and Matrix as evidence-based instruments for an evaluation of management quality issues.

We would like to thank our chapter contributors for sharing their expertise and knowledge. Also thanks to the contributor of our series foreword – Penny Humphris – and to Karen Middleton for her foreword to this book. Thanks to our publisher – Radcliffe Publishing.

We hope that *Managing Money, Measurement and Marketing in the Allied Health Professions* will be a helpful source of information, background, techniques and support which will be thought-provoking and a useful book for Allied Health Professionals and others involved in healthcare.

Robert Jones and Fiona Jenkins
June 2010

About the editors

Dr Robert Jones PhD, MPhil, BA, FCSP, Grad Dip Phys, MHSM, MMACP
Head of Therapy Services Directorate, East Sussex Hospitals NHS Trust

Robert has management responsibility for all therapy services in one of the largest Trusts in the UK. He leads a large team of therapy and support staff in acute services, primary care, external contracts and the independent sector.

A Physiotherapist by background, he is a former Chair and Vice President of the Chartered Society of Physiotherapy and registrant member of the HPC.

He was seconded to the Commission for Health Improvement for a year as the AHP consultant/advisor; he has represented AHPs on an NHS information authority project board. Robert has recently completed a five year term as a Governor of Moorfield's Eye Hospital NHS Foundation Trust, and is a member of the SHA Map of Medicine project board.

Robert has led a wide range of successful re-design projects and service innovations including national exemplars. He has published widely on management, clinical topics, IM&T in Allied Health Professions and is Honorary Fellow of the University of Brighton and Plymouth University. His PhD is in Management and MPhil is in Social policy.

Fiona Jenkins MA (dist), FCSP, Grad Dip Phys, MHSM, NEBS Dip(M), PGCO
Executive Director of Therapies and Health Sciences Cardiff and Vale University Health Board

Fiona is Director of one of the seven Local Health Boards in Wales, a new post taken up in 2010. Her responsibilities extend to the HPC registered staff, both AHPs and Health Scientists, in a large organisation including primary, community, secondary and tertiary care. She is Executive lead for a range of services including the Professional forum and Stroke services and Director of Therapies and Health Sciences lead for IM&T. Prior to this she was Clinical Director of Therapies in South Devon and lead for Map of Medicine and member of the national Map of Medicine co-ordination group. Fiona also previously held the post of Trust service re-design lead.

A former Council member and Vice President of the Chartered Society of Physiotherapy, Fiona has led and been involved with a large number of service improvement projects several of which have been award winning. She has extensive experience of care pathway development and service re-design across the health economy. She has also published widely. Fiona holds an MA (Dist.) in management and is currently undertaking research for a PhD in NHS management related to AHP services.

Fiona and Robert collaboratively lecture both nationally and internationally, lead masterclasses and workshops and give presentations on management and leadership topics and service re-design. They undertake AHP service management reviews and are commissioned for research and surveys.

They successfully completed the INSEAD NHS/Leadership Centre Clinical Strategists' programme at the Business School in Fontainebleau Paris and continue to undertake project work with the University. They have both been members of DH working groups for AHP information management and AHP Referral to Treatment projects.

They have a range of publications including the series of Allied Health Professions Essential Guides. Their website is: www.jjconsulting.org.uk.

List of contributors

Professor Gerry McSorley PhD
Senior Leadership Fellow NHSI
Interim Programme Director NHS National Leadership Council Board
Development Workstream
Visiting Professor, Healthcare Management and Leadership, University of
Lincoln
Former President of the Institute of Healthcare Management
Head of Board Level Development
NHS Institute for Innovation and Improvement
University of Warwick Campus
Coventry

Professor Rosalie A Boyce PhD, MBus, BSc, Grad Dip Dietetic, Grad Dip
Principal Research Fellow
Centre for Rural & Remote Area Health
University of Southern Queensland
Toowoomba
Australia

Professor Alan Gillies PhD, MA, MILT, MUKCHIP, Doctor Honoris Causa
Professor in Information Management
University of Central Lancashire

Margaret Hastings MBA (Dist), BA, FCSP
Physiotherapy Manager West Dumbartonshire CHP
NHS Greater Glasgow and Clyde Clinical Information/eHealth Lead
Chair National Clinical Data Development Programme NHS Scotland
AHP Information Advisor to Scottish Government Health Department
Chair of AHP eHealth Leads in NHS Scotland

Davis Ballestracci BS, MS
Harmony Consulting
Portland
USA

Professor Ann P Moore PhD, FCSP, FMACP, Grad Dip Phys, Cert Ed, Dip TP,
ILTM
Professor of Physiotherapy and Director of the Clinical Research Centre for
Health Professions
University of Brighton

Professor Stephen E Chick PhD
Professor of Technology and Operations Management
The Novartis Chaired Professor of Healthcare Management
INSEAD Fontainebleau
France

Professor Christoph Loch PhD
Professor of Technology and Operations Management
The GlaxoSmithKline Chaired Professor of Corporate Innovation
Dean of PhD Programme
INSEAD Fontainebleau
France

Professor Doctor Arnd Huchzermeier
Chair in Production Management of the WHU – Otto Beisheim School of
Management
Wissenschaftliche Hochschule für Unternehmensführung in Vallendar near
Koblenz, Germany
www.whu.edu/cms/index.php?id=535&L=1

Professor Jon Chilingerian PhD
Adjunct Professor of Organisational Behaviour
INSEAD Fontainebleau
France
Brandeis University
Heller School for Social Policy and Management
USA

Janice E Mueller NZRP, MNZSP, MNZCP, ADP(Paediatrics), MBA (Dist)
Director of Allied Health, Scientific & Technical
Auckland District Health Board
Auckland
New Zealand

Ian S Rowe
Management Consultant
Orion Health
Auckland
New Zealand

Julian Glover MA, BA Hons, DipIM, CIM
6X6 Creative Ltd
Canterbury
Kent

Julie Shepherd MCSP, DipMDT
Lead Physiotherapist
Gloucestershire Hospitals NHS Foundation Trust
Cheltenham General Hospital

Natalie Beswetherick OBE, MBA, FCSP
Director of Professional Development
Chartered Society of Physiotherapy
London

Dr Lesley Holdsworth PhD, FCSP
Head of Health Services Research and Effectiveness
NHS Quality Improvement Scotland
Glasgow

Zac Arif
Director
The Access Partnership
Middlesex

Dr Elizabeth Roberts PhD
Senior Associate and Independent Consultant
The Access Partnership
Middlesex

List of abbreviations

A&E	Accident and Emergency
AHP	Allied Health Profession
BAU	Business as Usual
BPPF	Best Practice Performance Frontier
BPM	Business Performance Management
CABG	Coronary Artery By-pass Graft
CEO	Chief Executive Officer
CHI	Commission for Health Improvement
CIP	Cost Improvement Programmes
CQC	Care Quality Commission
CRES	Cash Releasing Efficiency Savings
DEA	Data Envelopment Analysis
DH	Department of Health
DNAs	Did Not Attends
DRG	Diagnostic Related Groups
EBITDA	Earnings Before Interest, Taxes, Depreciation and Amortisation
ECDL	European Computer Driving Licence
EPR	Electronic Patient Record
FT	Foundation Trust
GDP	Gross Domestic Product
GP	General Practitioner
HIS	Hospital Information Systems
HPC	Health Professions Council
HR	Human Resources
HRG	Healthcare Resource Groups
ICD	International Classification of Disease
ICD-10	International Classifications of Diseases 10th Revision
ICF	International Classification of Functioning, Disability and Health
ICT	Information and Computer Technologies
IEA	Industrial Excellence Award
IHTSDO	International Health Terminology Standards Development Organisation
IM	Information Management
IM&T	Information Management and Technology
IP	Internet Protocol
IT	Information Technology
KPI	Key Performance Indicator
MFF	Market Forces Factor
MOH	Ministry of Health
MQM	Management Quality Matrix
NHS	National Health Service
NICE	National Institute for Health and Clinical Excellence
NLH	National Library for Health

NLOP	National Local Ownership Programme
NPfIT	National Programme for Information Technology
NPSA	National Patient Safety Agency
OH	Occupational Health
OPCS	Office of Population Censuses and Surveys
PACS	Picture Archiving and Communication System
PAS	Patient Administration System
PBC	Practice Based Commissioning
PbR	Payment by Results
PC	Personal Computer
PCT	Primary Care Trust
PDA	Personal Digital Assistants
PEST	Political, Economic, Social, Technological
PFI	Private Finance Initiative
PI	Performance Indicator
PR	Public Relations
PROMs	Patient Reported Outcome Measures
PROMIS	Patient Reported Outcome Measurement Information System
R&D	Research and Development
RBAC	Role-based access control
RFID	Radio-frequency identification
RSS	Really Simple Syndication
RTT	Referral to treatment Time
SFIs	Standing Financial Instructions
SHA	Strategic Health Authority
SLA	Service Level Agreement
SLR	Service Line Reporting
SNFs	Skilled Nurse Facilities
SMART	Specific, Measurable, Achievable, Realistic, Timed
SNOMED	Systematised Nomenclature of Medicine
SUS	Secondary User Service
SWOT	Strength, weakness, opportunity, threat
TCP	Transmission Control Protocol
TQM	Total Quality Management
TUC	Trades Union Congress
UK	United Kingdom
UPI	Unique Patient Identifier
USB	Universal Serial Bus
VAS	Visual Analogue Scale
WHO	World Health Organization
www	World Wide Web

List of books in this series

Chapter 1

The jigsaw of reform: pushing the parameters

Robert Jones and Fiona Jenkins

The jigsaw of reform

The Allied Health Professions (AHPs) are a key piece of the jigsaw of reform resulting from changes in global healthcare funding and provision. The pressure is on all of us to provide higher quality care for less cost. The focus of this chapter is an overview of the issues facing all of us, setting the scene for the detailed discussions which are presented in subsequent chapters related to money, measurement and marketing, to support our roles in successfully dealing with the challenges we are facing as healthcare managers and leaders.

Healthcare is fast moving and changing; the ways in which our services have been organised and managed are being challenged. The National Health Service (NHS), like other global health services, is facing a period of uncertainty – the only certainty being that cost savings are required. The NHS is required to make unprecedented savings. The scale is enormous and the pace that is needed is unprecedented. This is accompanied by the added pressure caused by service user expectations, the global economic downturn and 'credit crunch', together with public service pension deficit, demographic shifts and aging populations, developments in technology and innovation, the world wide web and ease of access to information, public services and the green agenda and many others. Organisational change is being driven by Governments worldwide in the quest to make public services efficient, effective and value for money. How will the global 'credit crunch' and the resulting enormous public sector borrowing requirement affect services and future funding allocations?

Is funding in your service assured? Do you, like most of the rest of the developed world, have growing requirements and a finite budget? One certainty is that AHP managers must be aware of politics, funding, technological change and the economics of healthcare in order to manage and lead their services effectively. The evidence base is growing and the effectiveness and contribution of AHP interventions is increasingly recognised. Our roles in assessment, diagnosis and management of acute and longer term conditions, as well as our growing scope of practice, places us well to contribute to this challenging agenda. Healthcare leaders and managers are increasingly being made accountable for the clinical, financial, corporate and information governance of the services they provide. Instead of providing care to patients there is a shift to engage patients in modelling the care they receive, putting patients at the centre of what we do, rather than just being the end point.

Providers of care – by whom to whom and where?

Our workforce is also changing, the different age profiles of our workforce have differing priorities and expectations. Whether starting a career, portfolio working, moulding it around family life, or whatever suits staff needs, jobs are less likely to be constant for a whole career. We need to ensure that our services meet the needs of individuals as well as service requirements, always looking ahead. Regulation is an increasingly important piece of the 'jigsaw of reform' and one that managers must be aware of in order to ensure compliance to safeguard patients. The ever increasing tendency for litigation requires practice to be of the highest quality supported by registration mechanisms. Careers are changing; they are much more competency based rather than skills and knowledge based, less profession specific with more blurring of old professional boundaries. Healthcare is moving towards a protocolised system to reduce variability and raise standards, this may be beneficial to service users and staff alike, but at the same time beware of the dangers of being over prescriptive. There are a number of workforce questions which will need to be addressed when developing a high quality workforce, for example:

1 Can the organisation afford all the staff needed?
2 Do your staff want to work the hours you need them for?
3 Do you provide a seven day service?
4 How skilled are your support staff?
5 Have you the right mix of grades and skills?

The 'baby boomer' generation – those born between 1945 and 1970 – have different aspirations from their parents. They have worked hard, are well informed, have high expectations from healthcare and want to remain fit. They do not want mixed sex wards, to wait for treatment or receive second best. They want the best, and they want it now! Their children have even higher expectations. The care we provide needs to fit our changing population, who they are and where they are, multicultural and acknowledging individual needs.

In the 21st century care is, and will increasingly be, provided in a wide variety of settings: hospital, multiple hospitals working in a network system, clinics, home, residential care, school, high street outlets, supermarkets, railway stations, health maintenance centres, aided living centres, devolved self-care models with clinical support, everywhere! There are many different models of health provision and commissioning, we work in different areas with differing needs. In England, for example, there are five levels of commissioning.

1 National commissioning schemes.
2 Regional group commissioning schemes.
3 Specialist care group commissioning schemes.
4 GP group commissioning schemes.
5 GP individual level choice.

Care purchasers will determine what is required, we must be prepared to diversify and meet the challenges of purchasing and provision.

Technology

Developing technologies are transforming many aspects of healthcare, from advances in imaging techniques, to telemedicine and the electronic patient health record. Information technology with advanced informatics and decision-making to support safer practices all require the use, storage and sharing of data. Rapid changes in technology be they clinical, educational or managerial are in place now and will be the shape of things to come. Technology is changing the way in which service users access care and how they can be supported through the use of multimedia. This is seen through the growing use of electronic appointment booking systems and the exchange of clinical information by electronic transmission between care providers. AHPs and their leaders must embrace this technological age or be left at best playing catch-up or at worst decommissioned.

Changes in organisation

Change in the NHS is a continual cycle, arguably too much change without 'bedding in' best practice and the benefits of experience. However, to stand still is not an option for anyone. Changes in healthcare are driven by financial, political, economic and social factors. Consumer changes, with increasing life expectancy, the increase in long term conditions, widespread access to health information and increasing demand for quality, quantity and immediacy of healthcare have required health strategists to re-evaluate the organisation and structure of healthcare services in the developed world. AHP managers have often been required to consider what might be the 'best' organisational structure for their services – this remains a recurrent challenge.

The importance of organisational structure cannot be ignored as the structure supports the context for the provision of the most effective clinical service, improved clinical outcomes and sharing of information, improved communication, clinical governance and the management of risk. Management structures should be defined after the functions of a service are determined.

Who is the profession for? Increasingly healthcare is developing workforces and capacity through the use of highly skilled and competent practitioners rather than depending on workforce development based on the traditional profession centred approach. Emphasis is increasingly on the patient's experience in health and social care with services provided by multi-disciplinary teams in vertical and horizontal integration models, not interrupted by organisational boundaries or professional barriers which might militate against streamlined working. This is likely to increasingly involve alternative patterns of employment in which staff are employed in multidisciplinary networks centred around specific clinical clusters such as cancer networks, children's services, elderly care services rather than uni-professional structures. However, the process is by no means complete, there is little doubt that the role and power of the profession has evolved in the context of rapidly changing needs.

Successful collaborative working places the patient or service user at the centre. Whilst working towards this objective we need to acknowledge and respect the backgrounds, skill, knowledge and competencies of one another from every professional background whilst at the same time forging new inter and multi-disciplinary structures.

Although we are embarking on a remodelling of organisational structures to support our service provision, there are many positive attributes which flow from our professional backgrounds and we can take forward into the future including: putting the patient first – subordinating self-interest; the pursuit of continual improvement and service re-design; collaborative team working; professional behaviour and a willingness to redraw and breakdown professional boundaries. The most important thing for our patients is the quality, responsiveness and affordability of our care and essentially the quality of outcomes we achieve working with our service users.

Clinical heads of clinical services

AHP managers and leaders provide clinical consultancy, work within a shared understanding, knowledge, skills and competence base. There are many good reasons why AHP managers and leaders bring benefits to organisations and patient care, such as:

- the understanding which flows from being educated and trained as a clinician
- education and development in leadership and management skills
- lead and manage by example from the clinical knowledge and skills base
- empathy with patients and professionals which flows from the clinical background
- ability to represent the clinical service from a background of coming from within it
- clinical leadership and consultancy giving credibility.

It is essential to use this expertise and experience giving managers and leaders authority, responsibility and accountability whether they are combined managers and professional leads or clinical leaders within a general management model. Heads of AHP services are clinical heads of clinical services and there is a link between the professional background and management and leadership. Whatever model is in place as always the patient must be at the centre of all our efforts whether our base is in healthcare, education or social care.

Culture

Culture defines not only who you are but how you operate, both as an individual and as a group. Culture is the social and psychological environment in which people operate. Staff read signals from that culture, often unconsciously, about how they should and should not behave, and how they can and cannot behave. If an organisation or service wishes to influence the behaviour of its staff in particular directions, it has to create and sustain a culture from which people will read the signals. If we wish staff to behave consistently, the cultural messages need to be consistent and coherent. Mixed cultural messages cause staff unnecessary stress and confusion and lead to inconsistent behaviours as they try to guess what the organisation really wants of them.

Pushing the parameters

In an environment of continuing and rapidly increasing change we need to be proactive and responsive to political, economic, social and technological imperatives. This requires the AHP manager to push the parameters of their services. Fundamental to the management quality and innovation necessary to thrive are:

- putting research into practice, both developing and implementing the evidence base
- rigorous use of information to support management and clinical practice
- reduction of waste
- risk taking to bring about innovation and new developments
- learning from other services and being able to adapt to improve
- sharing experience and knowledge, and supporting others
- workforce development at all levels
- facilitating expert clinical practice
- involving patients in service evaluation and development
- ensuring educational and professional development
- nurturing and facilitating clinical leadership
- robust management including performance management
- audit and critical evaluation leading to service improvement
- challenging traditional working patterns to provide better continuity, for example, seven day working and extended days
- commitment to quality improvement and cost containment
- being business 'savvy' as well as a healthcare provider
- having a business plan, know your market, know your competitors
- developing your strategy with your team.

AHPs can take a lead in pushing the parameters of integrated pathway design, the use of data and information to enable these developments and to create an evidence-base.

Other strategies may include re-profiling services through skill mix, peer review and developing the workforce in new and innovative ways, for example, developing the skills of non-graduate colleagues. There are also many examples of extended scope and expert practice such as supplementary prescribing, case-managing, imaging and injection therapy, which push the parameters and enhance our outcome focus. Importantly, engaging our service users in re-design will ensure the parameters of AHPs remain patient focussed.

Beware of pitfalls, fads and whims

In pushing the parameters and shaping tomorrow beware of pitfalls, fads and whims and do not forget the past by embarking on change for change's sake, not recognising what you have that works well; if it's not broken don't fix it. There are many service improvement techniques and methodologies available to managers and leaders. However there is sometimes a danger that individual approaches can be over-emphasised and adopted as the one and only method turning the process into single track management by whim.

Techniques such as quality circles, lean thinking, Six Sigma, continuous quality improvement, re-engineering, TQM and PDSA all have an important place, but not when used in isolation. It is therefore beholden for the AHP manager to be skilled, trained and competent in the use of a wide range of approaches.

Shaping tomorrow – break the rules that stifle change

Be sure to break the 10 rules which stifle change.

Box 1.1 The rules which stifle change, which MUST be broken.

1 Regard any new idea from below with suspicion
2 Insist a hierarchy exists
3 Criticise others' ideas
4 Treat problems as a sign of failure
5 Express criticisms; don't praise
6 'Name and shame'
7 Control everything
8 Plan change in secret
9 Delegate difficult decisions
10 Count everything that moves…frequently

These are rules that definitely should be broken. From time to time all of us will have been subjected to, or guilty of, one of these negative behaviours. In order to push the parameters effectively:

- make sure we are fit for purpose
- develop a vision
- value yourself
- ensure relevant roles for managers and leaders
- develop consultancy skills
- work together, respecting differences
- promote cross boundary multidisciplinary and interdisciplinary working.

Leadership

The reform jigsaw requires exceptional AHP leaders. Leadership in the NHS has traditionally been perceived as being hierarchical, defined by job title, position and grade or band. Though some of this remains true today there has been a growing acknowledgement that leadership is required at many levels and throughout the whole career of a healthcare professional. The key to leadership is using ways of thinking and behaving that effect change and bring about positive improvements regardless of position or rank.

Early in the 20th century it was suggested that successful leaders possessed certain inherent qualities. This so-called 'trait theory approach' attempted to identify personality-based characteristics. Later it was demonstrated that success was often achieved despite the application of less desirable styles and behaviour. These limitations led to the application of 'contingency theory', indicating that it was not leadership style as such that led to effective leadership but the ability of the leader to adapt their style to the needs of their followers. The balance between the needs of the team, its members and the tasks to be undertaken all need to be weighed up to obtain the desired outcomes. Therefore, the desired models of leadership are both transactional and transformational.

The NHS of the 21st century[1] requires a model that is 'not based on heroism, but on enabling others to lead themselves, not about being an extraordinary person; but being open accessible and *transparent*'.[2] A liberal measure of emotional intelligence,[3] with motivation, self-awareness, emotional resilience, integrity and consciousness is required to lead in the NHS at this time. Gantz,[4] describes leadership as:

   Enabling others to achieve purpose in the face of uncertainty.

Leadership cannot be taught through academic study alone or learned purely through experience, it requires a combination of the two along with reflection to develop future action. This therefore requires some inherent qualities, the desire to learn and the ability to adapt. AHP services need inspired, enthusiastic, disciplined and focussed management and leadership.

Social movements

Social movements have developed as the result of organisations and individuals asserting public values and forming new relationships rooted in those values to mobilise political, economic and cultural power and translate this into action.[5]

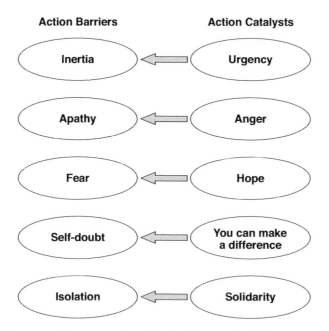

Figure 1.1 Values to action – emotions that facilitate and inhibit purposeful action.[4]

Social movements are strategically driven, involving large groups of people who are organised and passionate about the changes they want to make.

The NHS leadership community recommends that social movements could be the answer to the demanding health agenda enabling services to meet the challenge of possibility at a time of uncertainty.[6] The requirement to deliver transformational high speed change requires the workforce to be highly motivated and inspire action ensuring staff become emotionally charged and impassioned to deliver the scale of change needed.[7] The focus that will connect with staff to bring about change is about improving services for patients, with a focus on purpose, values and quality rather than cost. Shared values are a prerequisite for commitment. Techniques such as narrative and storytelling can trigger powerful emotional connection with values.

Key to making transformational change is the ability for leaders to turn values into action. This requires leaders to 'frame' the strategic messages in a way that connects with staff rather than one that demotivates and demoralises.

Is everyone the architect of their own future?

AHP managers and leaders might consider their personal building blocks necessary for influencing future patterns of working. Perhaps the key aspirations listed in Box 1.2 are worthy of consideration.

Box 1.2 Key aspirations.

1 Always ensure that patients are your top priority
2 Hold onto the healthcare expertise and excellence you have striven for
3 Be flexible, innovative, 'future proof' and be the solution not the problem
4 Be business minded and business skilled, aim to provide the service you would choose to use yourself
5 Nurture, develop and support your staff
6 Keep costs under control; be responsible but also entrepreneurial
7 Look at your processes, can you do better?
8 Ensure AHPs work collaboratively, leave professional 'silos' behind
9 Know and value yourself; holding onto your core values
10 Demonstrate value for money, compete in the market place and strive to be the best

---

The mastery of money, measurement and marketing are essential elements of the management and leadership process for AHPs. The purpose of this chapter has been to focus on some of the key pieces which form the jigsaw of reform, which AHP managers and leaders will need to address in framing their services to be fit for the demanding future.

References

1 DH. *NHS Plan*. London: DH; 2000: www.dh.gov.uk/en/Publicationsandstatistics/Publications/PublicationsPolicyandGuidance/DH_4002960.

2 Alimo-Metcalfe B. *Effective Leadership*. London: Local Government Management Board; 1998.
3 Goleman D. What makes a leader? *Harvard Bus Rev*.1998: Nov/Dec; 94–102.
4 Gantz M. *What is Public Narrative?* Harvard University; 2008: www.hks.harvard.edu/about/faculty-staff-directory/marshall-ganz.
5 Rochon T. *Culture Moves Ideas, Activism and Change Values*. Princeton, NJ: Princeton University Press; 1998.
6 Bevan H. *How do we mobilise the NHS leadership community and workforce at scale for cost and quality improvement? A call to action, a provocation and a proposed was forward*. Draft consultation. Warwick: NHS Institute for Innovation and Improvement; 2010.
7 NHS I 2009. *Living our Local Values: the value of values;* 2009: www.institute.nhs.uk.

Chapter 2

Money, money, money: fundamentals of finance

Robert Jones and Fiona Jenkins

Introduction

As the largest employer and service organisation in Western Europe, the NHS consumes vast financial resources. Although the NHS has been subject to constant change since its inception in 1948, there is much that has remained unchanged such as:

- the principle that the service is free at the point of use or provision. Wanless[1] confirmed the view that funding the NHS through taxation is 'fair and efficient'
- the requirement to manage within overall funding limits determined annually by the Government
- the need to match finite resources to infinite demand
- the policy that ongoing efficiency savings will be made, for example, through Cost Improvement Programmes (CIP) and Cash Releasing Efficiency Savings (CRES)
- scrutiny of the NHS through constant public and media interest.

Health is always an important priority for any government and as such the NHS receives a major share of funding from the public purse. Spending on healthcare in the UK is the second largest budget after social protection/welfare; it is larger than defence, education, public order and safety. The main source of NHS funding is taxation; National Insurance with other sources of funding such as private healthcare provision, charitable donations, money voted by parliament – including the research and development levy – and supplementary sources such as car parking charges. During recent years – before the 'credit crunch'– healthcare spending increased at a significantly higher rate than in other government programmes. More than 99% of spending on healthcare comes from public funding.[2] The development of the NHS reflects a cyclical pattern of change, but there are important differences in emphasis between each cycle. New terminology comes to life with each new phase of development adding to, and sometimes replacing, the previous language and the practices reflected by this.

  The main focus of this chapter is to set out an overview of key issues in NHS finance in relation to policy, procedures and practice changes and business developments including briefing notes and definitions to support AHPs to 'negotiate' the way around the maze of financial and business functions.

NHS funding and key policy developments

In 2006 the total spending on healthcare in the UK was £120 billion, representing 9.4% of Gross Domestic Product (GDP).[3] The GDP is the value of all goods and services provided in the country by residents and non-residents. This corresponds to the total sum of expenditure – consumption and investment – in the private and public sectors. The total expenditure on healthcare is the sum of general government and private health expenditure in a given year on healthcare. Within the NHS Operating Framework for 2009 there was a predicted spend of £74.2 billion (annex to main operating framework), on top of that there would be significant other expenditure bearing in mind that not all funding is channelled through the PCT commissioners.

The allocation of funding by the government rests with the Chancellor of the Exchequer who is the government minister responsible for heading up the Treasury. The mechanism in place for funding allocation is through periodic spending reviews which lay down fixed three year government department spending limits. In recent years the comprehensive spending reviews have taken place in alternate years. Following a special review of NHS funding in 2002 a five year plan was put in place following the Wanless review[1] which was intended to put the NHS on a sustainable financial footing. Government spending reviews are further examined twice each year at the pre-budget review in the late autumn and in the budget. Funding allocation for healthcare in Scotland, Wales and Northern Ireland is included in separate block grants. Changes in planned spending on the NHS in England are matched by increases in these block grants, but the individual Administrations may flex this spending to a level above or below the grant depending on their own priorities.

The flow of funding from government sources is:

- Parliament sets the broad policy, decides structures and allocates the funding
- the DH sets overall policy on healthcare and social care – responsible for high quality healthcare provision through the NHS
- Strategic Health Authorities (SHAs) are required to provide leadership, co-ordination and support in defined geographical areas; they are not providers of healthcare services. There are ten SHAs in England which act as the 'local' headquarters
- there are a number of Special Health Authorities such as National Patient Safety Agency (NPSA), NHS Institute for Innovation and Improvement, NHS Litigation Authority, NHS Blood and Transplant. These organisations have a national remit rather than a local or regional one
- there are other 'arms length' bodies such as the National Institute for Health and Clinical Excellence (NICE) and the regulators. The duties of these organisations include, for example, setting and improving standards, inspection, regulation and promoting public welfare across health and social care.

What is the money spent on?

Approximately 80% of NHS funding is allocated by the DH to the PCT commissioners of healthcare services where it is further allocated to hospitals,

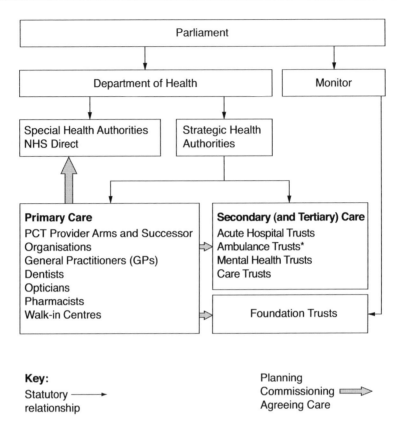

Key:

Statutory ——→
relationship

Planning
Commissioning ⇒
Agreeing Care

*Ambulance Trusts also work with NHS Direct and via the 999 system to respond to emergencies – this is regarded as part of Primary Care.

Figure 2.1 The structure of the NHS in England – funding flow. Adapted from 'An Introductory Guide to NHS Finance in the UK'.[2]

community and family health services – secondary, tertiary and primary care. Together with this there are a range of smaller budgets, for example, for dental and ophthalmic services, support to the voluntary sector and the running costs of the DH itself.

In summary, the government – advised by the Treasury – allocates money to the DH. The annual allocation or budget is made up of a revenue allocation which is for current expenditure, that is the day to day money for salaries and consumables and a capital allocation for expenditure on large long life items such as land and buildings. The running cost of the DH is 'top-sliced' from the NHS budget for its own running costs, for special allocations and centrally funded projects. Some of this is allocated to Trusts undertaking teaching and research. Funding is also made available to the SHAs for running costs and development support for organisations within their local boundaries.

The 80% funding for PCT commissioning is calculated to reflect local differences based on a weighted capitation formula. The formula includes a base which is the total population covered by a PCT and the total is then adjusted to take account of the age distribution of the population, additional needs, social problems and morbidity and unavoidable geographical variations in the cost of services.

The allocation is designed to fund:

- commissioning of hospital and primary care services
- providing some community services directly
- improving the health of the population
- PCTs own infrastructure and running costs
- the commissioners – purchasers – use the majority of their funds to set up Service Level Agreements (SLAs) with providers – NHS Trusts and Foundation Trusts (FTs). The PCTs purchase hospital services and also purchase services from the private or independent sector.

Key policy developments relevant to NHS financial resource allocation include:

- purchaser/provider split
- Practice based Commissioning
- payment by results
- foundation trusts
- contestability
- independent treatment centres
- NICE recommendations
- new technologies and developments in diagnostics and treatments.

Costing and pricing

Relatively little work has been undertaken on costing and pricing AHP services in the NHS. There are many reasons why work in this area is now taking place with increasing urgency. Within the NHS and healthcare services worldwide there is increasing emphasis on value for money, accountability for the use of resources, the need to adopt a business-like approach, for all clinical services to be able to demonstrate 'added value' and the requirement for effective and efficient service provision.

Perhaps the most important initiative in the context of robust financial management within the NHS has been the introduction of the purchaser provider split in which provider functions have been separated off from purchasing (*see* Chapter 3).

The recently enacted health service reforms under which commissioners purchase services from a variety of providers increases the urgency for sound costing and pricing mechanisms to be put in place. AHP managers and leaders will undoubtedly become increasingly involved in this work. An important element in the implementation of costing and pricing mechanisms is robust data collection analysis, interpretation and conversion to meaningful information. AHP managers will need to be aware of data use; this issue is explored in detail in Chapters 6 to 9.

It may be that some purchasers and providers will decide that it is easier to cost and price AHP services as overheads to larger service contracts. However, meaningful AHP costing and pricing mechanisms will provide opportunities for these services to be recognised in their own right, for the essential contributions they make to overall healthcare provision. In a system where money is supposed to follow patients, this should be a positive step for the AHP services, even though it might be 'painful' arriving at a workable and satisfactory solution. AHP services are core to healthcare provision just as medicine, nursing and drugs. It stands to reason, therefore, that these services are properly costed and priced and that levels of service are clearly identified and agreed.

Costing and pricing mechanisms in AHP services are not yet fully developed; however, many of the 'tools' needed are already available, but there is no universally agreed methodology, although mechanisms are gradually being put in place in several locations around the country.

Service costing may be set up on the basis of:

- *cost per contact*, under this system, payment is made for each individual item of activity – contact – and income is dependent upon the activity provided. In other words, increased activity equals increased income and vice versa
- *cost per episode of care*, in this system the provider is paid for the completed episode of care
- *cost and volume*, in which there are indicative activity levels and as soon as the agreed level is exceeded extra income may be generated by agreement
- *block contracts*, where block sums of money are made available to deliver an indicative activity level. This can be set up in such a way that if the activity varies above or below the agreed activity level by a certain percentage, the income may be flexed accordingly.

Reference costs are calculated annually in respect of NHS service providers. NHS organisations are required by the DH to submit a schedule of costs of Healthcare Resource Groups (HRGs) to facilitate direct comparison of the relative costs of different service providers. This annual exercise for all Trusts in England and Wales provides a quantum of costs divided by the total activity within the Trusts. The activity is divided, for example, between patient types, elective cases, day cases, non elective cases, out-patients and others. In the case of physiotherapy, for example, reference costs for direct access GP referred out-patients will be the cost of service provision divided by the number of patients seen within the period. Reference costs include all costs – including overheads – to service lines and down to HRGs. It is essential to have good quality data, whether computerised or manual, to provide accurate, timely and relevant information for this purpose.

At the end of the reference cost exercise, each organisation has a reference cost index constructed from the calculation; 100% is the national average. Any percentage above the 100% level, means that your service is more expensive than the national average. Below this level, the service is more cost efficient. It is generally acknowledged throughout the NHS that the reference cost system is flawed for a variety of reasons. However, it is used as an important factor in calculating funding allocations for services.

Definitions

When the authors started out as AHP managers the 'learning curve' for financial management was steep and there was little help available for managers of clinical services such as ours. Even though this has greatly improved recently, we thought that some guidance on definition of key terms would be useful. We do acknowledge that the topic of finance can be 'dry'; however understanding finance is a fundamental part of the AHP manager's role. We also acknowledge that finance departments in all NHS organisations are the experts in this field and can be called upon to support and advise AHP managers, but it is important in the context of present day healthcare provision and business that AHP managers and others are familiar with the language and use of key terms.

Budget

> **Box 2.1 Budget.**
>
> A budget is an organisation or individual's plan or target for income and expenditure. It's not always money, it can represent budgeted activity.
>   There are three main types of budget:
>
> 1 *Incremental:* where last year's budget is allocated and incremental changes added for the new financial year. AHP budgets are often incremental, starting from last year's position with changes to reflect required savings such as CRES, pay increases and uplift to reflect agreed increases in activity. Benefits of this method are that the system is easy to maintain and administer. However, inaccuracies become apparent very quickly when services alter, and the system is not flexible enough to change in response to variations in activity.
> 2 *Activity based budgets:* where the budget is 'flexed' in relation to changes in activity. The more activity, the greater the funding. This can also occur in the opposite way so that decreases in activity result in decreased funding. An example of this in AHP services is funding on a cost per contact basis, in out-patient physiotherapy or podiatry services. A benefit of this method is that changes in activity levels are recognised and in-year changes in activity are therefore reflected in funding changes. A disadvantage of this system is the difficulty of obtaining suitable and agreed accurate activity measures as a foundation for 'flexing' the budget. This method of budgeting requires clarity about fixed costs, semi-fixed costs and variable costs and is not yet widely used within the NHS, but it may become more common as funding and financial flow changes.
> 3 *Zero-based budgeting:* where the starting point is a blank balance sheet. All budgets are calculated on agreed activity levels and costs associated with them. This method requires a clear statement of objectives or intended outcomes, identification of ways to achieve them, ability to foresee and identify all resources and the costs needed to achieve the outcomes. This system uses benchmarking techniques to identify best clinical and financial practice. The main benefit is that zero-based budgeting is accurate in relation to what is going on at any given time. It has good 'ownership' from budget holders as it is an important pre-requisite that they are essential to the budget setting process. An important disadvantage is that the method is time consuming and it is often argued that it increases the budget too much. Zero-based budgeting is used most often in the context of planning new services and service reviews.

The finance department will provide monthly, quarterly and annual budget reports. Generally, the report identifies each department and the period to which it refers. The report is set out in four main sections:

1 pay
2 non-pay
3 recharges
4 income.

Figure 2.2 shows an example of a budget sheet.

Line number	Budget WTE	Actual WTE	Annual budget	Budget in month	Expenditure in month	Variance in month	Budget to date	Cumulative expenditure	Variance

Figure 2.2 Example of budget sheet layout.

The columns usually come in the following order from left to right: the line number, budget whole time equivalent(WTE), actual WTE, annual budget, budget in month, expenditure in month, variance in month, budget to date, cumulative expenditure, variance.

1 Pay includes all items of remuneration; including monthly salaries, overtime, on-call and standby payments, locum agency payments and so on.
2 Non-pay includes payments to suppliers for goods and services, travel expenses, uniforms, equipment, maintenance, consumables, study leave costs, travel and so on.
3 Recharges are made up of cross-charges between different departments/ organisations to ensure the purchaser of the service bears the cost.
4 Income includes budgeted income such as SLA income and funds received from, for example, income generation projects.

Budget reports can be illustrated graphically (*see* Figure 2.3).

The reports enable financial control, monitoring of the financial position and corrective action to be taken. It is the responsibility of the budget holder and budget manager to keep the financial position continually under review, to manage cost pressures and to take decisions about the affordability of planned changes, to balance the budget and improve value for money and ensure improvements.

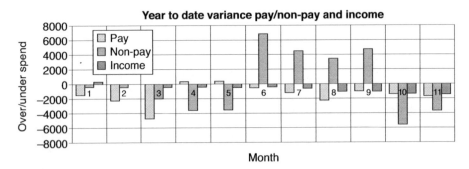

Figure 2.3 Monthly budget summary.

Cost

> **Box 2.2 Cost.**
>
> Cost is taken to mean the expenditure incurred to produce goods or provide a service. The cost of providing a service in healthcare must take into account expenditure on workforce, equipment, drugs, facilities and various overheads. The cost of a service to a purchaser is the measurement in cash terms of what the purchaser must spend in order to obtain that service. When a service provider sells a service, they will normally sell at the price sufficient to cover full costs, plus profit where this is appropriate.

Hierarchy of costs

The hierarchy of costs (*see* Figure 2.4) sets out some overheads; corporate functions such as finance department, human resources and payroll; support services such as facilities and housekeeping, as well as indirect costs such as radiology and clinical support services.

In the NHS therapy in-patients are often classed as indirect costs. Direct costs are for example, ward costs, nursing pay, non-pay such as consumables, medical staff pay.

Costing: the system by which the cost of service provision is calculated.

Marginal costs: the additional cost incurred by producing just one more unit of production or treating one more patient over the agreed volume.

Variable costs: costs which vary according to level of activity, for example, materials.

Fixed costs: do not vary when activity increases or decreases. In some respects, pay costs are fixed because of manpower and contract constraints. Even if a hospital

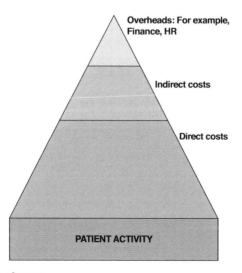

Figure 2.4 Hierarchy of costs.

is empty, there would still be fixed costs in terms of capital charges or rates for example. Fixed costs will probably increase each year.

Semi fixed costs: difficult to identify; for example, in an empty facility just opening its doors to service provision, as patients started using the rooms, electricity consumption would increase. Clearly, this varies with increasing use. Semi-fixed costs are also known as 'step' costs. The costs remain fixed within a given level of activity, but change takes place if activity falls below, or rises above, a certain level. A semi-fixed cost is a cost whose magnitude is only affected by the level of activity, although there is a relationship between activity and spending, it is not directly proportional whereas a variable cost is one in which the magnitude varies proportionally with the level of activity.

Opportunity cost: in the NHS scarcity of resources is an everyday challenge for managers, providers and commissioners in all areas. Limited resources necessitates 'trade-offs' and this results in opportunity costs. While the cost of a service is most often thought of in financial terms, the opportunity cost of a decision is based on what must be given up – the next best alternative – as a result of the decision. Decisions which involve two or more options have an opportunity cost. This concept is useful when undertaking an options appraisal.

Overhead costs: incurred by the service provider over and above the direct cost of providing the service itself and the material associated with this. Examples of such costs will be building maintenance and administration.

On-costs: the costs of employing a member of staff over and above their salaries including for example employer's National Insurance and superannuation contributions.

Standard costs: planned target costs for an area of activity or unit of production, for example, a standard cost per case could be calculated, assuming the average costs incurred in treating a certain type of condition. In practice, the actual cost of treating each case may turn out to be more or less than the pre-calculated standard.

Recurrent costs: any item that is payable year after year, such as staff pay.

Non-recurrent costs: in place for a fixed time only for specific projects or schemes. An example of non-recurrent might be 'deep cleaning' of hospital wards and financial allocations which take place on a relatively ad hoc basis.

Capital charges: a mixture of depreciation on fixed assets and an interest charge on the 'book value' of those assets. In effect, capital charges are a device for ensuring that there is a cost associated with owning capital. A charge is made to the income and expenditure account of the organisation on all capital assets except donated assets and those with no net 'book value'. The rate of return is set by the Treasury.

Price: this represents the sum at which services are bought or sold. It is a measure of what a purchaser must spend in order to obtain the service.

Payment by results (PbR)

PbR was set up to bring about change in the way finance moves between commissioners – purchasers – and providers of services. It does not relate to the way commissioners receive their funding as this is received from the DH and is based on capitation. PbR is intended to be a method by which providers are paid for the actual work they do at a national pre set rate. It is not practical to construct a separate price for every single treatment/procedure, so activities are grouped together according to 'typical' treatment episodes in which they occur and a tariff price is set for each grouping. However, not all activities are included in PbR; it has been an important policy in Government reform of the financial framework and funding streams within the NHS. The overriding objective is that money flows with the patient enabling a further key element of government policy; strengthening choice for service users. The theory is that by introducing standard tariffs, the need for negotiations at local level on price is minimised or eliminated so that the focus can be on quality and service responsiveness. In summary, this method was introduced in 2003–04 to support patient choice and plurality of provision by fixing a national tariff for acute hospital activity, whereby the discussion should take place on quality of care rather than price. PbR accounts for the majority of hospital care with the remainder of funding going on local tariff or block contracts. The system is based on reference costs.

Market forces factor

Within the PbR regime there is one tariff nationally for much acute care. However, recognising that the costs of individual care arise according to the location of the organisation, each Trust receives a Market Forces Factor (MFF) adjustment, paid centrally by the DH. This supplements the tariff. The MFF is paid each month and at the end of the year a final return is adjusted up or down.

Staff establishment

This is the agreed level of funded staffing.

Cross charging

A method of funding indirect cost centres or support departments for the inputs they make. This can be managed informally by financial adjustments within the month, or managed formally with specific SLAs. They describe not only the likely activity units to be provided but also the quality standards and other targets. A disadvantage of this system is that it can be overly bureaucratic.

Cost improvement programmes (CIP)

The identification of schemes to reduce spending and increase activity. The Treasury expects the NHS to become more efficient every year.

Private finance initiative (PFI)

This scheme was introduced by the government in the early 1990s. It is a scheme which enables investment in new buildings and property. It is public/private partnership designed to fund capital projects without depending on public money in the short term. The NHS works with private sector partners who are contracted to design and build the facilities required.

Charitable funds

Donations from the public both individuals and organisations.

Standing financial instructions (SFI)

SFIs are the rules governing financial probity including how individuals need to operate in purchasing and all other financial transactions. AHP managers are required to adhere to SFIs and to sign off annually that they have read and understood the documentation.

EBITDA

Earnings before interest, taxes, depreciation and amortisation. This has recently been introduced into the NHS, having been used widely in the private sector. It is a method of comparing organisations without distortion of the financial position. This represents what profit or surplus is available before interest, tax and depreciation. Meaningful comparison is made possible by comparing profits at the 'bottom line'. It is regarded as a 'good proxy for operating cash flow. As such, it provides an indication of the organisation's ability to reinvest in asset replacement and service innovation and to meet financing charges and dividends'.[4]

There are six main steps in calculating EBITDA, these are:

1   to calculate net income, obtain total income and subtract total expenses
2   determine tax owed
3   compute interest charges
4   establish the cost of depreciation
5   ascertain the cost of amortisation, the reduction of the value of assets by prorating its cost over a period of years. In respect of intangible assets it is identical to depreciation which relates to tangible assets
6   add all of these components: the resulting figure is then subtracted from total expense. The final figure is then subtracted from the revenue to arrive at EBITDA.

EBITDA is in effect, operating profit after adding back the specific non-cash items of depreciation and amortisation.

For AHP managers, this is relevant to profit available from contract activity for services provided as part of an organisation. For example, in direct access service provision which is the subject of GP referral, income is derived from each item of service provided. The EBITDA can be interpreted as profit on such activity. Organisations have a target percentage for EBIDTA and a plus figure in excess of this indicates a profitable situation; it is another way of identifying the financial performance.

Service line reporting (SLR)

This measures a trust's profitability by each of its service lines, rather than just an aggregate for the whole trust. At service line level it is possible to monitor cost, income, activity and resources separately. Effective SLR requires good leadership at service line level, a clear strategy for the goals that the service will achieve, effective operational planning and budgeting through which annual targets are set against all key metrics, effective financial controls for delivering against plan, and effective operational management.

SLR enables a trust to increase its productivity by giving the necessary financial information to:

- make informed decisions
- manage performance against agreed levels of financial performance at the service line.

Patient level costing

Traditionally, the NHS has used average costs – reference costs – to look at specific procedure costs such as hip replacement, emergency care or the cost of accident and emergency attendances. Under patient level costing, costs are identified to individual patients. This method 'pulls' information from a range of systems within the organisation, to identify the cost of providing care to a single patient. For example: two patients have a hip replacement operation. One patient has hip prosthesis 'A' and the other prosthesis 'B' from another source; one takes 2 hours, the other three hours. Hip 'A' cost £2,000 and hip 'B' £3000. Under the original system both patients might be costed at £2,500 – the average costs – and the theatre cost would be averaged out between them also. Under patient level costing, patient A would be costed at £2,000 plus two hours theatre time and patient B at £3,000 and three hours theatre time; in other words the actual cost per patient. This system requires input from many information systems within the organisation and requires accurate patient level data which is consistent across all systems to enable calculation of costs.

Practice based commissioning (PBC)

PBC is a policy under which the responsibility for commissioning healthcare services is devolved from PCT commissioners to GP practices. Practices are given budgets which they use for purchasing services and may join up with other practices to develop PBC consortia. The process includes identification of needs, designing effective and relevant service responses and allocation of resources against competing services' priorities and demands. The role of the PCT is to act as agent for the practices to procure services.

> 'Practice Based Commissioning is about empowering GPs and other clinicians such as nurses, pharmacists and Allied Health Professions to shape the health and healthcare of local populations.'[5]

The objective is that GPs are given greater control of resources so that they can better respond to local need. The DH guidance[5] sets out a vision of the benefits of PBC as:

- greater variety of services from a greater number of providers
- services will be in settings closer to home and more convenient for patients
- bringing the decision-making process closer to communities

- more efficient use of services, for example, eliminating unnecessary hospital admissions
- greater involvement of frontline staff in commissioning decisions.

The DH[6] suggested that over time the Government expected that PCTs would extend indicative budgets to individual practices for the full range of services.

This might be seen as a 'throw back' to the previous Conservative Government policy of GP fundholding in the early 1990s.

PBC is integral to the World Class Commissioning programme[7] under which PCTs have developed strategic plans for their catchment areas, mapping out priorities for improvement in local health and wellbeing. It is a PCT's role to strategically lead the commissioning of the right services to provide health improvements.

Figure 2.5 shows the commissioning process through PBC, the various stages in how practice based commissioners and PCTs work in collaboration to identify and commission services:

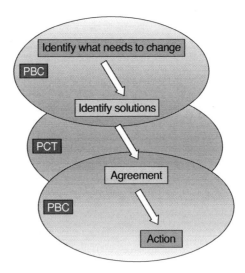

Figure 2.5 The commissioning process: practice based commissioners and PCTs.

Foundation trusts

The NHS 10 year plan[8] introduced the concept of a hospital trust which would have more freedom than conventional hospitals trusts to run themselves. FTs provide the entity known as a Public Benefit Corporation bringing together aspects of 'conventional' corporate bodies, together with the principles of mutual organisations operating for public benefit. FTs are not accountable to the SHA but are regulated by Monitor which was set up specifically to be the independent regulator of NHS FTs. Unlike conventional trusts, FTs have members drawn from local communities, staff and patients. Contracts between the FTs and PCTs are legally binding which they are not with 'ordinary' trusts. FTs can also keep surpluses and sales of assets for their own use and can reinvest surpluses. In creating FTs it was the government's objective that staff would be motivated to increase the quality and efficiency of their services, improving innovation and making secondary care more responsive to local needs and communities. FTs have boards of governors comprising members from patients, staff, carers and the local population.

There is an application process for trusts to become FTs. The trust applies to the Secretary of State for Health for support and approval to apply for FT status; if approved the trust prepares its formal application having been recommended to Monitor. The trust then completes a development phase to:

- show commitment and leadership to modernising services
- show that staff and local stakeholders are involved
- undertake a public consultation on strategy and governance
- be subject to a historical due diligence report by an accounting firm which includes analysis and interpretation of finance, commercial, legal and marketing information
- undertake a five year business development plan.

The original government plan was that all trusts suitable for FT status should have completed the process during 2008. However, this objective was not achieved and the timescale was extended several times.

Monitor

Established in 2004, Monitor is the independent regulator of FTs, its role is to make sure that NHS FTs are 'professionally managed, legally set up and run, and have their finances in good order'.[9] Monitor is responsible for regulating FTs in proportion to the risks they face, placing responsibility for performance on Trust Boards. The role is to ensure NHS FT Boards discharge their responsibilities effectively and to take remedial action if they do not. 'Our belief is that well managed Foundation Trusts are best positioned to deliver high quality care, responsive to patients and commissioners'.[9]

NHS FTs are free from central government control – the Boards having authority to run the FT as they judge best – but is accountable for the success or failure of their organisation. This is an important cultural shift intended to foster improved leadership and innovation.

Summary

In summary, finance embraces a complex set of inter-related topics and the fundamentals of finance are rapidly becoming a key area of work for AHP managers in common with all managers throughout the NHS. The field is rapidly expanding and becoming of greater importance in an increasingly business-minded NHS. AHP managers facing the demands of preparing business plans, service specifications, contracts for their services and responses to tendering exercises, for example, must be 'business savvy', proactive in learning about and understanding financial matters in the broadest sense. Not only is this area of work important in its own right, but it is crucial in the wider context of AHP managerial and clinical development.

References

1 The Wanless Report, 2002: www.dh.gov.uk/en/Publichealth/Healthinequalities/Healthinequalitiesguidancepublications/DH_066213.
2 Healthcare Financial Management Association in association with the Audit Commission. *Introductory Guide to NHS Finance in the UK*. 8th ed. Bristol: HMFA; 2006.
3 Griffin A. UK nears European average in proportion of GDP spent on health care. *BMJ*. 2007; 3 March: 334–442.
4 Healthcare Financial Management Association. *Foundation Trust: an Introduction*. HFMA E-Learning. Bristol: HMFA; 2007.
5 DH. *Practice Based Commissioning in Action, a Guide for GPs*, 2009: www.dh.gov.uk/en/publicationsandstatistics/publicationspolicy and guidance.
6 DH. *Practice based Commissioning*, 2007: www.dh.gov.uk/en/Publicationsandstatistics/Publications/PublicationsPolicyAndGuidance/DH_4098564.
7 DH. *World Class Commissioning*, 2008: www.dh.gov.uk/en/Publicationsandstatistics/Publications/PublicationsPolicyAndguidance/DH_080956.
8 DH. *NHS Plan*, 2000: www.dh.gov.uk/en/Publicationsandstatistics/Publications/PublicationsPolicyandGuidance/DH_4002960.
9 Monitor. *Briefing for Commissioners*, 2008: www.monitor-nhsft.gov.uk/sites/default/files/_publications/Briefing_for_commissioners0608.pdf.

Chapter 3

Commissioning for health improvement: policy and practice

Gerry McSorley

Introduction

Healthcare policy in the UK is placing an increasing priority on the innovation and creativity of healthcare commissioning – purchasing – for health improvement and the skills and competencies of those charged with its leadership and management. Before reviewing these critical issues any consideration of the current state of strategic commissioning of healthcare in the UK must be framed within a number of key contextual issues:

- the divergent approaches to health policy and its implementation being taken by each of the four different government departments in England, Wales, Northern Ireland and Scotland[1]
- the history of health funding and current financial climate will always play a great part in the demands placed upon those responsible for health commissioning and the relative scope for health improvement that enhanced or deteriorating levels of funding create[2]
- the broader approach to public services and public services management of the Government in power.[3, 4, 5]

The approach to health policy implementation within the four countries of the UK

With the advent of increased devolution of power to the devolved administrations of Scotland, Wales and Northern Ireland, the UK has no single unified approach to health policy or its implementation.[1]

Box 3.1 Health policy implementation in the UK.

- Scotland has bet on professionalism, reducing layers of management, placing NHS Trusts within integrated Boards along with clinical networks and increasing the role of professionals in rationing and resource allocation.
- England has gone for markets, hoping that competition between independent trusts (similar to private firms) and between trusts and

> privately run treatment centres, will drive up standards and efficiency. It is hoped that this model will rescue the Government from responsibility for every detail of health service delivery
>
> - Wales has relied on a professionalist and localist approach, integrating health and local government to improve coordination of different forms of care at local level and to raise standards. It is hoped that this will increase local participation in healthcare.
> - Northern Ireland has resorted to permissive management, in and out of devolution, concentrating on keeping services going in tough conditions.
>
> Adapted from Greer.[1]

In this chapter particular emphasis is given to the position in England. This is not because it has the right or wrong solution but as the majority of the population of the UK live in England this is where the greatest impact of health policy reforms falls.

Background to the position in England

The Labour Government's position on the NHS since 1997 went through a number of initiatives and changes. On election the key attribute was fiscal prudence, largely accepting the previous Conservative Government's spending policy. General practice fundholding, a major plank of the Conservative Government's reform programme was scrapped. A new Commission for Health Improvement (CHI) was created to enhance the drive for quality. Many have argued that these early reforms were a stop-gap programme pending agreement on the future.[6]

The first major directional vision was contained in the NHS Plan[7] published with considerable professional support, which laid out a ten year strategy to modernise health services.

The key tenets of the NHS Plan were:

- investment accompanied by reform – was the mission phrase
- extra acute hospital beds
- new hospitals funded through the PFI
- extra staff who were paid more money
- created the concept of 'earned autonomy' for hospitals providing those judged as successful with greater scope to innovate
- created the Modernisation Agency to spread best practice
- local Municipal Social Services and the NHS to come together with new agreements to pool resources. Care Trusts could be created to commission health and social care in a single organisation
- extended roles for AHPs and nurses
- set up Patient Advocacy and Liaison services in each healthcare organisation, and a national patients survey
- reached a concordat with private sector providers with a view to end the historical divide between the private and public sector providers
- set new waiting time targets
- new investment and service delivery programmes in cancer, coronary heart disease and older people's services.

However over the next two years the sense at governmental level was that, whilst the NHS Plan had considerable support, the NHS was not moving quickly enough to modernise and meet patients' and public expectations of care and access. The NHS Plan was therefore followed up with the NHS Improvement Plan in 2004[8] which added new reform components.

Box 3.2 Components of the NHS Improvement Plan.[8]

1 Introduced the concept of Foundation Trusts
2 Introduced patient choice
3 Revised the role of the Commission for Health Improvement to an inspectorate role as Commission for Healthcare Audit and Inspection
4 Set challenging new targets for access time for diagnosis and treatment
5 Advocated the adoption of the triangle of care, with self management of health by far the most potent proportion of care, followed by disease management appropriate where more proactive support is offered, and finally case management for the smallest group of patients with complex needs requiring active and specialist care

---

The recognition of the divergence of the supply and demand sides embodied in the purchaser-provider split indicated the need for vision and skills on both sides if major progress was to be made in healthcare reform, efficiency and productivity.

The final pieces of the reform 'jigsaw' *Creating a Patient-led NHS,*[9] the merger of regulators of social and healthcare into the Care Quality Commission (CQC) in 2009 and the advent of World Class Commissioning in 2008 which saw the culmination of growing concerns about the unbalanced nature of the power of the NHS supply side in the absence of assertive and skilled commissioning, illustrated by the following:[9]

'Our main focus since 1997 has been the acute sector, incentivising it to reduce waiting times and improve its services. It has responded magnificently to this...'
'But there is a clear risk that a strong, vibrant, incentivised hospital sector will suck all investment into hospital care unless it is balanced by an equally strong and vibrant commissioning function.'
'This commissioning function will represent patients; focus on prevention and public health, and management of hospital providers to ensure good value for money.'
'...a Patient-led NHS focuses...specifically on the importance of expert, imaginative commissioning...'

The resulting model, based on the reforms of the early part of the decade is captured in Figure 3.1.

This framework was based on the political need to devolve power at the same time as introducing market style incentives stimulated by giving patients choice over which provider to go to, whether not-for-profit, or for profit private hospitals, or public hospitals in the shape of FTs.

In order to provide that better balance of skills on the Commissioning side of the equation, the DH devolves 75% of the NHS budget directly to the PCTs with

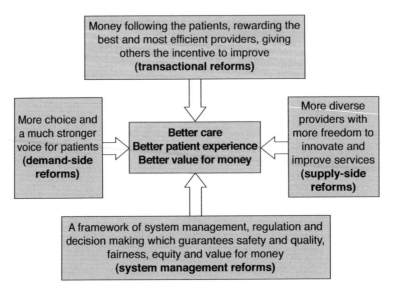

Figure 3.1 Organising Framework for NHS Reform. HFMA.[10]

a further level of devolution to individual practices in the form of PBC. The unit of currency in this new model was the patient. The method of payment, the Tariff, a fixed price for individual procedures based on the Diagnostic Related Groups (DRGs) but adapted to UK clinical practice and renamed HRGs.

This combination of demand and supply side reforms (FT and private sector involvement) resulted in the NHS in England being in transition from a public monopoly insurer and provider of healthcare, governed from Whitehall, to an insurer with devolved commissioning from a mixed market of providers.

One perspective of such a multi-dimensional approach to health policy is offered by Stevens[11] describing the need to overcome the inertia inherent in all human systems as 'constructive discomfort'.

Finally, the Organising Framework for NHS Reforms considered the need for system management reforms. Organisationally *Creating a Patient-led NHS* required changes to the structures underpinning excellent commissioning, and the mechanism by which the DH devolved market management to regional level. New SHAs and PCTs were formed with the functions shown in Figure 3.2.

Strategic commissioning

In any debate about the value of commissioning clear definition is required:

- what is 'commissioning'?
- what does it involve?
- what does it seek to achieve?

The DH definition of commissioning (DH, 2006)[12,13] is:

Commissioning is the means by which we secure the best value for patients and taxpayers. By 'best value' we mean:

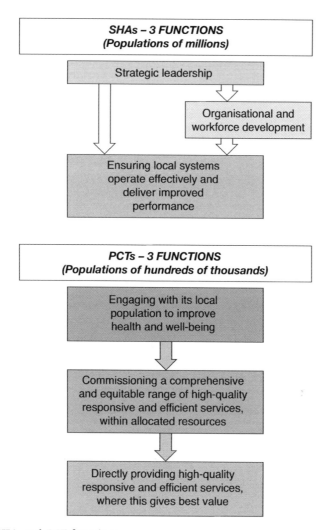

Figure 3.2 SHA and PCT functions.

- the best possible health outcomes, including reduced health inequalities
- the best possible healthcare
- within the resources made available by the taxpayer.

Øvretveit[14] some years earlier, provided an alternative definition – that it is a sophisticated and strategic process of assessing health needs, developing new services or providers, contracting for services, and undertaking a range of strategic efforts to improve population health.

Work by Smith and Mays,[15] gives a final illustration of the perspective on commissioning:

- it has a conscience – setting out 'how things should be' – what the system aims to achieve and how
- it has eyes and ears – observing and reporting on 'how things are' – what the system is currently delivering

- it has a brain (having processed information from both sources) – identifying and implementing the optimal solutions for delivering stated objectives.[16]

The arrival of World Class Commissioning [13]generated a further definition – 'adding life to years and years to life through better health and well-being for all; better care for all; better value for all'.

The similarities and differences of these definitions underscore the debate about the role and purpose of commissioning. In particular they question what emphasis to be put on each of the elements of successful commissioning. Smith[15] emphasises the visionary and transactional components, whilst Øvretveit stresses the health gain outcomes. The DH model adds the concept of 'value for money' or 'better value' as an essential element in a publicly funded system.

The criteria for judging what successful commissioning would add to the health of a local population are less clear. This may reflect the continually changing expectations of healthcare of the public, staff, and politicians.

Developing strategic commissioning

Strategic commissioning may be defined as 'a form of commissioning that gives PCTs more effective instruments to shape local services more actively in a way envisaged in the commissioning framework'.[13] There are many possible refinements to the framework that can minimise such consequences for example, moving from annual to longer term contracts and paying the full tariff only for contracted volumes of activity and at a standard marginal cost thereafter.

Such an approach can have many advantages:

- commissioners can be seen as having real 'teeth' through their ability to shift resources
- providers would be more likely to support the 'care closer to home' agenda as their ability to expand beyond contracted volumes became more muted
- medium term contracts provide greater certainty for providers
- this may be less destabilising for both providers and commissioners as marginal costs have less impact
- the incentives for providers to improve efficiency would be greater because of marginal income only from extra work.

Some observers may however see some disadvantages:[17]

- that in a market based system these matters should be left to the market
- that lower marginal prices for above contract volumes reduces the incentive to expand supply, an important characteristic of a system with lower access times and patient choice.

Practice based commissioning

The final act of devolved decision making within the framework for NHS reforms is to devolve purchasing to the lowest organisational level – individual GP practices. PBC is where funds from the PCT are passed to individual GP practices for them to commission services for their practice population as they see best and within the overall strategic aims of the PCT.[8] The English NHS is unusual in its continuing faith in primary care based organisations to carry out effective purchasing of healthcare services.[18]

The aim of PBC[19] is to enhance prospects of:

- improved patient pathway design
- better working in partnership with PCTs to create convenient community based services
- GPs taking responsibility for a budget delegated from the PCT covering acute, community and emergency care
- budgets being managed more effectively.

Studies reviewing the efficacy of commissioning by primary care[20] indicate that the factors shown in Box 3.3 are important:

Box 3.3 Primary Care commissioning efficacy.

1   Stability in health organisations
2   Time for clinical engagement
3   Policies that support choice for patients
4   Policies to allow shift of resources between providers and different sectors
5   Incentives for GPs to develop new forms of care
6   Effective management support and information
7   Regulations to minimise potential conflicts of interest from GPs being both commissioners and providers

---

The greatest challenge will be to create a set of incentives that will engage GPs, enable the development of new forms of seamless services for people with long term conditions that have eluded previous forms of primary care led commissioning.[12]

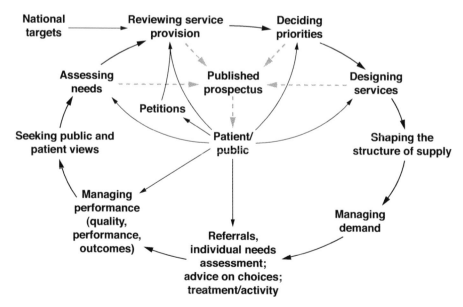

Figure 3.3 The commissioning cycle for health services.

In addition to these organisational factors there are also profound changes in the skills and competencies needed by commissioners, whether clinical or general management. The most radical exponent of commissioning skill sets – Simon Stevens, President of United Health in the UK and previously health advisor to the then prime minister – has identified a number of 'tools' needed by commissioners in this 'new world':[12]

- actuarial design of risk pools and incentives
- utilisation and equity auditing
- elective care demand management
- emergency care subsystems redesign; including out of hours and community hospital usage
- profiling primary care performance
- medicines management to ensure appropriate prescribing
- skill mix re-design especially at primary/secondary, health/social care boundaries
- patient and public engagement including self-care
- strategies for changing clinical practice including clinical decision support methodologies.

The commissioning cycle

Assessing needs. This will increasingly be based on more rigorous analysis involving population segmentation and risk stratification and will involve public health professionals, local authorities, GPs, patients and local communities.

Reviewing service provision. Practices will identify gaps and the potential for improvements in existing services. PCTs will use aggregated intelligence of their practices and their local needs assessment to identify gaps or inadequacies in provision, as well as broader requirements for service development.

Deciding priorities. The PCT should produce a strategic plan for the health community based on needs assessment data collected from practices and on choices patients are making. Practices and PCTs will work collectively to reinvest resources that have been released through service re-design where these would achieve greater impact. PCTs should ensure patients and the local community, as well as local government and other partners, are properly involved in the process of deciding priorities.

Designing services. Practices will work individually or in groups to develop strategies and service models to improve healthcare services and address the priorities of the public.

PCT prospectus. PCT prospectuses will signal the strategic direction for local services highlighting commissioning priorities, needs and opportunities to service providers, offering a focus for discussion with patients and local communities and an opportunity to open dialogue with potential providers.

Shaping the structure of supply. PCTs will be clear about the services and service specifications they and their practices and patients want to see developed and will give strategic support to proposals where necessary. They will seek to develop new services and will work with NHS Trusts and FTs, expanding GP practices, neighbouring PCTs and private and third sector providers to ensure the best services for local people. Incentives and 'levers' will be available to PCTs to stimulate the supply of services. PCTs will agree contracts with local secondary care providers within a new national contracting framework with the involvement of Practice Based Commissioners. For a few very specialised services contracts will be held at National level, while for other specialised services, PCTs will group together to set contracts.

Managing demand and ensuring appropriate access to care. Practices and PCTs will establish strategies for care and resource use to ensure that patients receive the most appropriate care in the right setting, ensuring that healthcare resource is maximised.

Clinical decision-making. Clinicians undertake individual needs assessments, make referrals and advise patients on choices and the treatments available to them; each referral is effectively a micro commissioning decision. Practices will work with social services and other agencies where appropriate to assess the needs of their patients. It will be important to facilitate the opportunity for patients to make their choices with the benefit of good advice from their GPs. PCTs and local authorities will need to work together to develop an environment in which integrated working between practices and social services is the 'norm'.

Managing performance. Practices will seek to manage their indicative budget to maximise the benefits from the resources available to them. To assist PCTs will provide support programmes, including training and development, and will develop systems to allow practices to monitor the services their patients receive through accurate, relevant and timely data. PCTs will be responsible for the aggregated financial position and ensuring financial balance.

Patient and public feedback. PCTs will be responsible for measuring and reporting patients' experience. Practices will also want to monitor patients' satisfaction. Robust mechanisms for collecting and understanding patients' views will need to be developed by PCTs and made available to practices. Throughout, PCTs will ensure that the public voice is heard in the development of priorities and shaping services.[12]

Understanding the information needs of commissioners. The emphasis on commissioning at all levels demands strong information to continually assess progress. This may be in many forms and for many uses ranging from public health improvement to contract monitoring. This spread of information suggests the importance of some underpinning principles.

Box 3.4 Underlying principles for information.

All information should be:
- clearly and simply presented
- forward looking, presenting trends
- updated in a timely manner according to its purpose and potential volatility
- directing attention to significant risks, issues, and expectations
- providing the level of detail that is appropriate to the Board's role

Strategic information should:
- show trends in health needs, provision and the satisfaction of patients
- provide forecasts and anticipate future performance issues

- encourage an external focus and understanding of the context for reform and local action

Information for monitoring performance should:

- provide an accurate and balanced picture of current and recent performance, including financial, clinical, regulatory, activity and patient expectations
- focus on the most important measures of performance and highlight exceptions
- be appropriately standardised in order to take account of known factors that affect outcomes, such as the age profile and deprivation factors
- enable comparisons with the performance of similar organisations and health economies

The key tests of the success of any information resource for the Commissioner will be the extent to which it:

- prompts relevant and constructive challenge
- supports informed decision-making
- is effective in providing early warning of potential financial or other problems
- develops an understanding of the organisation, the local health economy and its performance.

Leadership in commissioning

This agenda highlights the significant leadership task for commissioners. The complexity of the task and the prevailing financial climate creates a 'hothouse' climate for accelerating progress. The successful management of change and harnessing the various interests, both organisational and professional, is critical. Such leader attributes will require development throughout the organisations not just in the most senior levels.[15] This organisation-deep leadership function mimics the move away from the 'heroic leader' model so prevalent over recent decades to a more empowering and engaging style of lead behaviour and change leadership – though no less transforming in its ideology.[20, 21]

Within the public sector additional leadership behaviours are useful.[22]

1 Showing genuine concern.
2 Enabling.
3 Being accessible.
4 Encouraging change.
5 Being honest and consistent.
6 Acting with integrity.
7 Being decisive.
8 Inspiring others.
9 Resolving complex problems.
10 Leading the organisation.
11 Networking and achieving.
12 Focussing effort.
13 Building shared vision.

14 Supporting a developmental culture.
15 Facilitating change sensitively.

The development of clinical leadership in commissioning is critical to success. Clinical leaders add knowledge, experience and skills to the commissioning map. Their leadership development must not be left to chance but supported with personal coaching and organisational development nested within a framework of patient and public engagement in the commissioning process and anticipated outcomes.

What if the model as conceived does not deliver?

Speculating about 'what if' may seem a little advanced when the reform programme has so little maturity of experience. However, work commissioned by the Health Policy Forum has touched on the alternative, and perhaps more radical options, should these be needed.[14] These include, for example, holding commissioners more to account to their local populations. In addition whilst providers compete under patient choice, commissioners have 'locked in' populations, competition amongst commissioners may also be required.

Conclusion

Commissioning within the English NHS is still in its early days. There are hopes and dangers in equal parts. The divergence of health policy approaches within the UK's four countries will allow important comparisons to be made.

The complexity of the reform agenda, the newness of the commissioning organisations and the need to accelerate organisational and personal development to deliver the health gain expected by the public and politicians is not risk free.

Influential and visionary leadership with focussed organisational development will be needed to secure the potential in the system. Clinical participation is an integral part of that leadership drive.

The reform agenda, if successful, can deliver benefits to individuals and communities. Looking into the future furthermore, radical reform may be required to optimise those benefits.

References

1 Greer S. *Territorial Politics and Health Policy*. Manchester: Manchester University Press; 2004.
2 Wanless D. *Securing our Future: taking a long-term view*. London: HM Treasury; 2002.
3 Kelman S. *Unleashing Change: a study of organisational renewal in government*. Washington, DC: Brookings Institution Press; 2005.
4 Pollitt C. Clarifying convergence: striking similarities and durable differences in public management reform. *Public Manag Rev*. 2002; **4**: 471–92.
5 Osborn R, Gaebler T. *Reinventing Government: how the entrepreneurial spirit is transforming the public sector*. Reading, MA: Adison Wesley; 1992.
6 Klein R. *The New Politics of the NHS*. Harlow: Prentice Hall; 2001.
7 DH. *The NHS Plan*. London: Department of Health; 2000.

8 DH. *NHS Improvement Plan: putting people at the heart of public services.* London: Department of Health; 2004.
9 DH. *Creating a Patient-led NHS: delivering the NHS Improvement Plan.* London: Department of Health; 2005.
10 HMFA: www.mdlinx.com.
11 Stevens S. Reform strategies for the English NHS. *Health Affairs.* 2004; **3**: 23–37.
12 DH. *Health Reform in England: Update and commissioning framework.* London: Department of Health; 2006.
13 DH. *World Class Commissioning: Vision,* 2007: www.dh.gov.uk/en/Publicationsand statistics/_Publications/PublicationsPolicyAndguidance/DH_080956.
14 Øvretveit J. *Purchasing for Health: a multi-disciplinary introduction to the theory and practice of purchasing.* Buckingham: Open University Press; 1995.
15 Smith J, Dixon J, Mays N, *et al.* Practice based commissioning: applying the research evidence. *BMJ.* 2005; **331**: 1397–9.
16 Wade E, Smith J, Peck E, *et al. Commissioning in the Reformed NHS: policy into practice.* Birmingham: University of Birmingham/NHS Alliance; 2006.
17 Palmer K. *NHS Reform: getting back on track.* London: King's Fund; 2006.
18 Smith J, Lewis R, Harrison T. *Making Commissioning Effective in the Reformed NHS.* London: Health Policy Forum; 2006.
19 Crisp N. *Commissioning a Patient-Led NHS.* London: DH; 2005.
20 Smith R. Needed: transformational leaders. *BMJ.* 2002; **325**: 1351–44.
21 Higgs M, Rowland D. All changes great and small: exploring approaches to change and its leadership. *J Change Manag.* 2005; **5**: 121–51.
22 Alimo-Metcalfe B, Alban-Metcalfe R. Under the influence. *People Management.* 2003; **9**: 32–5.

Chapter 4

Striking the agreement: business case and service level agreements

Robert Jones and Fiona Jenkins

Introduction

The key focus of this chapter is guidance on developing effective business cases and service level agreements for AHPs with the object of 'winning and marshalling' business, and having clear effective agreements resulting in the provision of quality services which achieve identified and agreed outcomes. The ability to demonstrate value for money is a continuing and crucial element of the work of AHP managers, it is not only about quality of clinical outcomes – essential though this is – it is also of paramount importance that AHP managers contribute to the NHS commissioning process through demonstrating the contributions their services make to cost effective, relevant and improved services for patients. NHS service provision is increasingly pluralistic in a landscape of contestability, practice based commissioning, payment by results, mergers of health and social care services, the move to community based care and a wide range of other developments in policy and practice within the NHS business environment. It is increasingly necessary for AHP managers and services to communicate the anticipated impact, relevance, efficiency and effectiveness in business terms based on robust evidence.

> A business plan is not just a corporate formality, it's a test to see if your idea stands up – and an ongoing reference point once you are up and running.[1]

Different organisations have different templates for business planning and service level agreements. They both require up to date, relevant, accurate information which needs to be thoroughly researched. All the salient points must be included in order to 'hit the spot'. We acknowledge that there are many possible formats for putting together business cases. Our aim is to provide guidance and a checklist for business case and service level agreement development to signpost a methodology to support managers in striving to achieve successful outcomes.

There are many contributory factors underlying business planning and making effective business cases which are discussed in detail throughout this book. Important 'building blocks' include, for example, finance, activity analysis, marketing, project management, information, commissioning, management quality and others all of which are relevant and form the foundation of successful business cases.

Guidance for business case development

This outlines the key elements required in a business case to enable the organisation and commissioners/purchasers to make decisions that achieve fair and efficient allocation of resources to projects and sound appraisal and approval of investment decisions.

The level of detail required for each key element of the business case will depend on the size and scope of each proposal. The larger and more complex the proposal the greater the detail needed.

The financial appraisal and affordability sections may need input from finance departments.

Purpose of the business case

The purpose of the business case is to:

- put forward proposals for change or development
- consider possible options
- assess the benefits of change – benefits realisation
- assess the cost of change
- establish the timescale of change
- judge the value of the proposal against competing bids for resources.

Joint Strategic Needs Assessment Scorecards are a valuable resource for any data or intelligence which may help with projects and business case submissions. Scorecards show data at different levels of health and local authority geographies.

1 Health geographies: data at Primary Care Trust, Practice Based Commissioning Cluster, GP practice levels.
2 Local Authority geographies: data at county council, district/borough council, electoral ward levels.
3 Children's Services geographies: data at county council, district/borough council, Local Partnership for Children.

Option appraisal

An option appraisal should be completed for every project, capital or revenue, in order to identify the preferred option which best meets the identified objectives, it should be at the heart of the decision- making process. Option appraisal is a technique for setting objectives, creating and reviewing options and analysing their relative costs and benefits. It should help develop a value for money solution that meets the objectives of the project. Option appraisal starts with the identification of the options available to be considered. There are several processes involved including benefits appraisal, which identifies the benefits to be met by the project and against which the outcomes achieved will be measured and financial appraisal to identify the most cost effective solution.

A simple example of a method for undertaking an option appraisal might be:

1 set out each of the possible options in turn and number each one
2 describe each option in outline

3 identify cost
4 analyse the pros and cons of each option
5 evaluate the option through a scoring or weighting mechanism or in text description
6 compare options; rank them in priority order making recommendations for preference with reasons.

Key elements in a business case

Different organisations may have their own template for business case submissions, however if there is no set format the following is a useful guide. You may need to apply for project funding at some time; the better laid out your application, the better your chance of success!

Ensure essential information is included, such as: name of the organisation, name of the service, author(s), contact details and date. Presentation is of paramount importance as is the accuracy and relevance of the contents.

The following suggested template may be useful as a guideline setting out the headings for a business case including option appraisal, to give an idea of the process required.

Box 4.1 Key elements in a business case – an example.

Date:
Name of Division:
Business Case for:
Business Case Author(s):
Divisional Clinical Director:
Executive Summary:
  A brief overview of the Business Case, current situation, options, preferred option, financial details and recommendation.

Introduction and purpose of the Business Case:
  This includes an explanation of what the Business Case is about and why it has been prepared, what service(s) you are aiming to provide for whom, where, when and why. Set out an outline of the Business Case content and mention the option appraisal, stating that the preferred option for the Directorate is.................
Description and Analysis of Reason(s) for the Business Case:

Local Context:
  Explain what services are currently available, what the issues are, why something new, different or extra is required, what the gaps are and what would be needed to improve services or resolve the problem. This might include, for example, delays in access to treatment, long waits, no service available, waiting list information, service only available in other areas, information about relevant audits which have been undertaken, clinical governance issues, expertise available and so on.

Strategic Context and Headlines:
   Include a range of relevant information for example:
• fit with the organisation's strategy
• high impact changes
• therapy Referral to Treatment times
• National Service Frameworks
• NICE recommendations
• local or national guidelines
• targets set by the organisation, commissioners or nationally
• summary of the challenges and what the outcome is likely to be if the challenges are not addressed
• cancer strategy
• Trust strategy and objectives.

Options:
   For the option appraisal number and provide headings for each option. This could be set out in columns for example:
• Option 1:
   • column 1 – Description of Option – might be do nothing
   • column 2 – Advantages of Option – brief list of advantages
   • column 3 – Disadvantages of Option – brief list of disadvantages
   • column 4 – Total cost per annum – revenue and capital.
• Option 2:
   • similar format, except that column 1 will describe a specific option
   • columns 2, 3 and 4 as above.
• Option 3:
   • column 1 – description of a further option
   • columns 2, 3 and 4 as above.

Generally the options appraisal will include three or four options.

Ranking and Preferred Option and Benefits:
   In this section rank the options in order of preference and provide an explanation of why a specific option is preferred, benefits and so on.

Analysis of Risk:
   Outline the risks involved in implementation of each option and the risks involved in not implementing.

Impact on Other Divisions/Directorates within the Organisation:
   Give an outline of whether the proposal impacts on other Divisions, Directorates or Services within the Organisation in terms of, for example:
• staffing
• use of facilities and equipment
• timetabling
• funding
• patient flows.

Plan for Preferred Option Implementation.
To include for example:
- staffing required
- consumables and materials required
- facilities and equipment
- location
- timetable for implementation
- possibly include a plan of the week's/month's work envisaged in the form of a calendar.

Financial Impact Summary.
Full financial summary for the preferred option and runners up.
Annual revenue costs fully explained:
- pay
- non pay.

Capital costs fully explained:
- income.

Alternatively, funding arrangements could be set out in columns headed for example:
- description of option
- summary of costs
- financial impact
- total cost.

Conclusion:
Outline the main arguments for the preferred option.

Recommendation(s):
A clear and concise statement of recommendation.

Appendices:
Include relevant appendices as appropriate.

Signature of Sponsors..
The Business Case should be signed off by senior staff within the Directorate/Division, for example:
- Clinical Director, Senior General Manager and Director/Head of Therapy Services.

Service level agreements

If you provide services for another organisation you should have an SLA to set out exactly what is required and provided. Sometimes there may be benefits of establishing internal SLAs with other divisions or directorates. There are several templates than can be used,[2] our suggested format and worked example is given.

Memorandum of agreement

Between XX Trust and YY Trust
1 April 20XX to 31 March 20YY
For the provision of: Podiatry services

Schedule 1

Service Fee and Activity Level

1   Service fee
1.1   The service fee for the year will be £xxxx

Podiatry	£xxxx

1.2   The fee shown in 1.1 will remain fixed from 1 April 20XX to 31 March 20YY.
       It will be reviewed towards the end of the financial year and will be subject
to adjustment in line with NHS guidelines as indicated in Clause 8.4 of the
Memorandum of Agreement.
       The service fee shown in 1.1 for the year 1 April 20XX to 31 March 20YY
will be paid in twelve equal parts throughout the year as indicated in Clause 8.2
of the Memorandum of Agreement.
2   Activity level
2.1   The Level of Activity to be provided under the terms of this Agreement for
the period 1 April 20XX to 31 March 20YY based on:
       New patient (initials contacts) during year:

Podiatry	xxxx

Total contacts during year:

Podiatry	xxxx

2.2   The Service Fee will be based on the Level of Activity shown in 2.1 and will
not alter within a tolerance of +/− 3%.
2.3   Levels of activity outside the 3% tolerance will be subject to urgent
resolution between the Service Provider and Service Purchaser subject to Clauses
6.3, 7.1, 11.3, 13, 14 and 15 of the Memorandum of Agreement.
2.4   Agreed levels of activity will not be adjusted in year without the formal
agreement of both parties
2.5   There will be no downward adjustment of the Service Fee in year should XX
Trust fail to refer an adequate number of patients for treatment.
Directors:
For and on behalf of: XX NHS Trust
Signature: _____   Date: _____
                  XX Director of Finance
For and on behalf of: YY Trust
Signature: _____   Date: _____
                  YY Director of Service Delivery

Authorised managers/Head of Service:
For and on behalf of: XX NHS Trust
Signature: _____ Date: _____
           XX Head of AHP Services
For and on behalf of: YY Trust
Podiatry Services Manager Signature: _____ Date: _____

Schedule 2

Provision of facilities, utilities and services by:

X denotes which Trust will be the provider, inclusive of all associated costs.

	XX Trust	YY Trust
Accommodation (clinical and office)	X	
Administration support (not reception)		X
Clinical/medical records	X	
Clinical/non clinical waste disposal	X	
CSSD podiatry instrument packs	X	
Disposable linen	X	
EME support		X
Equipment replacement/repair	X	
Equipment servicing non electro medical engineering	X	
Estates services	X	
External postage	X	
Facilities services	X	
Health and Safety (clinical staff)		X
Health and Safety (accommodation / fabric)	X	
Health education materials		X
ID name badges	X	
Internal post (collection and delivery)	X	
Internet accounts		X
IT equipment		X
IT networking and support	X	
IT sundries (printer cartridges, etc.)		X
Laundry	X	
Medical gases		X
Non stock		X
Office equipment and furniture	X	
Paper hand/couch towels	X	

	XX Trust	YY Trust
Patient transport	X	
Petty cash		X
Pharmacy (in-patient and diabetes centre)	X	
Pharmacy (out-patients)		X
Photocopying	X	
Podiatry instruments for CSSD packs	X	
Portering	X	
RDC		X
Reception staffing (where currently exists)	X	
Repair/replacement of podiatry instruments	X	
Risk/H&S (clinical and staffing)		X
Risk/H&S (accommodation and fabric)	X	
Sharps bins (provision and disposal)	X	
Splinting materials		X
Staff training/updating		X
Staff travel expenses		X
Telephone	X	
IM&T (hardware, software and support)	X	
IM&T inputting	X	
Uniforms		X
Utilities (heating, lighting, electricity and water)	X	

Schedule 3

Podiatry services specification

1   Objective:
To provide a high quality comprehensive range of podiatry services to patients at the XX Hospital site. All service delivery will be based on individual need, established professional standards, ethical practice and national guidelines including NICE guidelines.

2   Services to be provided:
- Out-patient clinics
  - Podiatry out-patient clinic
  - Diabetes centre podiatry clinic
  - Surgical appliances out-patients
  - Department of psychiatry
  - Staff occupational health (monthly)
- In-patient ward based care
  - DGH
  - Department of Psychiatry

- Ward staff training in the cutting of toenails
- Operational management of Podiatry staff
- Professional support to Podiatry staff
- Professional advice to XX Head of AHP services.

3 Staffing:
- Whole Time Equivalents:
  - xxWTE   -   Podiatry Out-Patients / Wards
  - xxWTE   -   Diabetes Centre / Diabetes Clinic
  - xxWTE   -   Surgical Appliances Department
  - xxWTE   -   Department of Psychiatry
  - xxWTE   -   Management / Professional support

  Total staffing = xxWTE
- Gradings:
  - xxWTE Band 6
  - xxWTE Band 7
  - xxWTE Band 8a
- Cover for annual leave, short-term sickness or study leave is not provided for within this SLA.
- Management and Clinical Supervision is incorporated for all staff within their contracted hours

4 Service locations/hours available:
- Podiatry Out-Patients, XX, Podiatry Clinic:
  Clinic times:
  - Monday   9:00 – 12:15 & 13:30 – 16:30
  - Tuesday   9:00 – 12:15 & 13:30 – 16:30
  - Wednesday   9:00 – 12:15 & 13:30 – 20:00
  - Thursday   9:00 – 12:15
  - Friday   9:00 – 12:15 & 13:30 – 16:30
- Diabetes Centre
- Podiatry Clinic
  Clinic times:
  - Tuesday   13:30 – 20:00
  - Wednesday   13:30 – 16:15
  - Saturday   10:00 – 16:00
- All the above times are when appointments / clinical care will be booked. These times include In-patient ward based care and administration time (record keeping and collection of activity data).
- They do not include clinic preparation, appointment/ diary management, clinical correspondence/feedback that is undertaken outside of the above hours.
- There is no provision for any part of this service to be delivered on Bank Holidays.

5 How to access service:
- Self-referral, GP or Consultant referrals are accepted.
- For all clinical In and Out-Patient care on XX site, referrals should be sent to the Podiatry Our-Patient Clinic within XX.
- All referrals regarding footwear or in-shoe devices should be sent to the Surgical Appliance Department via email.

- All In-Patient referrals should be submitted on the Podiatry In-Patient referral form, and emailed to the department
- XX monthly staff clinic is by referral through Occupational Health only.

6   Quality:
- All podiatry staff will:
  - comply with the Society of Chiropodists and Podiatrists 'Guidelines on Minimum Standards of Clinical Practice'
  - work within the principals of Clinical Governance in order to maintain and improve patient care, quality and efficiency
  - be subject to annual appraisal and regular review
  - be subject to regular management and clinical supervision
  - will hold current registration with the HPC
  - will receive regular mandatory training in:
    - fire safety
    - moving and handling
    - resuscitation
    - anaphylaxis
    - infection control.
  - will have time identified for self directed professional development
  - will be subject to Standard disclosure check by the Criminal Records Bureau.
- Audits on access to Service, User satisfaction, developments in line with NSF's and NICE guidelines, together with other local clinical governance initiatives will be undertaken as agreed with the Head of Therapy Services.
- All advice sheets will be reviewed annually and updated as required.
- Annual Risk and condition assessments will be undertaken of the Podiatry Clinical Accommodation and equipment within Out-Patients, Diabetes Centre, Department of Psychiatry, together with equipment used for undertaking care on wards.

All complaints will be handled in line with XX Trust Complaints Procedure.

7   Contact details:
- Podiatry services manager: XXXX
- Address:
- Phone:
- Email:

Schedule 4

Podiatry services agreement

The underlying principles supporting this Agreement are:
- the specification is intended to provide a framework for the service to be provided rather than a precise operational manual.
- both parties agree that they will not undermine either organisation through withholding a Service or payment and that neither party will be unfairly disadvantaged by default of a service.

1   Agreement
This agreement shall cover the provision of, Podiatry and services as detailed in the attached specifications for the period from 1st April 20XX to 31st March 20YY

2   Definitions

2.1 In this Agreement the following expressions shall have the meaning shown:
   - 'The Parties' are XY
   - 'The Service Purchaser' means XX
   - 'The Service Provider' is YY

3   Service specification

3.1 The services to be provided under the terms of the Agreement are defined as individual specifications in Schedule 2, these being: Schedule 3 Podiatry Services

3.2 The aim of both Parties will be to provide a service of high quality to NHS patients and their carers aimed at resolution, reduction or control of the condition, through informed choice and evidence based practice.

4   Authorised officers

4.1 For the purpose of the overall control of this Agreement, the powers of both Service Provider and Service Purchaser shall be vested in the Service Manager/Head of Service.

4.2 Both parties shall endeavour that the Service Manager/Head of Service or a nominated representative duly authorised to act on their behalf is available for consultation during normal business hours.

5   Agreement period

5.1 The period during which these services shall be provided is defined in Clause 1 above.

5.2 The Agreement may be rolled on past the end date stated in Clause 1, if agreed in writing by both parties

6   Notice period

6.1 In the event of one party deciding not to continue with the Agreement after the completion of the Agreement period, that party shall provide a minimum of six months notice to the other party.

6.2 A minimum of six months notice in writing must be given by either party of an intention to terminate an individual service or service element before the end date of the Agreement period.

6.3 In the event of service activity falling materially below acceptable levels, written notice of this fact should be given to the Director of Service Delivery; XX. This notice has the effect of instigating the notice period in 6.1 and 6.2 above and enables the Service Provider and the Service Purchaser to agree upon either restitution or effective alternative arrangements. For the purpose of this Agreement acceptable levels will be determined by the mutual agreement of both parties through service monitoring mechanisms.

6.4 Any information or communication given to the Service Managers/Head of Service shall be deemed to have been given to the organisation concerned.

6.5 Any notice required to be given by either the Service Purchaser or the Service Provider, one to the other, under the terms of the Agreement shall be in writing and addressed to the relevant Director or Service Manager, as identified in Schedule 1.

7   Variation /additional services

7.1 Services requested which are over and above those provided for in the attached Service Specifications that would require additional staff or other resources will be subject to a supplementary charge by the Provider and may only be provided if formal approval in writing has been given by the Service Purchaser.

7.2   Either party may initiate discussion to vary the terms of the Agreement at any time. Any changes to the Agreement that are mutually agreed will be subject to a formal Variation to be issued by the party initiating the discussion.

7.3   Both Parties may agree minor changes from time to time which do not significantly affect the service provision and by mutual agreement will not necessitate issue of a formal Variation.

8   Service fee/payment conditions

8.1   The Service Purchaser shall pay the Service Provider the agreed amount set out in Schedule 1 of the Memorandum of Agreement.

8.2   Subject to compliance with this Agreement and presentation of an invoice, the Service Purchaser shall pay the Service Provider in twelve equal parts throughout the year making payment no later than the third Thursday of each month.

8.3   Should the Agreement end in whole or any Service or part service be terminated other than at the end of a complete month, the sum payable by the Service Purchaser shall be that amount due pro-rata to the period involved.

8.4   The Service Fee will remain fixed throughout each year of the Agreement period but will be subject to annual increase to cover pay rises and inflation. Any other increase will be by negotiation between the parties.

8.5   The activity tolerances and thresholds that justify a review of the Service Fee will be shown in Schedule 1 of the Memorandum of Agreement.

9   Use/provision of facilities and services

9.1   Where the Service Purchaser has traditionally provided facilities, utilities and services supporting the individual clinical services this will continue to be made. See Schedule 2

9.2   All facilities provided by the Service Purchaser will conform to national guidance / Department of Health Estates standards and be maintained and cleaned to a level required for the procedures undertaken and to comply with current infection control directives.

9.3   All clinical equipment provided by both the Service Purchaser and Provider will be fit for purpose, serviced as per Department of Health or manufacturers guidance and repaired or replaced without delay in the event of breakdown or condemnation.

9.4   Where it becomes necessary to make changes to any accommodation or facility/utility/service provided, the Service Purchaser shall give notice to the Service Provider of such changes and reach agreement with the Service Provider for the re-provision of suitable alternatives at no cost to the Service Provider.

10   Information

10.1 The Service Provider will collect relevant patient and activity data using systems agreed with the Service Purchaser, in a format suitable for data entry into the Service Purchasers information systems.

10.2 Data entry will be the responsibility of the Service Purchaser

10.3 The Service Purchaser will be responsible for ensuring that the statistical returns required by the Strategic Health Authority and Department of Health are collected and provided.

10.4 The Service Purchaser will make quarterly summaries of activity available to the Service Provider.

10.5 Quarterly staffing details provided at set dates by grade and hours will be provided by the Service Provider.

10.6 The Service Purchaser will use its best endeavours to ensure that the Service Provider is kept up to date with local Trust policies and procedures together with any other relevant communications. This may be provided by giving access to electronic copies via the Trust Intranet.

11 Monitoring/review

11.1 Bi-monthly meetings will be held between the Manager/ Head of Service of both parties for the purpose of reviewing service delivery and information sharing.

11.2 An annual meeting will be held between the Managers of both parties to review:
- service delivery over the past twelve months
- achievement of agreed activity levels
- achievement of quality/clinical governance objectives
- finance (inflation levels, cost improvements)
- developments /changes for coming year
- further development of SLA as an accurate working document.

11.3 The Service Provider shall inform the Service Purchaser without delay of any issues, which might jeopardise delivery of services within this Agreement such as: inability to obtain sufficient staff cover, absence of key staff, major equipment failure etc. Notification under this clause does not necessarily mean that the issue(s) so notified fall within the scope of 'exceptional circumstances' outlined in Clause 14.

12 Performance

12.1 The Service Provider will use its best endeavours to comply with all relevant legislation, statutory instruments, Department of Health Notices and Circulars, Professional Bodies guidance, National and local trust policies and procedures.

12.2 The Service Provider will make all reasonable endeavours to employ staff with the appropriate level of training and current skills required to deliver the service as per the individual service specifications.

12.3 The Service Provider shall allow persons nominated by the Service Purchaser to have reasonable access to the Service Provider's staff, facilities and records for the purpose of verifying or monitoring work undertaken by the Service Provider.

12.4 The Service Provider will ensure that all staff from disciplines covered by the Health Professions Council have current registration.

13 Service developments

13.1 The Service Provider will provide notice to the Service Purchaser of any service developments, which have a fundamental effect on the provision of any service incorporated in this Agreement.

13.2 The Service Purchaser will provide notice to the Service Provider of any service developments, which will have an effect on the required volume, frequency, timing, location, (or any other variable attribute) of services to be purchased.

14 Exceptional circumstances

14.1 During the period of this Agreement exceptional circumstances may arise which are beyond the reasonable control of the parties and prevent performance of the Agreement. In this context exceptional circumstances can be defined as events, which are unpredictable, out of the ordinary and not easily recovered without undue cost or difficulty. In such circumstances the terms and conditions of the Agreement may be set aside subject to the agreement of both parties, for a period not to exceed six weeks. In the event of such circumstances arising, both parties to the Agreement shall meet to agree appropriate interim working arrangements and possible additional financial commitments.

15   Staffing

15.1 Staffing levels purchased within this agreement, provide services across the year, but do not provide cover for annual leave or short term absence due to sickness or study leave.

15.2 In the case of long term absence of designated staff due to sickness or maternity leave, the Provider agrees to only charge actual costs incurred. Any savings remaining will in the first instance be used to purchase the services of additional staffing to help cover the absence period.

15.3 If the Provider is unable to purchase the services of additional staff or the Purchaser does not wish the Provider to take this action, then the Provider will only charge actual costs incurred (net of any savings).

15.4 In the event of a vacancy arising and the provider being unable to fill the position, then the Provider will only charge actual costs incurred (net of any savings).

15.5 In the event of Bank or Agency staff being used to cover any period of long term absence. The level of additional manpower purchased by the provider will mirror the level of funding released through the staff absence after actual costs incurred.

16   Best endeavours

16.1 In the event of a disagreement or dispute between the Service Purchaser and the Service Provider, the authorised officers shall use their best endeavours to resolve the issue.

16.2 Should this course of action not be successful the Service Purchaser's Chief Executive and the Service Providers Chief Executive shall meet and use their best endeavours to resolve the issue.

17   Arbitration

17.1 Both parties believe that it would be in the best interest of the local health services for any disagreement to be resolved locally.

17.2 However in the event of an unresolved dispute between the parties the issue shall ultimately be referred to a mutually agreed arbitrator. Both parties shall consider the decision of the arbitrator final. Both parties in all circumstances will meet their own costs.

18   Assignment and sub-contracting

18.1 The Service Provider shall not transfer or assign the Agreement or any part thereof and shall not sub-contract any party of the provision of the Services to any party, NHS or otherwise, without the Service Purchasers prior consent in writing.

18.2 In the event of any transfer, assignment or sub-contract taking place the conditions of this Agreement will continue to apply in full to the further party.

19   Indemnity

19.1 The Service Provider shall be liable for and shall indemnify the Service Purchaser against any liability, loss, claim or proceedings arising from the negligence of his employees in the course of or in connection with provision of the Services detailed within the Agreement (unless attributable to negligence by the Service Purchasers Officers, Servants or Agents).

Editors' note

The editors would like acknowledge input and advice given by Adrian Lever former Head Podiatrist at East Sussex Downs and Weald PCT, for his insight into Podiatry SLA development.

Conclusion

The ability to ensure that AHP services are at the forefront of planning within the organisation requires AHP managers to develop the essential skills of business planning, business cases and the development of SLAs.

References

1   Ford E. *How to Write a Business Plan*. Timesonline, 27 September 2007: http://business.timesonline.co.uk/tol/business/career_and_jobs/graduate_management/article2537485.ece.

2   www.service-level-agreement.net.

Chapter 5

Thriving in the cash strapped organisation

Rosalie A Boyce

Allied Health Professionals (AHPs) make valuable contributions to the health of their patients, clients and communities as expert clinicians. Work priorities are often dominated by managing large caseloads and meeting complex client needs. Less well appreciated is the need for a range of non-clinical skills that support and amplify the health professional's clinical outcomes. Competence in management, leadership and finance, come to the fore in environments where resources are declining, unstable or where political and organisational politics dominate the allocation process. Resource allocation processes are inherently competitive and the financial status of AHPs in terms of their ability to acquire resources depends on being able to obtain and manage money creatively.

The focus of this chapter is the art of acquiring resources, particularly in the 'cash strapped' publicly funded healthcare sector. The rationale is that firstly, although AHPs work across many settings, the publicly funded health sector in many western industrialised countries is the majority employer. Secondly, compared to the private sector, the publicly funded health sector is often more constrained by the methods and techniques that can be used to secure resources. Bureaucratic controls and public accountability standards typically act as limiting factors on public sector management and financial behaviour.[1, 2] The priorities for health professionals in the public sector are usually expressed as a requirement to concentrate on the 'core business' of meeting client demand, not on generating innovative revenue streams. Despite these priorities health professional managers need to exercise strategic thinking about how to acquire additional funding. Where resource environments are unstable, service providers also need to use the same strategic thinking to ensure they maximise the available resources and opportunities. This is especially the case for the AHPs. Marginalised or 'Cinderella' services in the health system are often targeted for deeper cuts, so AHP managers need to be especially skilled in the finance and leadership area.

Financial autonomy and professional power

In terms of relative power to garner new resources, or to defend the prospect of budgetary cuts, the AHPs often lack the same strategic power as the medical and nursing professions. Marks[3] described this relative deficit in organisational positional power and clinical standing as due to misunderstandings about the role of the AHPs in modern healthcare organisations. The role of the therapist is 'often misinterpreted as just the jam between the bread-and-butter roles of nursing and medicine'.[3] In competitive resource allocation environments it becomes very important that the AHPs use strategic thinking approaches and controlled risk-taking to redress the difficulties that arise from their often 'inferior' relative organisational position in the hierarchy of professions.[4]

Public policy regarding the desirability of public sector health professionals actively seeking to be innovative, entrepreneurial and aware of commercially-oriented funding alternatives is highly dependent on the government of the day.[5] Professionals are frequently portrayed as reluctant or resistant when government policy requires them to play an active and strategic role in organisational leadership and financial management.[6, 7, 8] However, health professionals can also be receptive to engagement with new funding methodologies and service models when positive shifts in autonomy are possible.[9,10,11,12,13,14,15,16] Øvretveit[17, 18] argued that professional autonomy for the AHPs increasingly depended on financial independence in the policy environment of competition and 'internal market' reforms. He labelled this as 'business autonomy' arguing that generating income from service contracting, especially stand-alone services, was:

> one way of acquiring the business autonomy which is necessary to maintaining and extending professional autonomy…contracts are the main way in which physiotherapy services secure their independence and future.[17]

Irrespective of the particular funding model in place or the national policies circumscribing funding behaviour, there are often 'soft' funding opportunities to exploit in order to obtain income that can be used in a discretionary way. Fundamental to success is a finely developed sense of strategic opportunity that is grounded on cultivating relationships with those that either have the money you want – direct influence – and with those who influence the decisions of those with the money that is wanted – indirect influence. It is the capacity to see how an entrepreneurial business case can be developed across a range of scenarios that will reveal opportunities and set out the path of networking until the right mix of strategies to deliver the funding required is identified.[19]

Competencies in management, leadership and strategic financial thinking and practice are of crucial importance for AHP and other managers in modern healthcare. In many locations, particularly the larger urban based professional departments, the requirement for post-graduate management and finance skills as a condition of appointment to senior and leadership positions is becoming routine. However, these skill demands also exist for professionals in centres with smaller departments and for new graduates or experienced professionals who undertake 'solo' positions in rural areas or locations with persistent staff recruitment and retention issues.[20, 21] Before exploring the creative strategies that can be deployed to obtain 'soft funding' formal financial systems particularly the interplay between funding models and politics are explored.

Finance models and the politics of value

Health systems typically evolve more sophisticated financial management and control arrangements as the political need to demonstrate value from the allocated resources increases. Black[22] reported on healthcare productivity in the NHS showing that the assumptions that underpin different financial modelling frameworks can dramatically affect the assessment of the direction and quantum of productivity changes in the system. In other words, the assumptions underpinning the model will affect determination of the 'value' that is being derived from the resources used. Despite the limitations of highly assumption-based modelling, the political necessity of producing productivity estimates, and their linkage to patterns of resource allocation, suggests that further shifts in financial modelling and payment systems will continue.

> While achieving a meaningful measure of the productivity of the NHS might be a forlorn hope and not worth pursuing, the contemporary political environment makes it a necessity.[22]

It is precisely because resource allocation processes are inherently political, and therefore open to influence, that AHPs need to master both the rational and formal processes of finance and accounting models, as well as the creative possibilities that arise from taking a strategic and entrepreneurial approach to generating revenue. All health financing systems provide opportunities for working more effectively within the rational models[23,24,25] through exploiting knowledge of:

1 the underpinning frameworks that effect budget yield
2 the funding cycles and the timing of influence points
3 the shifts to new funding approaches before they become established – becoming an early adopter or supporter of change, for example, a demonstration site.

More effective working within the formal funding processes can generate greater resource allocation. For example; gaining early knowledge of funding cycles enables better preparation than rivals when competing for funding. Alternatively, when there is a shift in funding models, for example from historically allocated budgets to a purchaser/provider model or output-based model, early adopters often secure more favourable terms of engagement than the more cautious who wait several funding cycles before entering the new system.[26] Late entrants may find that the terms of participation have 'tightened' compared to those available to the early adopters.

Drivers for change in financial models

There are several 'drivers' for change in the financial models used within health systems. One is the increasing availability of reliable and valid data to underpin the development of new funding models. The quality of data has progressively improved for clinical budgeting approaches leading to the development of:

- patient classification systems
- case-based funding systems
- output funding models and outcomes based funding
- service/patient line reporting

The political push for greater healthcare productivity and the demand by Government for proof that further investment in the health portfolio yields quantifiable improvement in health outcomes has also driven shifts in funding methodologies. However, all methodologies are only as rigorous as the data upon which they are built. Quality of data, and the cost of gathering data, remains a primary limiting factor in funding model developments and application. Health professional managers need at least a rudimentary understanding of the weaknesses of alternative funding and costing methodologies so that they can exploit the application of such models to their services.

From a period of relative stability and historically-based annually allocated budgets several decades ago, health professionals today have to deal with a mix of funding models that include, but are not limited to, payment by results, population-based funding, practice based commissioning, output-based funding, activity-based costing as well as the idiosyncrasies of internal organisational budgetary and reporting cycles. These models have their visible face in frameworks such as 'internal market' reforms, purchaser-provider split, contracting, outsourcing, commercialisation, commissioning and so on.[27, 28, 29, 30]

Equally important to internal formal financing systems, is gaining an understanding of payment models used by bodies external to the organisation that provide financial support. Many countries use a mix of public-private funding in their health systems and as private sector funding increases so too does the importance of understanding 'third-party' payment models, such as those of insurers and their impact on professional practice patterns.[31, 32] For example, in Australia, where private patients can be treated in public hospitals under controlled arrangements, 'third-party' payers in the form of private health insurance companies, and their payment models are increasingly influential.[23]

Irrespective of seniority or location, many AHPs find the demands of competent leadership and financial management amongst the most stressful of their role responsibilities.[3, 33, 34] This is particularly evident in times of financial downturn or when budgets are under pressure at either departmental, organisational or system levels. AHP services are too often perceived as 'soft' non-core services or easy targets for additional cuts when the organisation is reducing its expenditure. When the internal financial environment becomes hostile or unstable, AHP managers need to examine their potential services and products to see what they can 'sell' to reduce dependency on internal resource allocation systems. They need to look to other sources of funds as a way of augmenting declining organisational income. In addition, they need to assess the commercial potential for a new array of services or products in terms of revenue generating activity to support core services and to pay for 'Cinderella' items like professional development, which are typically the first activities to lose organisational funding support.

Several strategies to help AHPs sharpen their skills in extracting funds from cash-strapped health services are explored. A worked example called 'A negotiation unfolds' traces alternative possibilities with finance managers when attempts to obtain funding are unsuccessful. Several of the strategies outlined can also be used to 'win' funds from other organisations, for example charities or voluntary organisations. A further approach to funding; gaining money through applications for formal research grants is another important strategy for obtaining funds.

Technical and creative skills as complementary elements – style and substance

The primary focus is 'creative' and 'entrepreneurial' skills in increasing resource allocation from potential funders; this includes the mix of communication techniques, marketing, business development and relationship networking skills.

Proficiency in the basic techniques of finance management, service costing, budgeting, cash flow and business case development are also important in the quest for greater resources.[23,25,30,35,36,37,38] Managerial, technical and creative skills are essential and complementary to each other. Success in resource acquisition, particularly when moving beyond traditional funding sources requires a complimentary mix of style and substance.

The funding scenario

For the purposes of this discussion a single example is used. £15 000 is needed for an item of rehabilitation or treatment equipment however the organisation has no spare capital to spend. The strategy for approaching the task of obtaining the funding is vitally important to success. It may be tempting to think that £15 000 is unobtainable, and it will be impossible to raise. 'Negative thinking' equals negative results. In a curious paradox, sometimes the more funding requested, the greater the chance of success. A well constructed business case enhances the funding request and likelihood of success, increasing awareness within the organisation. It is essential that the strategies used to pursue the funding are credible, measurable and innovative. The decision to support funding is managerial, clinical and commercial on the organisation's part, particularly as there are likely to be a range of competitors for funding.

It is necessary to adopt a positive mindset, taking the attitude that the equipment is attainable and the funding will be forthcoming. Resource acquisition is a highly competitive process. Many business cases do not succeed at the first attempt. It is important not to give up or be discouraged after the first attempt if the request is to be taken seriously. To submit a business case that is weak, incomplete or unconvincing may be harmful in terms of credibility and reputation.

Thorough preparation and a good case is the key to gaining success. Trying to extract money from organisations 'strapped for cash' is difficult but not impossible. There will be many competing good quality bids for finite resources within all organisations. If your service has not been successful in attaining additional funding for equipment previously, it will have to compete with services that have a successful track record. Persuasive arguments, astute marketing plans and a good communication strategy are essential elements of the planning stage. An important marketing tool and strategic 'weapon' is yourself, it is vital to be well prepared and as knowledgeable as possible about financial terms and processes. Portray your service as essential to the success of the organisation with a reputation for excellent service provision. Important aspects to include are:

- service re-design
- service development
- revitalising infrastructure
- improving patient care
- responsiveness to service users.

For the business case to be successful, 'investment partners' are required to accomplish the goals. It is essential to work closely with colleagues in the organisation, particularly the finance department.

Getting the preliminaries right

Alternative approaches should be mapped out before commencing a funding 'campaign' in order to sustain influence if not successful at the first attempt. Some things that must be prepared before formalising funding requests will seem obvious, others less so. Examples of points to consider include the following.

1 The major decision is whether to seek external or internal funding or a mix of both. This will have a bearing on marketing and strategy. When sourcing funds internally the issue is mostly financial. For external bodies a persuasive selling 'angle' is required.

2 For external funding there are four main possibilities:
   - philanthropic trusts give community grants related to health and welfare. There may be a local or national directory listing charities which could be applied to for funding support
   - special purpose government grants. Examples include:
   - www.governmentfunding.org.uk/ in the UK
   - www.grantcanada.com in Canada or
   - www.grantslink.gov.au in Australia
   - www.beehive.govt.nz/release in New Zealand.
   - be aware of special funding programmes offered by the SHA or DH. Sometimes professional bodies will know about various opportunities in advance of formal advertising. Networking with experienced colleagues could be beneficial. Employer permission may be necessary before applications to external organisations can be lodged
   - other local examples include the League of Friends and Women's Royal Voluntary Service.

3 Have specifications of the equipment costs, including maintenance and servicing with purchase quotes, product reviews and supplier(s). It is a useful strategy to phase equipment requests, when more than one piece of equipment is required. Incremental development proposals may be worth considering. Annual capital development plans clarify the strategy within the organisation.

4 Identify evidence-based arguments supporting the use of the equipment in clinical practice. It is important to prepare convincing arguments that relate to the expected benefits. The request is likely be strengthened by patient support for the case.

5 Business projections about use of the equipment must show that it will be central to practice. If the equipment is to be used for a high frequency clinical condition, argue that the service is central to the treatment or rehabilitation. Argue the case further by contending that with a relatively small outlay to purchase equipment it will be possible to increase efficiency and clinical outcome. It may be possible to show that the equipment will pay for itself over time, according to your projections.

6 Know where the nearest example of the equipment is in travelling time for patients. Undertake a survey to find out how many pieces of equipment there are in the area; local provision may be a powerful justification for the purchase recommendation.

7 Creating a good news story for the community may pay dividends. Have a story in the local newspaper about obtaining the equipment when it is supplied. Publicity on one funding success may have a beneficial effect on future requests.

8 Up to date equipment is a positive attribute for the recruitment and retention of staff. Health professionals are more likely to stay in departments that are well resourced and equipped with modern facilities.

9 A good understanding of the financial reports of the organisation is essential. Finance information is published with the Annual Report and is usually also available in monthly trust performance reports. Developing strong working relationships with the finance department is helpful. Ask questions so that funding possibilities can be 'unlocked'. It may be useful to know:
   • what 'special' account funds, such as charitable trust funds, exist and the operational limitations
   • how much money the volunteers/friends raised last year and what was purchased.

10 A good understanding of financial processes is essential. AHP managers with responsibilities for budgets should undertake training in this area.

11 When negotiating equipment funding requests it is worth emphasising the non-recurrent nature of the expenditure. Funding bids with recurrent commitments – such as staff or annual maintenance contracts – will be much more difficult to obtain and funding streams are likely to be different.

12 Timing of requests is important. An understanding of the capital planning cycle within the organisation is essential or the planning timetables of voluntary organisations.

13 Understand the decision-making process. Identify any 'natural allies' for the type of funding request. The more support garnered, the greater the chance of success.

14 It will be necessary to write a submission in support of the request. Treat this as a marketing 'tool' and a business case. Lay out the justification but remember, those making the decisions in the organisation will give weight to high quality business cases.

15 If, despite the best efforts, funding requests are unsuccessful use the opportunity to negotiate high priority for the following financial year.

Listed below are a series of strategies that might be used in the quest for funding. Combine the various approaches to find the strategic mix that is most likely to work locally. The strategies are mainly orientated towards an internal organisational request for funding. In this example the strategies have been devised for a piece of 'must-have' equipment worth £15000 as the scenario. However, before presenting the strategies it is necessary to examine a worked example of a negotiation where funding is requested. As an exercise, develop a funding example and write out a model template using your own word preferences.

A negotiation unfolds

It is recommended to have several alternative strategies fully developed when commencing a negotiation. Use a worked example as the first strategy to show how a financial negotiation might unfold.

Notice that as the negotiation continues and funding is refused each of the different approaches involves a decreasing amount of money the organisation would have to pay at any one time. Keep in mind however that there is a corresponding rise in the paperwork for the finance department; the transaction costs increase as the payments become more frequent due to the additional work generated.

Box 5.1 A worked example.

Assume that you are in a meeting with the finance manager to hear the result of the proposal to purchase equipment outright for £15 000 (Plan A). You are told that it was a good submission but unfortunately 'we just don't have the money'. You must immediately come back with a counter plan (Plan B) while still in the meeting: 'Yes I know money is tight so I have an alternative strategy that involves a payment plan of five payments of £3000 spread over 18 months to reduce pressure on the bottom line.'

Hopefully this will have gained their attention with this response. If they knock Plan B back then come back with another alternative, (Plan C). 'My alternative is that I can organise a lease plan from the supplier based on a monthly payment of £700 over two years. [Your suppliers may not normally trade this way but try negotiating an option that will give them a sale and you the equipment.] I think the transaction costs of this option are higher for the organisation but I am happy to go with it if that is your preferred option. The plan for this equipment has strong support from the Director of Rehabilitation and we are anxious to get the equipment in place by October to help us reduce the referral to discharge time.'

Hopefully they will agree to Plan A at this point. If they reject Plan C, 'hold your nerve' and shift the conversation to new ground. By now they will realise that they have said 'no' three times and may be looking for a way that makes you both feel that a resolution is in sight. It may then be possible to agree that your equipment request will be given high priority in the purchase programme for next year.

A smorgasbord of strategies

Several of the strategies suggested below are based on building support networks internally and externally. It is necessary to undertake an analysis of potential stakeholders to 'map' the likely sources of support. Other strategies are based on manipulating the process and others focus on utilising patient and community support. Check what organisational permission or ethical clearance requirements are needed when involving the public.

1 A strategy may be to have multiple payment options.
2 If the funding request is dismissed and it is not possible to increase pressure without damaging relationships, put all the effort into securing high-priority funding status for the next financial year.
3 If it is possible to obtain half the money through fund-raising, ask if the organisation will contribute the other 50%.
4 Offer to give a seminar to staff about a clinical condition that is dependent on the use of the equipment. Clinical support is a powerful pressure on the local hospital.

5 Demonstrate how the equipment will 'pay for itself' over 'N' years. Ability to demonstrate how the equipment has multiple positive impacts on service flows, patient satisfaction, staff expertise, waiting lists and so are major selling points.

6 Is it possible to charge providers from other local organisations to use the equipment on a sessional basis as a way of raising money?

7 Can a charity be persuaded to undertake a funding drive?

8 Know the process by which the organisation decides on equipment financing.

9 Review departmental records on previous equipment purchases. Point out that the service has not been supported to purchase equipment for 'N' years.

10 Engage the support of service users to participate in a publicity campaign ensuring ethical permissions have been obtained where appropriate.

11 Enlist the support of local media to raise awareness.

12 Enlist the support of other discipline(s) in the organisation for purchase of the equipment on the basis that they will utilise it as well.

13 Ask the hospital League of Friends to nominate your item as one of their preferred funding projects during the year.

14 Would colleagues in an adjacent service share the equipment and costs?

15 Would it be possible to share across the private and public sector if there is a private provider nearby?

In conclusion, it is important to be clear about what the service needs, why it needs it, and the financial implications. Develop strategies and prepare a thorough well written business case with an accompanying presentation. Network and gain support for the proposal using both formal and informal approaches, be assertive and flexible. If unsuccessful do not give up, learn from the process, work on alternative strategies for the future and success should follow.

References

1 Boyne GA. Public and private management: what's the difference? *J Manage Stud.* 2002; **39(1)**: 97–122.

2 Poole M, Mansfield R, Martinez-Lucio, *et al.* Change and continuities within the public sector: contrasts between public and private sector managers in Britain and the effects of the 'Thatcher Years'. *Public Admin.* 1995; **73** (Summer): 271–86.

3 Marks AL. MAPS for PAMS: managerial and professional solutions for professions allied to medicine. In: Marks AL, Dopson S, editors. *Organisational Behaviour in Health Care.* Basingstoke: MacMillan; 1999.

4 Chilingerian J. The discipline of strategic thinking in healthcare. In: Jones R, Jenkins F, editors. *Managing and Leading in the Allied Health Professions.* Oxford: Radcliffe Publishing; 2006.

5 Osborne SP, Flynn N. Managing the innovative capacity of voluntary and non-profit organizations in the provision of public services. *Public Money Manage.* 1997; **17(4)**: 31–9.

6 Hoque K, Davis S, Humphreys M. Freedom to do what you are told: Senior management team autonomy in an NHS Acute Trust. *Public Admin.* 2004; **82(2)**: 355–75.

7 Griffiths L, Hughes D. Talking contracts and taking care: managers and professionals in the British National Health Service internal market. *Soc Sci Med.* 2000; **51(2)**: 209–22.

8 Dopson S. Why is it so hard to involve doctors in management? Seeking to understand

processes of managed social change. In: Fincham R, editor. *New Relationships in the Organised Professions: managers, professionals and knowledge workers.* Aldershot: Avebury; 2000.

9 Cook S. The future of occupational therapy in health and social care markets: report of a professional workshop. *Brit J Occup Ther.* 1994; **57(7)**: 284.

10 Calnan M, Silvester S, Manley G, *et al.* Doing business in the NHS: exploring dentists' decisions to practise in the public and private sectors. *Sociol Health Ill.* 2000; **22(6)**: 742–64.

11 Ristevski E, Gardner H, Tacticos T. Altruism or entrepreneurialism: competing ideologies in the voluntary sector. In: Liamputtong P, Gardner H, editors. *Health, Social Change and Communities.* Melbourne: Oxford University Press; 2003.

12 Stone DA. The doctor as businessman: the changing politics of a cultural icon. In: Peterson MA, editor. *Health Markets? The new competition in medical care.* London: Duke University Press; 1998.

13 Lewis JM, Marjoribanks T. The impact of financial constraints and incentives on professional autonomy. *Int J Health Plan M.* 2003; **18(1)**: 49–61.

14 Forsberg E, Axelsson R, Arnetz B. Effects of performance-based reimbursement on the professional autonomy and power of physicians and the quality of care. *Int J Health Plan M.* 2001; **16(4)**: 297–310.

15 Rowe PA, Boyce RA, Boyle MV, *et al.* A comparative analysis of entrepreneurial approaches within public healthcare organisations. *Aust J Publ Admin.* 2004; **63(2)**: 16–30.

16 Ennew C, Feighan T, Whynes D. Entrepreneurial activity in the public sector: Evidence from UK primary care. In: Taylor-Gooby P, editor. *Choice and Public Policy.* Basingstoke: MacMillan Press; 1998.

17 Øvretveit J. Issues in contracting occupational therapy services. *Brit J Occup Ther.* 1994; **57(8)**: 315–8.

18 Øvretveit J. Changes in profession-management, autonomy and accountability in physiotherapy. *Physiotherapy.* 1994; **80**: 605–8.

19 Reiter KL, Kilpatrick KE, Greene SB, *et al.* How to develop a business case for quality. *Int J Qual Health Care.* 2007; **19**: 50–5.

20 Adamson BJ, Lincoln MA, Cant RV. An analysis of managerial skills for the current and future health care environment. *J Allied Health.* 2000; **29(4)**: 203–13.

21 Lopopolo RB, Schafer DS, Nosse LJ. Leadership, administration, management, and professionalism (LAMP) in physical therapy: a delphi study. *Phys Ther.* 2004; **84(2)**: 137–50.

22 Black N, Browne J, Cairns J. Health care productivity. *BMJ.* 2006; **333(7563)**: 312–13.

23 Courtney M, Briggs D. *Health Care Financial Management.* Marrickville, Australia: Elsevier Mosby; 2004.

24 Kaufman K. *Finance in Brief: six key concepts for healthcare leaders.* 2nd ed. Chicago: Health Administration Press (ACHE Management Series); 2003.

25 Zelman WN, McCue MJ, Millikan AR. *Financial Management of Health Care Organizations: an introduction to fundamental tools, concepts, and applications.* Malden, MA: Blackwell Publishers; 1998.

26 Majeed A. New formula for GP prescribing budgets: general practitioners in England need to understand its implications. *BMJ.* 2000; **320(7230)**: 266.

27 Boshoff K. Utilisation of strategic analysis and planning by occupational therapy services. *Aust Occup Ther J.* 2003; **50(4)**: 252–8.

28 Boyce RA. Internal market reforms of health care systems and the allied health professions: an international perspective. *Int J Health Plan M.* 1993; **8**: 201–17.

29 Brown K, Ryan N, Parker R. New modes of service delivery in the public sector commercialising government services. *Int J Pub Sector Manage.* 2000; **13(3)**: 206–21.

30 Lian PCS, Laing AW. The role of professional expertise in the purchasing of health services. *Health Serv Manage Res.* 2004; **12(2)**: 110–20.

31 Anthony D. Changing the nature of physician referral relationships in the US: the impact of managed care. *Soc Sci Med.* 2003; **56(10)**: 2033–44.

32 Uili RM, Wood R. The effect of third-party players on the clinical decision making of physical therapists. *Soc Sci Med.* 1995; **40(7)**: 873–9.

33 Healy K. Managing human services in a market environment: what role for social workers? *Brit J Soc Work.* 2002; **32**: 527–540.

34 Llewellyn S. Boundary work: costing and caring in the social services. *Acc Org Soc.* 1998; **23(1)**: 23–47.

35 Waters HR, Hussey P. Pricing health services for purchasers: a review of methods and experiences. *Health Policy.* 2004; **70(2)**: 175–84.

36 Øvretveit J. The quality of health purchasing. *Int J Health Care Qual Ass.* 2003: 116–27.

37 Secretariat BI. *BRI Inquiry Paper on Commissioning, Purchasing, Contracting and Quality of Care in the NHS Internal Market.* BRI; 1999.

38 Ellwood S. Full-cost pricing rules within the National Health Service internal market: accounting choices and the achievement of productive efficiency. *Manage Acc Res.* 1996; **7**: 25–51.

Chapter 6

Information is power: measure it, manage it

Robert Jones and Fiona Jenkins

For many years computerised information systems have been developed in order that organisations become more aware of their own performance and that of others. In a rapidly developing technological age, information systems within healthcare are evolving. Information systems, their development and management are complicated areas of work reflecting the complexities of healthcare provision. There are always difficulties in making Information Technology (IT) 'fit' for purpose. It is all the more important that AHPs get involved in this work to ensure that information systems support their work, both clinical and managerial.

The need to provide more detailed and relevant information than ever before is fundamental to the many changes being brought about by national and local priorities. There are many possible approaches to the development and use of computerised systems for the AHPs; it is the purpose of this chapter to focus on some of the important issues and to provide guidelines on some of the aspects to be considered. This is not a 'prescription', nor do we claim that the approaches outlined are the only or 'best' way forward. This chapter, together with the following three chapters form a solid foundation and reference point for AHP managers and staff to build a wider understanding of this increasingly important aspect of their work.

The development of IM&T for AHPs

The primary function of the AHPs is the provision of clinical services. However, over recent years information systems have become increasingly more important in the NHS and consequently, also in our services.

Computers were first used in medical records departments for the Hospital Activity Analysis, which summarised selected basic information held in medical records on, for example, admission and discharge, but no AHP information.

For many years, statistical returns for AHPs asked only for data on new patients and attendances by in and out-patients. The returns were often based on estimates or 'finger in the wind' rather than accurate data. There was no feedback to managers on local or national activity trends which resulted in very little managerial or staff commitment to the quality of data submitted.

The initial impetus for the development of information in the AHPs was provided by Körner as long ago as the 1980s.[1] The data collection requirements set out in the Körner Reports for England and Wales gave rise to a variety of paper-based and computerised systems to capture and process information.

Körner noted that much 'lip-service' was paid to the crucial and central importance of high quality statistics and that few health authorities, management teams or heads of departments analysed data expertly or used them intelligently in the performance of their management tasks.[2]

The 1990s saw the development of costing mechanisms, development of pricing for contract purposes, of care profiles for clinical and managerial audit purposes, introduction of case mix systems and computers, improved coding systems, balancing organisational development and clinical information systems – the basis for much of current information systems work.

The main themes were:

1 development of specialty and consultant costing systems in detail
2 development of case mix measures for planning and management purposes
3 development of advanced nursing dependency and management systems
4 financial and staff activity systems linked together
5 future budget setting based on planned activity levels and case mix costs
6 regular report generation and on-going monitoring against budgets and planned activity
7 the development of costing systems
8 comparison of actual and predicted use of resources to allow monitoring of clinical performance and deployment of resources.

The basis of case mix systems was intended to be the bringing about of implementation of a comprehensive record of every patient with data about every event occurring during a complete episode of hospital care. The record was to include: the patient's personal details, diagnosis and operative procedures together with diagnostic events and therapeutic interventions. All of these events had resource use implications in manpower, materials and facilities. Therefore, costing was to be an important element of the case mix equation.

For the first time in the NHS a strategy for IM&T was initiated requiring active participation and implementation by the entire service.[3]

NHS Connecting for Health

The NHS Plan,[4] outlined the need for information systems to support patient-centred care and services.

In 2002[5] recommendations for the development of IT in the NHS were:

• a doubling and protecting of IT spend
• stringent nationally managed standards for data and IT
• a national programme for IT.

This laid the foundations for the National Programme for IT, to develop and implement modern, integrated IT infrastructure and systems for all NHS organisations in England.

NHS Connecting for Health is an agency of the DH with a main purpose of delivering the National Programme for IT (NPfIT). The origins of the programme was the Information for Health Strategy.[6] The most important commitment was that the programme would provide lifelong electronic health records for patients, round-the-clock 'on-line' access to patient records for clinicians and information about 'best' clinical practice for all. In Wales Informing Healthcare[7] was set up, and in Scotland, eHealth Scotland.[8]

In 2008, Connecting for Health became responsible for NHS Choices – a personalised website supporting patient healthcare acting as a portal to 'Choose and Book'.

NPfIT has evoked a huge amount of controversy, debate and public interest. *Improving safety with information technology*[9] reported benefits for patient safety using IT as:

- substantially improve the safety of medical care by structuring actions, catching errors, and bringing evidence-based, patient-centred decision support to the point of care to allow necessary customisation
- the use of decision support for clinical decisions can also result in major reductions in the rate of complications associated with antibiotics and decreased costs and the rate of nosocomial infections
- 53–83% reduction in serious medication errors.

NPfIT encompasses a range of parameters, though the future configuration of NHS IT services is likely to change.

Box 6.1 Examples of Connecting for Health applications.[10]

- Creating an NHS website
- Choose and book
- Data quality
- Electronic prescription service
- Enterprise wide arrangements
- E-prescribing
- GP2GP
- Health space
- Map of Medicine
- N3 – connectivity for networking anywhere
- NHS care records service patient website
- NHS mail
- NHS number
- Picture Archiving and Communications Systems
- Personal demographic service
- Secondary uses service
- SNOMED
- Spine (which stores personal characteristics of patients such as demographic information)

Computerised systems for AHP services

AHP managers facing the clinical requirements and the demands of preparing service specifications, business plans, service level agreements (SLAs), tendering documentation, pricing and costing mechanisms, capacity management including supply and demand, activity, outcomes, caseloads, case mix, skill mix must be proactive in the development and/or choice of relevant information systems and linking mechanisms with the wider demands of connecting for health.

Not only is this important in its own right, but it is crucial in the wider context of AHP managerial responsibility and clinical autonomy which could be undermined if these services were treated as an 'add-on' to other services such as nursing. The AHP input to patient care is wide-ranging and complex and differs from other services and, therefore, AHP managers must be involved in contributing their specific expertise, managerial and clinical requirements and management and business needs.

In order to be able to achieve all this – to be able to show what we are doing and how much of it, how effective and efficient it is and what it all costs – AHPs need powerful computerised information systems capable of bringing together managerial and clinical information.

IM&T is crucial in an ever increasing business-minded NHS in which the clinical requirements for data and information systems support are paramount. When considering which computerised systems might be suitable for AHP services or contributing to development and specification the principles which we set out below form a useful checklist.

Principles for computerised information systems for AHP services

1 **Information use.** All information collected should be for identified and agreed use. Computerised information systems should provide information required for:
   - clinical, managerial and business purposes within AHP services locally, regionally or nationally
   - the employing organisation
   - commissioners and all other service purchasers.
2 **Local 'ownership'.** The computerised information system should be specific to the clinical and managerial needs of AHP services locally:
   - systems should be 'owned' by the AHP services using them locally, and part of the wider computer system within the organisation
   - information contained within the system is 'owned' by the AHP services and the organisation
   - AHPs should be involved in the choice of appropriate information systems for their own service.
3 **Computer hardware**. AHP services should have appropriate hardware to support their information systems, the hardware must:
   - have the capacity to handle the quantity of data required at present and be capable of expansion to meet future needs
   - be capable of supporting a wide variety of applications
   - be capable of supporting a variety of input devices and terminals including adaptive equipment for sensory impaired users
   - be compatible with hardware used by other services and departments locally
   - be capable of supporting a variety of data collection modes such as data collection in 'real' time, bar coding, Personal Digital Assistants (PDAs), paper systems, retrospective input and so on

- operate at the highest speed commensurate with the size of the information system locally
- be capable of processing data in 'real' time and batch modes.

4 **Computer software.** Computer software for AHP information systems should be appropriate to clinical and managerial practice, the software must:
- be specific to AHP managerial and clinical requirements
- be compatible with other programmes used locally in order to facilitate interfacing
- enable archiving and retrieval of archived data
- interface easily with other programmes such as Microsoft packages, programmes for clinical purposes and other databases
- interface with specialist software for sensory impaired users
- be capable of updating in line with changing requirements
- be designed to accommodate SNOMED, ICD and other coding systems.

5 **System security.** AHP systems must be secure so as to protect the confidentiality of patients, staff and others about whom data are held:
- data must be collected, processed and stored within the requirements of data protection legislation
- entry to the AHP system must be governed by a system of passwords
- staff must 'log off' from computer equipment when not using it
- there must be full backup of data on a daily basis.

6 **Data collection.** All data collected by AHPs should – where ever possible – be a by-product of clinical practice:
- all patient intervention data items are collected once only if possible
- the data system must facilitate the collection, processing and reporting of locally agreed clinical and managerial information as well as that required regionally and nationally – it must be possible to report on all parameters input to the system
- the system should facilitate the collection, processing and reporting of information about the use of AHP resources in: patient activity and non-patient related activity
- data input to systems may be undertaken by clerical, clinical or managerial staff.

7 **Reporting.** The computer system must be capable of producing standard and ad hoc reports for AHP clinical, managerial, research and business purposes, as well as meeting the agreed requirements of others:
- the system must be able to produce reports to support a wide range of business processes, such as service line reporting, costing and pricing, referral to treatment time (RTT) reporting, external contract requirements, practice based commissioning, staff activity and throughput, capacity and demand
- the system must be able to produce reports to support a wide range of clinical processes, such as: audit, research requirements, clinical case loads, case mix, outcome measurement
- computer reports must be available to AHP managers and clinicians as and when required
- reports are easily accessible from the system in a variety of modes; tabular, bar charts, pie charts, spreadsheets and so on
- the system should facilitate the design and generation of ad hoc reports as well as standard reports by AHP managers and clinicians as well as others within the organisation.

8 **Service agreements.** There must be service agreements with computer companies supplying the AHP system:
  - there must be service agreements for the computer software with agreed 'call-out' and support response times
  - agreements should include – for example, systems failure, maintenance, support, trouble shooting, further developments
  - it is helpful if there is a user group attended by the software company that the AHP manager can participate in.
9 **Computer system documentation.** There must be full documentation for the software:
  - comprehensive manual on the computerised information system software use
  - user manuals
  - coding manuals
  - report templates.
10 **Staff training.** Training at all levels on use of the system must be provided:
  - training must be provided for clerical and reception staff
  - training must be provided for AHP staff.

Using the information

Detailed, timely, accurate and relevant information is essential for and central to the quality management of healthcare in the AHPs and throughout the NHS as a whole. Data and information are important to underpin all aspects of management quality and clinical practice, to demonstrate achievement of performance indicators of all types and facilitate and enable management and leadership processes to be pro-active. It is difficult to comprehend how services could be managed effectively, without good quality data and information which must be part of the culture; relevant data and information are the 'life blood' of management – if you can't measure it, you can't manage it!

We have challenged ourselves to find areas of management work which do not require quality information as essential, however, this has not proved possible. Quality data and information are essential, for example, in all ten of our management 'domains' for effective, efficient and economic service provision.

Box 6.2 AHP management domains.[11]

  - Strategic management
  - Clinical governance
  - Human resource management
  - Clinical professional requirements
  - Operational/service management
  - Management of resources
  - Information management
  - Education and training
  - Commissioning
  - Service improvement and modernisation

Quality information is essential for the management of, for example: waiting times, audit results, clinical outcomes, patient throughput and activity, ratios of first to follow-up attendance, for case weighting, skill and case mix, for business planning and service re-design and development, individual caseload management and analysis, time-tabling and scheduling, finance and human resource work, service reviews and costing and pricing, tendering, referral sources, marketing, project management, research and development, complaint management, assessment of patient experience, analysis of patient satisfaction.

Reports

Reports can be of two types; standard or ad hoc. Standard reports are pre defined when the computer programme is written and the system set up, they can be incorporated at any time as a permanent feature of the programme. Ad hoc reports allow the programme user to choose or 'mix and match' a variety of criteria and parameters. Standard reports enable the user to obtain information from the system very quickly without having to input a details series of queries to the system. The data for the compilation of standard reports is calculated by the computer system on an 'on-going' basis so that a report can be generated when ever required as a result of a single command.

The ad hoc reporting facility allows search and extraction from the database, which is from the full range of data input on any aspect. There are many questions which might be asked using an ad hoc reporting facility. Any such queries might be made in isolation or in combination with other questions. An example of this might be to ask the system how many patients of a certain age were referred from Consultant 'A' with a particular diagnosis and treated in a particular location. Alternatively, a report may be needed on the number of patients referred by a specific GP or GP practice or the number of self-referrals.

Box 6.3 Examples of standard and ad hoc reports.

Some suggested examples of standard reports might be:
- reports required at defined intervals for your service, the organisation, regionally or nationally
- workloads defined by referral source
- waiting times for waiting list monitoring
- number of referrals, contacts and throughput
- numbers of open and closed episodes of care indicating the volume of activity within the service as a whole, inpatients, out-patients and community
- GP referrals by individual GP or practice
- service purchaser reports on a range of service provision
- trend reports on demand and service use

Some suggested examples of ad hoc reports might be:
- individual patient reports
- number of open and closed episodes of care
- patient sex and age ranges

- staff case loads – individual and team
- comparison of caseloads by sources of referral
- patient classification – NHS, Private, Overseas visitor
- diagnosis or reason for referral
- outcomes and audit information
- referral classified by individual or groups of consultants
- appliances provided and for retrieval
- aggregated patient reports by groups of for example, diagnostic, care group
- team based activity reports
- HRG clusters

Examples of reports

Example 1. Monitoring number of out-patients waiting

Table 6.1: Patients waiting per week.

Department name	Week 1	Week 2	Week 3	Week 4	Week 5	Week 6	Week 7	Week 8
Dept. 1	63	86	99	121	142	152	150	155
Dept. 2	125	130	144	140	129	111	98	78

Table 6.1 illustrates how waiting list might be monitored on a weekly basis for two Departments, recording the number of patients waiting. This could also be translated into line graphs, for example, to demonstrate the trend as in Figure 6.1.

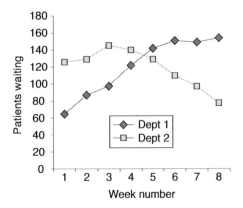

Figure 6.1 Waiting time in weeks: line graph to demonstrate trend.

Example 2. Monitoring activity

Your capacity plan – the amount of activity you are planning to provide for the year – needs regular monitoring. In Figure 6.2 an example is shown, where referrals in three areas in particular are higher than planned. This would enable the manager to discuss with referrers the extra capacity that is required to meet this demand and requiring action to align capacity with demand.

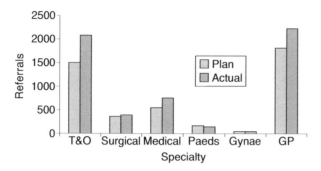

Figure 6.2 New referrals received per month.

Example 3. Monitoring out-patient new to follow up ratio

By monitoring new to follow up ratio, the departmental capacity can be controlled and where the number of follow up contacts increases further analysis of data on an individual therapist level can be undertaken. Figure 6.3 shows a monthly monitoring of first: follow up and would require further scrutiny on June and August to determine why these months have abnormal patterns.

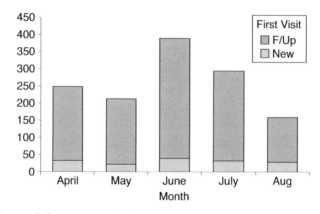

Figure 6.3 First to follow up monitoring.

Example 4. Research and audit presentation of results

Graphs can be a useful way of presenting research and audit data to enable easy interpretation of results. Figure 6.4 shows that the majority of services sampled did not provide self-referral.

AHP referral to treatment reporting

NHS Wales was the first home country to require the collection of RTT data for AHPs although targets are long. The DH Transforming Community Services[12] programme subsequently required national reporting for AHP RTT in England: 'The AHP RTT rules provide a framework within which the NHS has the

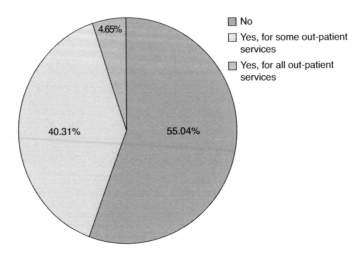

Figure 6.4 Percentage of services providing self-referral.

autonomy to make sensible clinically sound decisions about how to apply them, in a way that is consistent with how patients experience or perceive their wait.'

Mandatory reporting for AHP waits in England commenced on a voluntary basis from 2010, though no national target for length of waiting time was set. The beginning of a wait is defined as the date that the referral is received by the service. The end of the wait period being when first definitive treatment starts, or a clinical decision made that treatment is not required.

All NHS funded providers are required to report on a monthly basis to the DH. The AHP professions required to provide RTT data are:

- art, drama, music therapists
- chiropodists/podiatrists,
- dietitians,
- occupational therapists,
- orthoptists
- physiotherapists,
- prosthetists and orthotists,
- radiographers (diagnostic and therapeutic)
- speech and language therapists.

Time is money – how do we spend it?

AHP managers need to have an accurate picture of workforce activity: the throughput, exactly what work is undertaken, who does it, where it happens and what sort of service or interventions are provided. A thorough understanding of work activity is essential to service and workforce planning, development of staffing profiles for specific programmes such as the Consultant-led 18 weeks pathway and service re-design and for a wide range of other purposes such as for costing and pricing, evidence-based staff deployment, contract development, service level agreements, capacity and demand management and payment by results. Staff activity analysis also facilitates evidence-based service development and strategy, enabling critical evaluation of different staff activities, to support specific projects. This technique is essential for understanding management and administrative inputs and supporting analysis of patterns of work for capacity and demand management work. If carried out in collaboration with colleagues from other Trusts the approach can also be used for benchmarking exercises. Activity analysis is also important in monitoring and supporting a range of clinical governance parameters.

Activity analysis is a method of sampling volumes and types of activity undertaken by AHP staff in all grades and specialties on a regular 'snapshot' basis, using a sample activity data collection process based on a template form used for data extract to be input to a programme for reporting and subsequent analysis and interpretation. The different components of patient related work and non-patient care need to be understood for effective and efficient service provision and management in the increasingly business environment.

This approach has been used in our services and the data obtained used for management and clinical purposes and for benchmarking between locations.

Tips for implementation

- Ensure the data collection form is fully tested and piloted.
- Involve all team members.
- Computer support and analysis is essential.
- Forward planning for the sample enquiry is important.
- Thorough teaching of definitions of the data items.
- It is essential to share results and outcomes with all teams taking part in the sample.

Box 6.4 Therapy services activity sample form: briefing notes.

Understanding staff activity and the way we spend our working hours is important for management, clinical, and financial purposes and when developing new services and re-designing current ones. The activity sample can be run as a 'snapshot' for example a week or for a more comprehensive analysis a 13 week quarter can be used, doing one day per week, that is, week 1 Monday, week 2 Tuesday and so on. A consistent approach to completing the form is needed, so these briefing notes should be shared with all staff who are to undertake the survey.

The form is divided into four main sections:

1 general information
2 patient related activity
3 non-patient related activity
4 about your contracted working hours and caseloads
   - each member of staff completes a new form on each day of the activity sample whether working that day or not
   - the main activity sample takes place Monday to Friday inclusive, but members of staff working at the weekend will also be requested to complete forms for those days
   - the form should be completed by HPC registered staff and assistants.

Part 1 – general information

Professional group: the AHP professional group of which you are a member (including assistants), e.g. occupational therapy, dietetics, physiotherapy.

Date: the date on which the form is completed. All forms must be completed on the same day as the activity takes place. It is best to do this as you go through the day to be sure of accuracy.

Site: this is where you are working, e.g. DGH, community hospital, domiciliary, special school. If you work in more than one site on one day, a new form should be completed for each site.

Location: the place within your organisation where the interventions take place; e.g. wards, physiotherapy department, podiatry clinics, patients' homes.

Clinician code: the individual staff code (whatever is used within the organisation for your personal identifier.

Band: agenda for change grade.

Your post name/rotation: e.g. clinical specialist in...Band 5 in-patient rotation, out-patient department assistant.

Absent? Reason: why you are not working today, e.g. annual leave, part-time do not work today, study leave, sick.

Part 2 – patient related activity

Please enter hours and minutes spent on each activity accurately:
- face to face contact with individual patients
- face to face contact with patients in groups
- telephone contacts with patients, relatives and carers
- ward rounds
- case conferences
- liaison with other services related to patient care
- administrative work related to patient care, e.g. record keeping
- home assessment visits with or without the patient in attendance,
- clinics
- other patient related activity to capture others not included above (must be strictly patient related).

Part 3 – non-patient related activity

Please enter hours and minutes spent on each activity accurately:
- liaison with other services, not related to patient care, could be for a wide range of reasons
- administration; not patient related, e.g. sending out appointments
- management duties; all work involved in service management or management duties within the organisation
- study leave – you are on study leave yourself

- travel; in the community, between sites or locations, walking the corridors
- staff and team meetings
- in-service education/training; attendance (not leading or presenting)
- teaching and training; when you are leading, presenting or giving this for
  - your own professional group
  - students
  - others
- clinical supervision; providing or attending
- other non-patient related activities not captured above.

Part 4 – about your contracted hours and caseload

- *Your contracted working hours today:* the number of hours you are contracted to work that day, if part time and not working that day indicate this.
- *Number of group sessions you have done today.*
- *Number of patients on your caseload today:* how many patients did you see or should you have seen including did not attends or Unable to Attends (DNA or UTA).
- The total number of patients you have on your overall caseload; how many patients are registered to be seen by you at present.

Therapy services activity sample proforma

Professional group: _____

Date	Site	Location	Clinician Code	Band	Your post Name/rotation	Absent? Reason

Activity level	Hours	Minutes
Patient Related		
Face to face contact (individual)		
Face to face contacts (group)		
Telephone contacts with patient or relative		
Ward rounds		
Case conferences		
Liaison with other services – related to patient care		
Administration – patient related		

Activity level		Hours	Minutes
Home assessment visits			
Clinics			
Other (patient related)			
Non-Patient Related			
Liaison with other services – not related to patient			
Administration – not patient related			
Management duties			
Study leave			
Travel			
Staff/team meetings			
In-service training / education			
Teaching/training	Your professional group		
" "	Students		
" "	Other		
Clinical supervision			
Other (non patient related)			
Your contracted working hours Today			
No. of group sessions you have done Today			
No. of patients on your caseload Today			
The total number of patients currently on your caseload			

Example of reports from activity sample

The activity sample data can be analysed and the results shown in tabular or graphical formats as shown in Figures 6.5 to 6.7.

This is the aggregated activity for both patient related and non-patient related activity, these can be broken down to look at any specific parameter and make comparisons with any of the others. This type of analysis is an important and powerful 'tool' and needs to be used in association with qualitative measures. By understanding the way that staff spend their time and the division between patient contact time and non-patient contact time, the manager is able to workforce plan effectively to ensure efficient staffing.

Summary

Information management is an essential aspect of AHP management. IM&T offers many benefits to AHP managers, clinicians and service users including the following.

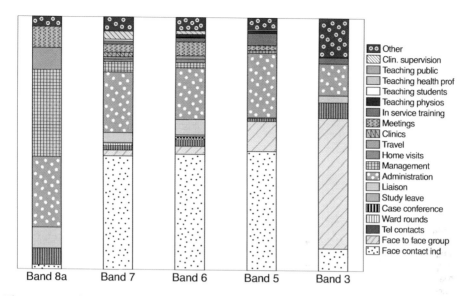

Figure 6.5 Sub-division of staff time by staff band.

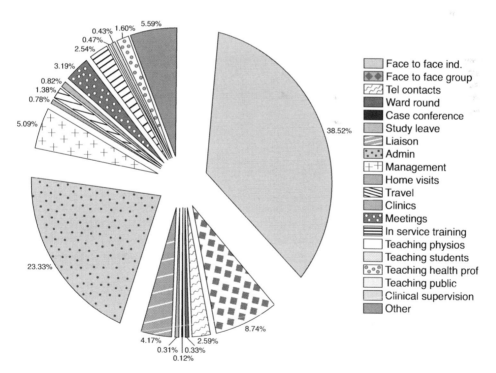

Figure 6.6 Sub-division of staff time; all staff.

- Support to strategic and operational management.
- Support to good business and staff management.
- Identification of trends.
- Warning of potential adverse events.

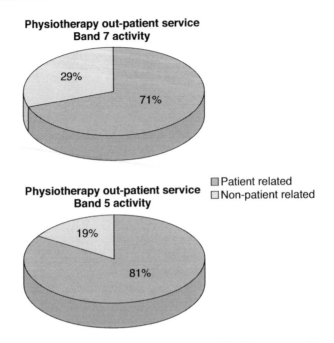

Figure 6.7 Comparison of out-patient staff: patient related to non-patient related activity by Band 5 and Band 7, physiotherapy out-patient service.

- More effective and efficient record keeping.
- Better management of patient care.
- Development of and access to the evidence base.
- Audit, research and development.
- Whether the service is in primary or secondary care, the private or other sectors, management of the service directly impacts on the quality of care provided. Information management and technology is an essential 'tool' to support all elements of quality management to enable service effectiveness and efficiency, management of change and service re-design. The effective use of data to manage services enables managers to contribute fully to business processes, performance management and clinical governance.
- Information is power and in the 21st century, all AHP managers and leaders must be increasingly involved in the use of IM&T for current purposes and future development.
- In order to thrive – or even survive – it is imperative that we have robust information management systems to ensure the evidence for our management, clinical practice and patient care.

References

1 Jones R. *Management in Physiotherapy*. Oxford: Radcliffe Medical Press; 1991.
2 Körner E. *Report on the collection and use of information about hospital clinical activity in the NHS (first Report)*. DHSS Steering Group on Health Services Information. London: HMSO; 1982.

3 IMG, NHSME. *Information Management and Technology Strategy*. London: HMSO; 1993.

4 DH. *NHS Plan*, 2000: www.dh.gov.uk/en/Publicationsandstatistics/Publications/PublicationsPolicyAndGuidance/DH_4002960.

5 DH. *Wanless Report*, 2002: www.dh.gov.uk/en/Publicationsandstatistics/Publications/PublicationsPolicyAndGuidance/DH_4074426.

6 Information for Health Strategy: www.dh.gov.uk/en/Publicationsandstatistics/Lettersandcirculars/Healthservicecirculars/DH_4005016.

7 Informing Healthcare Wales: www.wales.nhs.uk/IHC/home.cfm.

8 eHealth Scotland: www.ehealth.scot.nhs.uk.

9 Bates W, Gawande A. Improving safety with information technology. *New Eng J Med*. 2003; **25(348)**: 252.

10 Connecting for Health: www.connectingforhealth.nhs.uk.

11 Jones R, Jenkins F. *Managing and Leading in the Allied Health Professions*. Oxford: Radcliffe Publishing; 2006.

12 DH. *Transforming Community Services. Enabling new patterns of provision*, 2009: www.dh.gov.uk/en/Publicationsandstatistics/Publications/PublicationsPolicyAndGuidance/DH_093197.

Chapter 7

Information management for healthcare professionals, or what has IT ever done for us?

Alan Gillies

Introduction

There are many healthcare professionals that still regard information technology with suspicion. There are some valid reasons for this:

- historically, IM&T has been used to meet the needs of managers not clinicians or patients
- this has often involved clinicians in the use of a lot of their time, with very little benefit in return
- training for clinicians has often been inadequate and/or inappropriate.

However, this is not a sustainable position for the NHS as a whole or the individual clinician, as reported in the Wanless Report.[1]

> The Review's projections incorporate a doubling of spending on Information communication technology (ICT) to fund ambitious targets of the kind set out in the NHS Information Strategy. To avoid duplication of effort and resources and to ensure that the benefits of ICT integration across health and social services are achieved, the Review recommends that stringent standards should be set from the centre to ensure that systems across the UK are fully compatible with each other.
> The Review recommended that a more effective partnership between health professionals and the public should be facilitated, for example, by:
>
> - development of improved health information to help people engage with their care in an informed way.

The individual healthcare professional has a number of professional obligations around the use and management of information. These will be highlighted by extracts from the Code of Ethics for Occupational Therapists, but similar principles are defined in all professional codes of conduct for all healthcare professionals.

Box 7.1 Extract from code of ethics and professional conduct for occupational therapists.[2]

Each client is unique and, therefore, brings an individual perspective to the occupational therapy process. Normally, clients have a right to make choices and decisions about their own health and independence, and such choices should be respected even when in conflict with professional opinion.

- Normally, clients should be given sufficient information to enable them to make informed decisions about their health and social care.
- Information should be provided in a form which is capable of being understood by that client.
- Normally, reasonable steps should be taken to ensure that the client understands the nature, purpose and likely effect of the proposed intervention.
- It is the duty of occupational therapists to obtain sufficient information to enable them to determine the appropriateness of the referral.
- Occupational therapists shall accurately record all information related to professional activities.
- The prime purpose of records is to facilitate the care, treatment and support of a client. It is essential to provide and maintain a written record of professional intervention, advice given and outcome of decisions taken.
- Accurate, legible, factual, contemporaneous and attributed records and reports of occupational therapy intervention must be kept in order to provide information for professional colleagues and for legal purposes, such as client access and court reports.

Some clinicians may cling to the view that these standards have little to do with IT. However, clinical ethical codes are underpinned by the principle of beneficence, and its corresponding principle of non-maleficence. Beneficence and non-maleficence are summarised in the Hippocratic principle that care should seek to inflict no harm, prevent harm, remove harm and promote good.

Put simply, all healthcare professionals are required to embrace IT where it can be shown to have benefits for patients, and to ensure that when they do use it, they do so properly to ensure that no harm comes to patients.

In this chapter two questions are considered.

1 What can IT do for me and my patients?
2 What do I have to do to use IT properly?

What can IT do for me and my patients?

IT offers benefits to patients and clinicians, including:

- more effective and efficient record keeping
- access to best evidence
- warning of potential adverse events

More effective and efficient record keeping

Good record keeping is an essential part of healthcare and the responsibility of every clinician. Many clinicians feel comfortable with paper-based records, but there are a number of disadvantages to paper-based systems:

- ambiguity – language can be ambiguous, handwriting can be illegible
- transmission – paper records are difficult to transmit, methods such as fax are very insecure
- storage – paper records are bulky and vulnerable to damage from tear, fire, water, coffee
- sorting – paper records can only be sorted one way at a time, usually alphabetically
- searching – looking for information is time consuming
- sharing – in integrated care, paper records lead to incomplete data sharing across agencies and even within teams.

Problems can be most obvious at the interface. Consider discharge from hospital. Discharge summaries can take a while to emerge. For example, one hospital had a target of typing discharge summaries within two weeks. Worse still they had no target for how quickly summaries would reach the GPs. They were not meeting the target; recognising this was inadequate, faxes were used to transmit information in a very insecure fashion.

AHPs may be further distanced as information may have to reach them via the GP introducing delay.

Electronic records offer considerable potential benefits, such as:

- clarity – they are precise and legible
- transmission – they are simple to transmit and provide inbuilt protection methods such as encryption
- storage – they are compact and can be 'backed up' readily to protect from tear, fire, water, coffee damage
- sorting – they can be sorted in many ways
- searching – facilitated by the use of structured coding schema and query languages
- sharing – in integrated care, they facilitate data sharing across multiple agencies and within teams.

However, realising these benefits is a complex exercise and electronic records pose their own range of problems:

- ambiguity – sometimes the information for storage has a degree of inbuilt uncertainty, electronic records can be inflexible
- transmission – the ease of transmission of electronic data can pose a threat to confidentiality and offer potential routes for attack from hackers and computer viruses
- storage – although looking after electronic records is facilitated by the technology, many users do not do it, leaving records vulnerable
- complexity – the technology itself can be a barrier.

The proposed solution for the NHS in England is the National Programme for Information Technology delivered by Connecting for Health. More information can be found at www.cfh.nhs.uk.[3] Similar projects are underway in Scotland, Wales and Northern Ireland.

Connecting for Health is implementing a national data spine to which all clinical systems should be attached. Each local system will retain its full electronic patient record, whilst the core of the record will be made available to any care

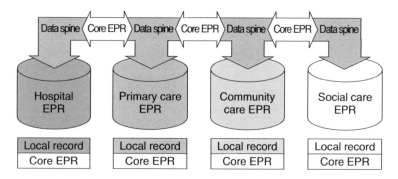

Figure 7.1 Schematic of National Programme for IT.

giver within the system, who has a need and a right to access the information. The schematic in Figure 7.1 shows how the system will work.

If the National Programme is to deliver it has a number of key hurdles to overcome:

- technological – whilst the system is big, it is not revolutionary. The technological issues are all about handling a huge number of transactions
- fitness for clinical purpose – the solution must demonstrably meet the needs of its users, the clinicians and their patients
- equipping and enthusing clinicians – there is need to both train and enthuse clinical staff: without this it is just a huge empty motorway system with no cars driving around on it.

The keys to an effective solution are a set of standards which users and developers must adhere to:

- clinical coding standards – the information must be stored in the same way across the whole system or the 'components' will not understand information from another part of the system: much like an English person abroad
- data standards – the data must be transmitted in a common format so that each system can extract the information it needs
- network standards – the links between the systems must be built to common standards or the transmissions will not work. The whole internet across the world uses the same network standards or protocols so that all machines can 'talk' to each other. The internet network protocol is known as TCP/IP.

The latter provides the evidence that the task can be achieved. The Internet is global in scope. It has the potential to link the entire world because everyone agrees to use the same standards. Hopefully the NHS can do the same.

Access to best evidence

IT can also provide rapid access to best evidence. There is a series of websites dedicated to help find the best treatments for patients. One of the most comprehensive is the National Library for Health (NLH), which can be found at www.nlh.nhs.uk.[4]

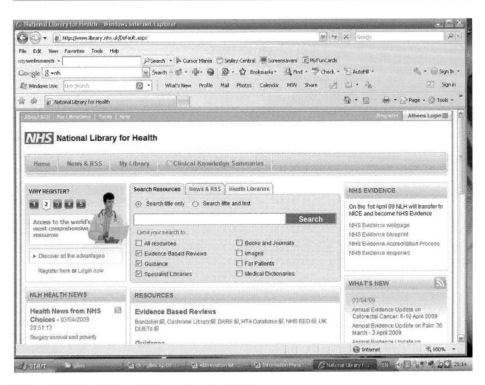

Figure 7.2 The National Library for Health homepage.

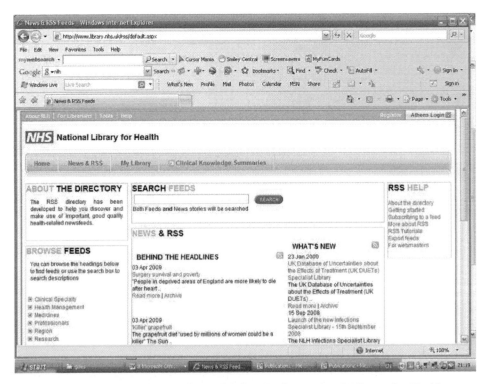

Figure 7.3 News and really simple syndication in the National Library for Health.

The NLH provides a huge library of resources. Access is via the NHSNet or Athens Password. As an example of how IT provides a much greater service than a paper-based solution, it is hard to think of a better one. On the other hand, the sheer quantity of information can be daunting. Local health librarians are an invaluable guide even in this electronic age.

One useful section is the 'News and RSS' section accessed via the tab on the screen. This feature provides the evidence behind current media stories about which patients may be anxious.

Reduction of potential adverse events

A major potential benefit from using IT is the prevention of adverse events, by prompting the clinician when a potential adverse event is about to happen. Many people suffer adverse events whilst within the healthcare system contravening the principle of non-maleficence: our first responsibility is not to do harm.

Computers are not psychic or even intelligent: they can prompt a clinician to act in one of two cases.

1 The records hold information that show that a proposed action would contra-indicate with an existing therapy. Most commonly, this is used with medication, because this is the area where most evidence is held. However, there is considerable potential to extend its use to a wide range of therapies.
2 The records hold information that show that a proposed action would contra-indicate with this particular patient due to an allergy or existing condition.

There is much interest in this area, not least because of the huge cost of adverse events in terms of patient wellbeing and healthcare system resources.

Box 7.2 Extract from Protti report 'A world view'.[5]

In his report, *Making Amends*, England's Chief Medical Officer reported that 10% of hospital in-patient admissions may result in some kind of adverse event and that 18% of patients reported being the victim of a medication error sometime in the previous two years. A study by the National Patient Safety Agency found that of 112 adverse incidents, 35 involved information not being available.

Dr Paul Aylin, a British researcher, reported that, on average, 2.2% of all episodes (over 276 000 per year) recorded within hospital episode statistics included a code for an adverse event. His study reported that the rate of adverse events recorded in UK NHS trusts ranged from 0% to 15%. He and his colleagues noted that other studies have found overall rates of between 1% and 36%, commenting that studies using administrative data tend to have lower estimates than those based on case note reviews or purpose designed systems. They were of the opinion that adverse events may be under-recorded within hospital episode statistics, noting that hospital acquired infections are poorly represented within the World Health's ICD-10 coding system (e.g. there is no specific code for methicillin resistant staphylococcus aureus). Similar evidence can be found in studies from elsewhere.

In Canada, according to Dr Robyn Tamblyn, drug-related adverse events are reported to be the sixth leading cause of death and contribute substantially to morbidity. Inappropriate prescribing has been identified as a preventable cause of at least 20% of drug-related adverse events. Elderly patients are at greatest risk of receiving inappropriate prescriptions. Because primary care physicians write approximately 80% of all their prescriptions for people 65 years of age and older, the Tamblyn study argued that effective interventions to optimize prescribing in primary care are a priority.

In America, according to Dr Blackford Middleton, over 98,000 deaths each year are related to medical error, 40% of out-patient prescriptions are unnecessary, and patients receive only 55% of recommended care. He noted that Medicare beneficiaries see 2–14 unique providers annually and on average 6 different providers/year. Patient's multiple records do not interoperate and providers have incomplete knowledge of their patients. In one study it was shown that patient data was unavailable in 81% of cases in one clinic, with an average of 4 missing items per case. Middleton's study estimates that 8% of medical errors are estimated to be due to inadequate availability of patient information. Like in many parts of the world, 90% of the 30 billion healthcare transactions in the US every year are conducted via mail, fax, or phone.

As information becomes more and more central to care, its potential for good or harm becomes greater. Therefore, the responsibility of individual professionals to act responsibly becomes more vital.

What do I have to do to use IT properly?

Clinicians have a number of obligations in respect of IT, including:

- competence in using IT to maintain records
- consent and confidentiality
- data protection.

Competence in using IT to maintain records

Competence in maintaining records has always been an assumed part of professional practice. However, jokes about doctors' handwriting suggest that in reality, such competence may not always be assumed.

Clearly, the use of electronic health records requires greater proficiency in some areas and this goes beyond simple IT skills.

There are at least three types of skills essential to a clinician if they are to fulfil their professional duty to maintain good records in an electronic age.

1 IT skills
2 Information Management (IM) skills
3 consultation skills.

IT skills are the ability to use the technology. The NHS has moved to address this through the introduction of the European Computer Driving Licence (ECDL) qualification to ensure all staff have basic IT skills. ECDL is an internationally recognised IT qualification that was adopted as the referenced standard by the NHS in November 2001 and was made available to all NHS staff in March 2003. During February 2005, the 100 000th NHS staff member registered for the course, so considerable rollout has been achieved.

However, whilst this is a welcome acknowledgment of the importance of training, ECDL is based around standard office applications and may not equip a staff member for the use of their clinical application. In particular, the most relevant module for many clinicians would be the database application and this module was simplified, reducing the requirements of students. Whilst this may increase overall pass rates, it may leave students less well equipped to deal with clinical systems that are usually quite complex database applications.

Once competence is achieved with technology, the next stage is to become competent in managing the information or in working in new ways with the technology. For example, the most common new skill needed is recording information as clinical codes or terms rather than using free text.

Computers process 1s and 0s: they do not like ambiguity. In order to deal with this, healthcare systems have developed coding schemas to allow computers to store clinical information. In primary care in the UK, for the last 18 years or so, information has been stored as Read codes. Epidemiologists use ICD10 or ICD 11, which is a disease classification system. A new system is being introduced across the NHS known as SNOMED (Systematised Nomenclature of Medicine Clinical Terms) to standardise the codes used.

Whichever coding system is used, working with codes is different from recording free text. When a computer searches, it only finds exact matches. In primary care, there have been many instances of problems caused by people using slightly different codes to record the same condition. Computer queries have failed to identify records with codes different from those expected.

In any sphere, when IT is introduced, changes in working practices are required and much of the benefit derives from the changes in working practices rather than the technology alone. Think of a word processor replacing a typewriter. Spell checking, use of document templates, mail and email merges are all new working practices that can bring great benefits, but require new ways of working and the skills required go beyond knowing which button to press to knowing how and when to use them to gain advantage.

The final skill type is an extension of the second. As far back as 1992, the NHS stated that information should be generated routinely from clinical consultations rather than from separate processes. Conducting a consultation whilst making use of evidence provided electronically, and recording information in the patient's electronic records, without excluding the patient is a skill in itself which will require learning.

Consent and confidentiality

Maintaining confidentiality and obtaining consent are professional responsibilities irrespective of the level of technology employed. However, there are different implications if a high degree of technology is employed.

Three specific areas are considered:

1 informed consent for a clinical procedure
2 maintaining confidentiality
3 obtaining informed consent for information sharing.

The DH produced guidance on what constitutes informed consent following the reports into Bristol[6] and Alder Hey.[7] This advice is shown in Box 7.3.

Box 7.3 DH guidance on informed consent.[8]

For consent to be valid, it must be given voluntarily by an appropriately informed person (the patient or where relevant someone with parental responsibility for a patient under the age of 18) who has the capacity to consent to the intervention in question. Acquiescence where the person does not know what the intervention entails is not 'consent'.

To give valid consent the patient needs to understand in broad terms the nature and purpose of the procedure. Any misrepresentation of these elements will invalidate consent. Where relevant, information about anaesthesia should be given as well as information about the procedure itself.

Clear information is particularly important when students or trainees carry out procedures to further their own education. Where the procedure will further the patient's care – for example taking a blood sample for testing – then, assuming the student is appropriately trained in the procedure, the fact that it is carried out by a student does not alter the nature and purpose of the procedure. It is therefore not a legal requirement to tell the patient that the clinician is a student, although it would always be good practice to do so. In contrast, where a student proposes to conduct a physical examination which is not part of the patient's care, then it is essential to explain that the purpose of the examination is to further the student's training and to seek consent for that to take place.

Although informing patients of the nature and purpose of procedures enables valid consent to be given as far as any claim of battery is concerned, this is not sufficient to fulfil the legal duty of care to the patient. Failure to provide other relevant information may render the professional liable to an action for negligence if a patient subsequently suffers harm as a result of the treatment received.

Mayberry and Mayberry[9] suggest that the following are essential elements of consent from a legal perspective:

- discussions of the interventions at an early stage
- a simple explanation of the procedure, including purpose, recognised complications and risks and alternatives
- checks with the patient with regard to how much they wish to know
- rechecking the patient's agreement at a later stage, prior to the procedure
- frequent checking at all stages that the patient has understood what has been said
- documentation of these discussions throughout the clinical record.

Through resources like the NLH, the clinician has a wide range of resources available to help inform patient choice.

We have already seen the professionals' duty to maintain confidentiality. The NHS[10] defines it as:

A duty of confidence arises when one person discloses information to another (e.g. patient to clinician) in circumstances where it is reasonable to expect that the information will be held in confidence. It:

- is a legal obligation that is derived from case law;
- is a requirement established within professional codes of conduct; and
- must be included within NHS employment contracts as a specific requirement linked to disciplinary procedures.

The official guidance makes a distinction between patient identifiable data and non-identifiable data. This creates its own set of difficulties.

Anonymised data may still be identifiable from other factors. For example, it would be difficult to identify a patient from a diagnosis of asthma, as this is very common. As the diagnosis is refined and combined with other factors such as age gender and ethnicity, it may quickly provide a unique profile of a patient who could be identified.

In practice, the duty of care on a clinician to protect the data is not removed by anonymising it. Some of the anonymised data used routinely for disease surveillance in public health, including for example sexually transmitted disease data, is amongst the most sensitive. Alternatively, if we diagnose a rare condition, that may be unique within a practice or PCT.

There is a mandatory requirement that all removable data including laptops, CDs and USB sticks for example must be encrypted and the movement of any unencrypted person identifiable data held in electronic format must not be allowed in the NHS.

When a patient discloses private information to their doctor, or another individual clinician, they do not necessarily expect that information to be available to another member of their healthcare team. They may go further and explicitly state that they wish it remain confidential to that individual clinician. In the modern healthcare system, however, care is often a team activity and may require information sharing amongst the team. The official advice[10] states:

Patients generally have the right to object to the use and disclosure of confidential information that identifies them, and the need to be made aware of this right. Sometimes if patients choose to prohibit information being disclosed to other health professionals involved in providing care, it might mean that the care that can be offered can be limited and in extremely rare circumstances that it is not possible to offer certain treatment options. Patients must be informed if their decisions about disclosure have implications for the provision of care or treatment.

There is a clear trade-off between disclosure of information to professional colleagues on a 'need-to-know' basis and the desire for patient privacy. However, there is a clear principle that patients' consent must be sought for disclosure and that consent must be properly informed.

The use of electronic patient records allows a range of things to happen which can facilitate better patient care:

- easier storage of patient information
- easier transmission of patient information
- easier sharing of patient information across a team.

Unfortunately all of these have implications for confidentiality and data protection and for every advantage there is a potential disadvantage:

- easier storage of patient information which is not for any legitimate purpose
- easier inappropriate disclosure of patient information
- easier inappropriate sharing of patient information beyond those with a need to know.

In the policy document that outlines the IT infrastructure to support the NHS,[11] the need for confidentiality and patient consent to disclosure is recognised.

Whilst it is essential that the infrastructure is designed to protect patient confidentiality, it is the users of the systems who must ensure that the confidentiality is protected. This places responsibility on individual clinicians to:

- ensure they understand their professional and legal obligations
- protect their patient's data against unauthorised access
- protect their patient's data against accidental damage
- protect their patient's data against deliberate damage.

Data protection

The use of IT changes the risks to patient records: it also provides new opportunities for managing risks. Paper-based records have always been at risk of accidental damage through the threats of fire and flood. Additional risks include loss due to incorrect filing.

Each of these risks has a corresponding risk for computerised records. Computers can be destroyed by fire or flood or even *in extremis* cups of coffee! Similarly, records may be filed under a wrong name or deleted accidentally. It is much easier to delete a computerised record accidentally than throw away a physical record accidentally.

Computers have additional risks due to their need for an external power supply and their technological complexity. Clinical coding makes incorrect data entry potentially more likely as different clinicians may wish to use different codes for the same condition.

However, the most significant difference is that the technology can provide a means of managing the risks.

Given our duty to keep patient information secure, so there is a need to make best use of technology to protect the information from accidental damage. Table 7.1 shows how we can protect against the identified risks.

A good backup strategy is essential, which might look like the example shown in Table 7.2.

Using this schedule gives daily protection against equipment or power supply failure or against accidental deletion. It means that you are never more than a week away from full data in the event of a major catastrophe.

Table 7.1 Protecting against risk.

Risk	Management
Flood	Regular backups
	Remote storage of backups
Fire	Regular backups
	Remote storage of backups
Power failure	Continuous power supply
	Regular backups
Equipment failure	Regular backups
Incorrect data entry	Data validation
	Data entry protocols
Accidental deletion of files	Confirmation dialog boxes

Table 7.2 Backup strategy.

Day	Task
Monday	Incremental backup
Tuesday	Full backup
Wednesday	Incremental backup
Thursday	Incremental backup
Friday	Full backup removed to remote secure destination
Saturday	Incremental backup
Sunday	Incremental backup

Procedures to make backup copies of the patient record system must be:

• appropriately planned to ensure that a valid recent copy can be recovered
• regularly, correctly and consistently carried out
• verified by checking the integrity of the backed up data – on every occasion.

Used backup hardware should be replaced with new media at regular intervals taking account of the manufacturers' recommendations on the anticipated working life of the media used. Old backup media should be re-formatted or physically disrupted so as to render any data on them unrecoverable. If the backup procedure offers a choice of backing up different parts of the system, the routine backup procedure should always include a backup of the audit trail.

The organisation should have a policy on data entry to minimise risks in this area. The policy may allow another person to make entries in the patient records on behalf of the responsible healthcare professional. The information on which such entries are based may be a written note, a dictated message or a verbal report by the healthcare professional responsible for the observations or interventions recorded.

Entries made in this way must be:

• transcribed to the computerised record by an authorised trained person who ascribes the entries to the healthcare professional who wrote or dictated the notes

- monitored in accordance with the practice policy on data entry to ensure the accuracy and correct attribution of the entries made.

The clinical system should record details of who, what and when, in an audit trail. Audit trails should be capable of detecting tampering and should be secured against deletion. If reports and correspondence are received electronically from outside the practice, the practice policy should include procedures to ensure that:

- all information received is seen by the person responsible for the original request or by another doctor acting on his or her behalf
- the information received is filed in the computerised record of the patient to whom it relates.

Finally, confirmatory dialogue boxes are an essential part of any system design. I call them 'Have you lost your presence of mind?' boxes. They are the prompts that ask you 'Are you sure you want to do this?' when you are about to delete a file or similar. They have a purpose. Ignore them at your peril!

Electronic records are at risk not only from people who want to read them, but people who think it is fun to see if they can.

Paper-based records have always been at risk of unauthorised access. In order to obtain access, however, the interloper has had to be in the presence of the records. Now with the advent of computer networks, people seeking unauthorised access can do so remotely. What is more, some people do it just for fun.

The first line of defence against unauthorised access is password protection.

The DH[10] code of conduct offers the advice in Box 7.4.

Box 7.4 DH code of conduct.

For all types of records, staff working in offices where records may be seen must:
- shut/lock doors and cabinets as required
- wear building passes/ID if issued
- query the status of strangers
- know who to tell if anything suspicious or worrying is noted
- not tell unauthorised personnel how the security systems operate
- not breach security themselves.

Manual records must be:
- formally booked out from their normal filing system
- tracked if transferred, with a note made or sent to the filing location of the transfer
- returned to the filing location as soon as possible after use
- stored securely within the clinic or office, arranged so that the record can be found easily if needed urgently
- stored closed when not in use so that contents are not seen accidentally
- inaccessible to members of the public and not left even for short periods where they might be looked at by unauthorised persons
- held in secure storage with clear labelling. Protective 'wrappers' indicating sensitivity – though not indicating the reason for sensitivity – and permitted access, and the availability of secure means of destruction such as shredding, are essential.

With electronic records, staff must:
- always log-out of any computer system or application when work on it is finished
- not leave a terminal unattended and logged-in
- not share logins with other people. If other staff have need to access records, then appropriate access should be organised for them – this must not be by using others' access identities
- not reveal passwords to others
- change passwords at regular intervals to prevent anyone else using them
- avoid using short passwords , or using names that are known to be associated with them such as children's or pet names or birthdays
- always clear the screen of a previous patient's information before seeing another
- use a password-protected screen-saver to prevent casual viewing of patient information by others.

Passwords should be longer than six characters and use a mixture of letters and numbers to make them as difficult to guess as possible. A truly random combination of five letters offers more than 10^{169} combinations, and including numbers increases this to 10^{186} combinations. This is increased further if upper and lower cases are used. However, it is difficult to remember a random sequence, the tendency is to use our pet dog's name or similar!

The other good practice is to change passwords regularly and always if you suspect that your password is no longer secure.

Paper-based records have always been at risk of malicious damage. Fire and flood may be initiated deliberately.

Computers are attractive objects in themselves, both to thieves and also to people who write viruses to attack computers. In Salford, Greater Manchester, one practice was so worried about theft from premises, that their entire computer system had to fit onto one laptop that could be removed at night.

Generally, however, whilst physical security is certainly an issue, the threat from viruses is a greater risk. In recent years, the NHS Net has been attacked and breached by the 'I love you' virus, and the Blaster worm.

The following advice is given to general practice:[12]

- disks received from outside the practice should be checked for viruses by effective and regularly updated anti-virus programmes;
- files received from outside the practice by electronic transfer should also be checked for viruses.

Every NHS organisation should have a security policy that takes full account of the need for confidentiality as well as authentication and integrity of the computerised patient record system. The security policy should take account of local circumstances and risks but should specifically address the points under the headings below:

- security policy
- security organisation
- asset classification and control
- personnel security

- physical and environmental security
- communications and operations management
- access control
- system development and maintenance
- business continuity management
- compliance.

The policy should recognise the need for data entry to be restricted to properly trained and authorised people. It must take full account of the need for entries to be accurate, complete and attributed to the person responsible for the observations or interventions recorded. When considering the issue of authentication, be aware that you may be held liable for the content and accuracy of information that appears to have been entered by you or on your behalf. It is therefore important that the security features of the system and procedures combine to minimise the risk of a record entry being accidentally or fraudulently attributed to the wrong user.

It may be necessary to prove that an entry was or was not made by the person to whom it is attributed. This means that, since most record entries are logged as being the responsibility of the individual whose password is currently entered, it should never be acceptable for an entry to be made into a record when someone else has logged into the system. More generally, it is essential to:

- have a unique user identity and password
- keep passwords secret and do not divulge it to other users for any reason
- change passwords at frequent intervals
- log out of workstations when their task at that workstation is finished and never leave a workstation logged in but unattended.

The policy should ensure that the organisation has a clearly laid out disaster recovery plan. This will need to address the temporary replacement of the organisation's electronic functions with paper-based alternatives, the retention and subsequent entry of these temporary records into the electronic record system when it becomes available again and the extraction of essential information from ancillary systems such as any electronic appointment book's backup.

In conclusion many clinicians feel that IT is not for them, that it is run for the benefit of the organisation or the senior management, not them and their patients. However, IT has major potential benefits for clinicians and patients alike.

In order to take advantage of these benefits, clinicians need to be prepared to take control of the IT agenda and make it work for them,[13] ensure that they have access to proper training and in some cases to adapt their ways of working to gain full advantage of the benefits of the new technology.

At the same time, in order to ensure that patients receive the best quality of care with minimum risk of harm, clinicians have a professional responsibility to ensure that they are competent with the new technology, maintain confidentiality and protect the data in their charge. There is no such thing as a free lunch!

References

1 Wanless D. *Securing Our Future Health: taking a long-term view*. London: HMSO; 2002.
2 College of Occupational Therapy. *Code of Ethics and Professional Conduct for Occupational Therapists*. London: COT; 2000.

3 Connecting for Health: www.cfh.nhs.uk.
4 National Library for Health: www.nlh.nhs.uk.
5 Protti D. 'A world view': www.cfh.nhs.uk.
6 Kennedy I. *Learning from Bristol. The report of the Public Inquiry into Children's Heart Surgery at the Bristol Royal Infirmary 1984–1995 Cm5207–1.* Stationery Office; 2001: www.bristol-inquiry.org.uk.
7 Royal Liverpool Inquiry: www.rlcinquiry.org.uk.
8 Department of Health, HSC 2001/023. *Good practice in consent: achieving the NHS Plan commitment to patient-centred consent practice.* London: HMSO; 2001.
9 Maybery M, Mayberry J. *Consent in Clinical Practice.* Oxford: Radcliffe Publishing; 2003.
10 Department of Health. *Confidentiality: NHS Code of Practice.* Information Policy Unit, London: HMSO; 2003.
11 Department of Health. *Delivering 21st Century IT for the NHS.* National Patient Record Analysis Service (NPRAS). London: HMSO; 2003.
12 BMA GPC/RCGP. *Good practice guidelines for general practice electronic patient records.* The Joint Computing Group of the General Practitioners' Committee and the Royal College of General Practitioners. London: BMA; 2000.
13 Gillies AC. *The Clinicians' Guide to Surviving IT.* Oxford: Radcliffe Publishing; 2006.

Useful websites

Department of Health: www.dh.gov.uk.
European Computer Driving Licence (ECDL): www.ecdl.nhs.uk.
The author: www.alangillies.com.

Chapter 8

Allied health records in the electronic age

Margaret Hastings

The use of electronic patient records has been a health service vision for the past 30 to 40 years.[1] Initially, technology could not support this vision, however technology advances now provide mobile, secure, functional solutions, but still AHPs stick to their pen and paper. If it is so much better to use technology,[2] why has this group of clinicians not gained from the advances in healthcare computing? In this chapter some of the issues and changes required by AHPs to achieve this vision are explored.

The majority of GPs are information and communication technology literate, using computers for clinical care recording and for business information. Perhaps here lies the key. The NHS in the UK has traditionally been based on medical specialty consultant episodes through HRGs and DRGs.[3] Where the economics of healthcare require business information – AHPs will use computer systems to provide accurate activity and 'billing' information. In places using cost per case methodologies there will be 'billing' systems which collect the contact data but may not be as rich on clinical information. Within the UK, GP systems are needed to deliver the annual Quality and Outcome Framework data [4] as part of the General Medical Service Contract, thus GP systems have data fields to record the information and reports to extract the information annually from the system to submit to the 'paymasters'. There is a purpose to using clinical systems which is well understood in General Practice and private healthcare. There are currently few such 'drivers' for change in Allied Health clinical practice in the UK.

Over the years AHPs will have had some exposure to IT systems and have found that they take too long to start up; find it difficult to record what needs to be recorded; systems require typing into boxes, not to draw; recording does not follow the normal structure of records; lots of data is recorded and nothing comes out, time is taken away from service user care.[5] All of these problems can be overcome by good system specification and a realistic expectation from AHPs, that system development takes time. It is better to start with the process improvement which will derive the greatest benefit to the service, rather than expecting an all encompassing Electronic Patient Record to be delivered overnight. Many IT systems projects fail as they are delivered under project methodology rather than transformational change in clinical practice. Changing clinical recording practice should not take another 40 years; realistically the timescale will be for the implementation of systems within UK national government timescales by 2012–2015.

Understanding systems

Current – paper, pen, filing cabinet. The majority of AHPs currently use a great variety of record cards, assessment forms, audit forms, medical notes and shared notes to hold the information they need to record using black ink pen, with every entry signed and dated. These records are then stored in a locked filling cabinet in a department or ward, and once no longer required stored in a records filing system for the required number of years under record retention policies.

Paper-lite systems. Some AHPs have access to IT systems which focus on clinical activity, allowing them to record contact information – appointments, attendances and demographics – with some clinical notes being held on the computer system and full assessment, care planning and clinical decision making being recorded on paper. The complete service user record will be a 'print-out' of the record held on computer, plus that on paper. AHPs should ensure that they are aware of their country's legal requirements for management and storage of such records.

Full electronic health records. There are a few systems available – both Hospital Information Systems (HIS) and AHP systems which provide sufficient functionality for AHPs to record a full electronic health record. When using these systems, great care must be taken to ensure the reliability of the security and integrity of the data contained in back-up files. Within health organisations this will be managed by the IT department. Small business and private practitioners should ensure that they do not neglect this area of their business.

The diversity of AHPs has them working in all clinical areas: in healthcare (hospital, community, independent and private providers); in social care; forensics and prison services; leisure services and sport; education services; housing associations; occupational health and the workplace; and the voluntary sector. This complexity of clinical networking and pathways is so variable that no one single IT solution meets the recording and sharing needs for every situation. Clinical records should be contemporary and data input solutions need to offer choices that meet service delivery needs. For example, Orthoptists take eye measurements with special instruments which output graphical data on special paper. In the electronic age this will have to be a stored digital image. Speech and language therapists may want to capture a voice recording; physiotherapists may need to store a gait video.

Infrastructure requirements. The speed of technological change has increased access to Information and Communication Technology through the reduction in cost and size of mobile devices. AHPs can be an itinerant workforce working across different health, social and leisure service buildings and people's homes. Paper and pen are easily carried to write clinical notes; the challenge to IT is how to easily capture the clinical record in the variety of different formats that AHPs use, without increasing the time it takes to complete the task. More time spent recording data, means less time to carry out direct clinical interventions. For all data capture there is a cost, the benefits of collecting data using IT must outweigh these costs. Figure 8.1 displays some of the different devices currently available to input data into an electronic system. AHPs working patterns mean that some professionals will record directly during the clinical intervention; others will be able to sit at a desktop after the intervention and record the data into the system. There will still be times when pen and paper are needed to take notes to be entered into a system later.

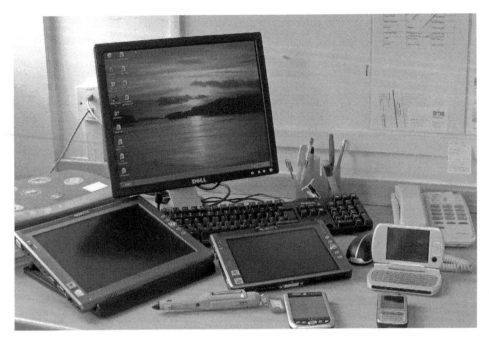

Figure 8.1 IT tools.

Within buildings, normal working practice and recording needs may allow the use of a standard 'hard wired' networked desktop solution. In a face-to-face clinical intervention in a busy out-patient department a wireless networked 'tablet' PC will allow, 'real time'– as it happens – clinical recording, including the annotation of body charts, without creating a barrier between clinician and client. Smaller portable devices such as PDAs can provide recording medium for ward and community staff. However the smaller screen size (6 x 10 cm) means that systems may need to be reconfigured to be used on mobile devices to avoid scrolling across and up and down the screen for data entry. For community use the development of Smartphones with PDA capability and the use of telephones have opened opportunities for 'real time' working in the community. However the on-line cost of data transmission can make these very costly to use and judgments need to be made about which clinical records need to be 'real time'. For the vast majority of community staff the ability to download the clinical record in the morning on leaving the office, storing the information in the mobile device – securely and encrypted , in case of loss – and synchronising through docking at a terminal, or downloading into the system over the Intranet at the end of the day, will generally suffice. Staff working in Mental Health with at risk service users, may be a clinical group who do require 'real time' connectivity.

A glossary of some information technology terms[6]

For greater detail search the world wide web for 'glossary of computer terms'.

Box 8.1 Glossary of some information technology terms.

- *Networks.* Join two or more computers together. From simply joining home desktop computer to a laptop computer or a broadband connection to global networks of computers within a worldwide organisation. Servers provide shared resources to the network and are attached to client computers – on the desk – either by cable in a wired network or via radio signals in a wireless network. Cabled networks require cabling to be run through walls and computers connected through fixed network points in rooms. Wireless networks have the advantage of being flexible and easier to use in clinical settings, but they are inherently less secure than a cabled network.

- *Personal computer (PC).* The equipment on the desk which has 4 parts; the computer system unit, a monitor, a keyboard and a mouse. A laptop (or notebook) PC has the screen attached to the system unit, a keyboard and a mouse, and is portable. A tablet or slab PC is similar to a laptop but has a screen and a digitiser pen which is used instead of the mouse and with appropriate software, writing with the pen on the screen records either the handwriting in a document or can convert the handwriting to text, storing the text in a document. This means that people without keyboard skills can write notes as normal and have them converted to text. Tablet PCs are often used where normal notebooks are impractical or unwieldy, or do not provide the needed functionality.

- *Input device.* The keyboard and mouse are the standard input devices to the computer. Every keystroke or movement of the mouse sends an input single to the computer. The digital pen in a tablet PC is an input device which replaces the mouse. Other devices which can be used to send input signals to the computer are joysticks, microphones, scanners, light pens, digital cameras, webcams, card readers, scientific measuring equipment. Any sensor which monitors, scans for and accepts information from the external world can be considered an input device.

- *Personal digital assistant (PDA).* These are hand held electronic devices which allow you to organise your schedule, take notes, do math calculations, play games, write memos, and even surf the Internet and send e-mail. Smartphones are mobile telephones with PDA functionality and web browser. These devices will all have removable storage devices which can be encrypted for safe storage of confidential information.

- *Software.* General term to describe computer programmes. The software contains lines of code developed by programmers which instructs the computer processor. The programmes may be applications, scripts and instruction sets, which allow the computer to undertake various processes.

- *Hardware.* This describes the physical parts of a computer. Internal devices include the motherboard, hard drive and Random Access Memory (RAM). External devices include mouse, keyboard, screen, printer and scanner.

- *Radio-frequency identification (RFID).* Is an automatic identification method, relying on storing and remotely retrieving data using devices called RFID tags or transponders.

- *Patient administration system (PAS).* An administrative system typically used in hospitals and community service settings, which contain essential non-clinical data, such as patient attendance lists, appointments and waiting times.
- *Role-based access control (RBAC).* Grants a view of a patient's record depending on the role the individual was assigned when they registered for their Smartcard.
- *Secondary uses service (SUS).* A single repository of person and care event level data relating to the NHS care of patients, which is used for management and clinical purposes other than direct patient care. These secondary uses include healthcare planning, commissioning, public health, clinical audit, benchmarking, performance improvement, research and clinical governance.
- *Portal.* Allows information access to many systems in a single screen that is personalised for the individual user.
- *Smartcard.* A plastic card containing an electronic chip – like a chip and pin credit card – used to identify those who are authorised to use a system. This is used together with an alphanumeric pass code. The chip on the Smartcard does not contain any personal information but provides a secure link between system and the database holding the user's information and assigned access rights.

Overall the system technology that supports clinical service delivery should:

- be easy to use
- be cost effective
- integrate with other systems where required, using standard terminology
- be secure
- derive clinical benefits to service user care though minimising clinical risk and facilitating best practice.

Table 8.1 has a checklist of the functional requirements that AHPs may require from an Information System.[7] Full specifications should deliver a useable electronic patient record. In an incremental approach from paper to electronic records, managers and clinicians may wish to identify the attributes that are essential to deliver the benefits they wish to gain from an electronic system. These factors should be weighted more highly in the functional specification to identify the system with the 'best fit'. Even with this it will only be as good as the integrity of the data entered into it.

Table 8.1 lists the functions which record systems should support for AHP clinical recording. AHPs should prioritise these requirements and question system providers about how the systems deliver these requirements.

Information management

IT supports the real requirements of clinical records which is information capture and sharing. Identifying the information needs before specifying a system will make it easier for IT to find a solution that meets clinical recording needs.

Table 8.1 Functions for record systems to support AHP clinical recording.

Function	Does the system?
Patient identification	Auto-populate with demographic information?
	Use Unique Patient Identifier (UPI) based numbering?
	Search on a variety of fields?
	Have links to required external agencies, e.g. NHS care record, birth, death registration
	Provide linkage between patients, e.g. families?
User identification	Provide secure authentication and access controls?
	Provide positive staff identification linked to registration bodies?
	Allow user demographics with user configurability?
	Have security services including encryption?
Clinical information capture	Allow multi device support?
	Allow multi modality support – text, voice, image, annotation?
	Accommodate digital input devices?
	Allow telemetry?
	Allow 'sticky notes'/Post-its?
	Allow wireless access?
	Allow mobile device download and synchronisation?
Care planning and pathways	Allow multi-disciplinary views of care plans?
	Provide time-lines to oversee care?
	Allow pathways to be developed to follow best practice?
	Provide structured records and clinical templates for care planning?
Workflow management and scheduling	Provide full clinic management requirements?
	Provide complex booking?
	Provide appointment management and outcome?
	Record procedures and interventions to meet regulatory body requirements?
	Schedule user-specific to-do lists and reminders?
Communication	Provide secure clinical messaging/access to messaging systems?
	Provide alerts to other service providers delivering care?
	Provide external, multi-modality telecommunications support for remote consultation/telemedicine?
Screening	Provide call-recall, surveillance for patients on screening, review or call back systems?
Tracking	Track patients?
	Track physical records?
	Track equipment and maintenance schedules?
	Track orthoses, prostheses and implants?
Decision support	Provide clinical alerts?
	Record patient information resources?
	Provide pathway support?
	Ability to evaluate learning?
Requesting	Request diagnostic testing?
	Refer on to other therapists?
	Request second opinion?

continued

Reporting	Are there links to diagnostic test results?
	Report adverse incidents?
	Provide activity reports by variety of fields?
	Provide audit reports?
	Provide clinical effectiveness reports?
	Provide caseload and case management reports?
Medicines management	Allow recording of prescriptions?
	Allow recording of dispensing?
	Allow recording of medication use?
	Allow recording of medicine stock management?
Image management	Allow links to radiology reports and Picture Archiving and Communication System (PACS) images?
	Allow recording of digital clinical images?
Document management	Save referral letters?
	Print appointments and patient contact letters?
	Print discharge letters?
	Print clinic specific reports?
	Allow storage of legacy records?
Patient contribution area	Facilitate consent management recording?
	Device support, e.g. telemetry, glucose monitoring
	Support a patient diary?
Secondary uses; audit, research, planning	Can anonymised reports be extracted for:
	• clinical audit?
	• clinical governance?
	• service management – activity and waiting times?
	• risk management?
	• regional and national statistics?
	• ad-hoc reporting?
	• research?
General resource management	Resources utilisation – room and equipment?
	Alerts, e.g. stock levels?
	Staff rostering?
	Clinical supplies?
	Decontamination requirements?
	User training?
	Out-of hours support?
Terminology	Support use of Systematised Nomenclature of Medicine (SNOMED)-Clinical Terms?
	Support use of drug and medical devices dictionary?
	Use national data sets, data standards and diagnostic codes?

Information governance

Information governance refers to the practice of handling information in a confidential and secure manner, following appropriate ethical and quality standards. Effective data protection, confidentiality and IT security practices are essential pre-requisites of modern healthcare provision. Every health and social care organisation will have effective and trusted arrangements for handling service user-identifying information and other sensitive data.

All AHPs require information governance competencies that demonstrate the knowledge, skills and understanding required for the competent handling of healthcare related information to recognised ethical, legal and quality standards.

Key principles of information handling are:

- **H**olding information securely and confidentially
- **O**btaining information fairly and efficiently
- **R**ecording information accurately and reliably
- **U**sing information effectively and ethically
- **S**haring information appropriately and lawfully (HORUS).[8]

Information Governance has six main components:

1 information governance management
2 confidentiality and data protection
3 freedom of information
4 records management
5 information security
6 information quality assurance.

Caldicott Guardian

A Caldicott Guardian is the senior person within an organisation who is responsible for protecting the confidentiality of service-user information and enabling appropriate information-sharing. The Guardian plays a key role in ensuring that the NHS, Local Authorities and partner organisations satisfy the highest practical standards for handling service user identifiable information. The Guardian actively supports work to facilitate and enable information sharing and advise on options for lawful and ethical processing of information as required. This role is particularly important in relation to the implementation of the National Programme for IT and the development of Electronic Social Care Records and Common Assessment Frameworks.

More information can be found from the Connecting for Health website especially NHS Confidentiality Code of Practice;[9] Information Security;[10] and a general overview at Patient UK website.[11] National Government websites will also provide guidance for healthcare practitioners within their jurisdiction.

Records management

Legal Duty

Dimond states: [12]

> The prime purpose of patient record keeping is the care of the patient: to ensure that each member of the health team is aware of the care and treatment which have been given or which have still to be provided in order to ensure that the service user receives all reasonable care.

Governing the patient record and the information held within are two legal requirements contained within:

1 Data Protection Act 1998[13] – the main piece of legislation which governs the protection of personal data in the UK

2 Freedom of Information Act 2005[14] – gives a general right of access, on request, on information held by public bodies.

In addition all health professionals have a duty to respect the confidentiality of information obtained from and about the service user.

In the UK the Health Professions Council[15] (HPC) is the regulatory body for AHPs. Their Standards of conduct, performance and ethics[16] states that the duties of a Registrant include keeping accurate records.

Box 8.2 Extract from Standard 10 of the HPC Code of Conduct.

10 You must keep accurate records.
You have a duty to make sure, as far as possible, that records completed by students under your supervision are clearly written, accurate and appropriate.

Whenever you review records, you should update them and include a record of any arrangements you have made for the continuing care of the service user.

You must protect information in records from being lost, damaged, accessed by someone without appropriate authority, or tampered with. If you update a record, you must not delete information that was previously there, or make that information difficult to read. Instead, you must mark it in some way (for example, by drawing a line through the old information).

Health Professions Council: Standards of Conduct Performance and Ethics, July 2008

Further detail, about the recording requirements for each profession to ensure safe and effective care, is given in Standards of Proficiency.[17] Clinical recording is covered in Identification and Assessment of Health and Social Care Needs. Key areas are being able to: gather, analyse and critically evaluate information; formulate and deliver plans and strategies for meeting health and social care needs; critically evaluate the impact of, or response to, the AHPs actions.

General record keeping principles

- Records should be completed as soon as possible after the contact/intervention.
- Clinical reasoning processes, care planning, interventions and outcome evaluation should be recorded.
- Records should be accurate, comprehensive and factual.
- Records should be written legibly, contain no jargon or abbreviations.
- Records should be signed and dated by the maker.
- Any alterations should be clearly visible with the original record crossed out and changes signed and dated.

Any information system must allow the AHP to keep clinical records to the standard defined by registration bodies. The UK Health Regulatory Body have aligned clinical recording standards across all professional groups. For AHPs this will include evidence of clinical reasoning and decision making which will include evidence from annotated diagrams of clinical findings to video/audio recordings of speech pathology. With the increased use of mobile technology including cameras the use of digital images is becoming routine in clinical recording.

About data

Clinical information is formulated by the clinician from the data that is collected about a service user. The collation of the data during the clinical reasoning process enables the clinician to make clinical judgments about the duty of care they have agreed with the service user. Data collected can be in the form of numbers, words, and images. Data tends to be unstructured, isolated and context independent. If it becomes separated from the context descriptor it becomes meaningless. The clinical reasoning process enables clinicians to develop the ability to read the clinical signs that come gradually together to form patterns on which clinical action can be based. The development of skills and knowledge takes time and requires the assembly of information and data into a linked, structured, format. This data will be assimilated by the individual to formulate the clinical diagnosis.

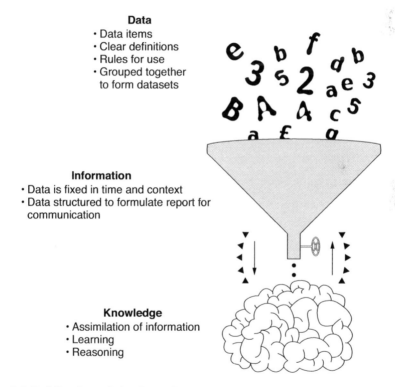

Data
- Data items
- Clear definitions
- Rules for use
- Grouped together
  to form datasets

Information
- Data is fixed in time and context
- Data structured to formulate report for
  communication

Knowledge
- Assimilation of information
- Learning
- Reasoning

Figure 8.2 Building knowledge from data.

The model in Figure 8.2 identifies the relationships between data, information and knowledge. Within clinical recording, AHPs will record **Data** such as history, subjective findings; objective measurements; observations; measures of outcome. As part of their clinical reasoning process they will build **Information** by analysing the data to formulate intervention plans; set goals and produce communication and clinical reports. AHPs will demonstrate knowledge and competence through appropriate selection and application of clinical skills and build new knowledge about clinical care through reflective practice, audit and research.

Healthcare is a complex, communications environment involving a large number of people and unexpected events. This complexity is increased with the need for AHPs to work closely with local authorities and other agencies to deliver integrated services. The unpredictability and complexity of this environment means that staff must constantly communicate with each other to be aware of the current needs of service users and up and coming care plans. Lack of access or not sharing information contributes to the significant duplication of data collection or time wasted looking for information. Apart from the obvious inefficiency this also reduces service users' confidence in the health services, may lead to repeated procedures being undertaken and raises service user safety concerns.

What data?

Arguably all clinicians have the same work processes and data flows, however the clinical terms and recording methods may be very specific to the professional group.

Data quality will be assured by:

1 data is recorded in the right service users notes – whether electronic or written
2 data standards and methods of recording the data are used to support consistency, validity and accuracy of data recorded
3 clinical data recording requirements are grouped in data sets which are accurately completed by the clinician within prescribed timescales.

Identifying the right service user

Data to be recorded will include demographics and unique patient identifiers – these will be specified by the local care system and must ensure in the electronic age that the right data is being recorded to the right service user. A unique patient identifier will help to pull together all records for this individual, from all the systems in which they have been stored ensuring the completeness of the record.

Consistent, valid and accurate data

Within the UK there is currently no national or country wide agreement on the structure of clinical records. This allows systems – including paper based – to devise their own structure. Many AHPs use the Subjective, Objective; Assessment and Plan (SOAP) note structure for recording free text notes. As clinical care moves to electronic notes, clinicians will need to agree standard formats for clinical records which can have the appropriate messaging data added to the electronic field, to ensure that it is always stored and retrieved in the right context.

Clinical language is complex and AHPs may use the same clinical term, but with a different meaning. All clinicians need to move towards using a common language, meaning and context across health and social care – and other partner agencies. AHPs need to use national data standards, including data definitions, data format and coding structures to support consistency and inter-operability of data within systems.

One of the main benefits of using electronic records is the ability to communicate information more rapidly to a wider group of people who need to access the information. With face to face or voice communication, non-verbal expression helps to define the meaning of the information. With the written word, whether hand written or electronic, the language used by the communicator has to ensure that the meaning is understood by the recipient without any non-verbal communication. Within individual health professions, language becomes highly specialised and shortcuts are taken using abbreviations and jargon. At times the same abbreviation may be used for different terms, which, when taken out of clinical context, will be very confusing and lead to misunderstanding of the information being shared. A primary concern for all healthcare professionals must be to safeguard service user care, thus sharing information that is understood by all, contributes to service user safety. Hence the requirement for a common NHS computerised language.

Terminology

SNOMED Clinical Terms® (SNOMED CT®)[18] is a comprehensive clinical terminology that provides clinical content and expressivity for clinical documentation and reporting. It can be used to code, retrieve, and analyse clinical data. SNOMED CT® resulted from the merging of SNOMED® Reference Terminology (SNOMED® RT) developed by the College of American Pathologists and Clinical Terms Version 3 developed by the NHS. The terminology comprises concepts of, terms and relationships with the objective of precisely representing clinical information across the scope of healthcare. Content coverage is divided into hierarchies, including:

- Clinical finding
- Procedure
- Observable entity
- Body structure
- Organism
- Substance
- Pharmaceutical/biologic product
- Specimen
- Special concept
- Physical object
- Physical force
- Event
- Environments/geographical locations
- Social context
- Situation with explicit context
- Staging and scales
- Linkage concept
- Qualifier value
- Record artifact

In 2007 the International Health Terminology Standards Development Organisation (IHTSDO)[19] acquired the intellectual property rights from, the College of American Pathologists. The UK Terminology Centre is hosted by NHS Connecting for Health and provides a central point for managing, distributing, supporting and controlling the use of SNOMED CT throughout the UK.

Classification

Traditional medical classification – coding systems – is needed for organisational purposes for service planning and commissioning. These classification systems have been based on the medical model of disease, with a range of codes for signs, symptoms, operations, procedures and disease. The most commonly used statistical coding system in medicine is the World Health Organization's International Classification of Disease 10th Revision (ICD).[20]

The International Classification of Functioning, Disability and Health (ICF)[21] classification complements ICD10 which contains information on diagnosis and health condition, but not on functional status. The ICD and ICF constitute the core classifications in the WHO Family of International Classifications.

The ICF is structured around the following broad components:

- body functions and structure
- activities (related to tasks and actions by an individual) and participation (involvement in a life situation)
- additional information on severity and environmental factors.

Functioning and disability are viewed as a complex interaction between the health condition of the individual and the contextual factors of the environment as well as personal factors. The picture produced by this combination of factors and dimensions is of 'the person in his or her world'. The classification treats these dimensions as interactive and dynamic rather than linear or static. It allows for an assessment of the degree of disability although it is not a measurement instrument. It is applicable to all people, whatever their health condition. The language of the ICF is neutral as to aetiology, placing the emphasis on function rather than condition or disease. It also is carefully designed to be relevant across cultures as well as age groups and genders, making it highly appropriate for heterogeneous populations.

Datasets

Clinical datasets will specify data items which should be collected as part of the information gathering process. Many professions have encouraged their clinicians to use standard recording pro-forma for recording clinical assessments, based on clinical datasets. The Single Shared Assessment, used to assess the care needs for older people throughout the UK, is an example of a structured record for assessment screening. Use of standardised forms, ensures that all data is captured in a standard way, making it easier for people to complete and for decision makers to have all the information they need to make a decision about a case. This ensures decisions made are equitable and fair. Data quality is improved as clinicians work with the outputs of the recorded data for analysis and reflective practice. Electronic systems can reduce transcription errors through allowing clinicians to enter data as part of clinical care, rather than recording on paper and have administration staff enter data retrospectively.

The DH has published an AHP Data set[22] which aims to help AHPs to collect data relevant to the patient journey. Data is grouped into data categories of patient, organisation, referral, waiting time, patient contact and discharge. The 80 items are not mandated and advice is given regarding the reason a service may want to collect this data. The Australian National Allied Health Casemix Committee[23] has developed a Health Activity Hierarchy to understand all the health activities undertaken by

AHPs as part of their workload. To provide standardised data to complete this hierarchy they have also developed the Australian Allied Health Minimum Dataset and Rehabilitation Outcomes.[24] Canada has a similar model of care provision to Australia and they collaborate on Rehabilitation Outcomes – both using the Functional Independence Measure[25] to evaluate functional outcomes. Data systems are highly developed through the Canadian Institute of Health Information.[26] Data sets are developed for acute care; home care and continuing care.

The development and agreement of national and international datasets for benchmarking Allied Health services will be a key professional 'driver' as services are required to demonstrate value for money and delivery of effective health and social care. Cost efficiency 'drivers' in other countries have ensured that AHPs evaluate their interventions much more frequently than in the UK and know the impact of changes in health state on the effectiveness and efficiency of the service. In several countries factors contributing to poor clinical outcomes will be assessed. Hart and Connelly[27] have demonstrated data input into predictive algorithms to identify the most efficient outcomes for clinical practice in USA.

Using data

Collected data will be structured to provide information for different purposes. Table 8.2 gives some examples of the different data items which will be provide information about clinical care; service management and secondary uses for planning.

Table 8.2 Data requirements for information needs.

Clinical information	Demographics; referral data; reason for intervention; objective assessments; lab findings; X ray findings; care plan; goal setting; clinical reasoning; appointments; intervention details; goal attainment; outcome measures; body charts – annotated; drawings; pictures; video clips; discharge data; data for clinical audit and report generation; risk management
Service management information	Waiting times; activity data; clinical governance data; manpower data; service utilisation data; resource utilisation; and others
Planning/secondary use information	Population data; resource and workforce data; activity data; historic trends; forward planning through estimate of demand and need

Benefits of moving to electronic records

Good information supports AHPs to:

- care for service users better by supporting their education and continuous professional development and by improving service user centeredness, effectiveness, timeliness, and equity
- share information across disciplines and agencies to improve service user safety, efficiency and timeliness of care within information governance requirements.

- compare information against standards and targets to advance clinical knowledge and practice and improve performance and the management of resources.

To achieve this they must use consistent language, terminology and data standards.

Apart from sharing information about service user care, AHPs must audit and evaluate the effectiveness and efficiency of this care – clinical governance – and to provide activity and management information about services delivered – service management. A well specified information system will deliver this functionality as a by-product of clinical recording and remove the need to keep numerous audit and activity sheets.

eHealth – the use of information, computers and telecommunications in support of meeting the needs of service users and the health of citizens[28] – has the potential to have a significant impact on the way AHPs work as they spend a large proportion of their time collecting, analysing, using and communicating information to support clinical decision-making. This information differs according to each profession's body of knowledge and the values or views that guide their practice. The overall aim in using information is to lead, co-ordinate, support and deliver safe, effective, service user centred care.

Key benefits of electronic records are to:

- make service user care safer and more effective by making available the right information in the right, place at the right time
- contribute to 'health literacy' to ensure that all citizens have the necessary skills, knowledge and confidence to manage their own health
- safeguard confidentiality by handling service user information securely
- enable more efficient use of healthcare resources through replacing paper-intensive processes and providing better management information
- provide 'real time' clinical data for service evaluation, audit and research.

Well designed electronic records improve the safety, efficiency and effectiveness of clinical care by reducing duplication of effort through repeated data collection and recording thus reducing the administration burden and improve information flows. The maxim should be:

Record once and use often to create more time for patient care.

References

1   Barnett D, Barber B. BCS involvement in health care informatics. In: Hayes G, Barnett B, editors. *UK Health Computing: recollections and reflections*. Swindon: BCS; 2008.
2   http://en.wikipedia.org/wiki/Electronic_health_record.
3   Jones RJ. Information systems and resource management. In: Jones RJ. *Management in Physiotherapy*. Oxford: Radcliffe Medical Press; 1991.
4   www.ic.nhs.uk/services/qof.
5   BSC. What's so different about electronic patient records? www.bcs.org/server.php?show=ConWebDoc.2972.
6   www.sharpened.net/glossary.
7   www.isdscotland.org/isd/4126.html.

8   www.connectingforhealth.nhs.uk/systemsandservices/infogov.
9   www.connectingforhealth.nhs.uk/resources/resources/nhs_code_of_practice.pdf.
10 www.nhsinformationsecurity@dh.gsi.gov.uk.
11 Records computers and electronic healthcare record patient UK, www.patient.co.uk/
    showdoc/40000769.
12 Dimond B. Legal issues arising in the management, leadership, and development of
    Allied Health Professions. In: Jones R, Jenkins F. *Managing and Leading in the Allied
    Health Professions.* Oxford: Radcliffe Publishing; 2006.
13 www.opsi.gov.uk/acts/acts1998/ukpga_19980029_en_1.
14 www.opsi.gov.uk/acts/acts2000/ukpga_20000036_en_1.
15 www.hpc-uk.org/registrants.
16 www.hpc-uk.org/assets/documents/10002367FINALcopyofSCPEJuly2008.pdf.
17 www.hpc-uk.org/publications/index.asp.
18 www.connectingforhealth.nhs.uk/systemsandservices/data/snomed.
19 www.ihtsdo.org.
20 www.who.int/classifications/icd/en.
21 www.who.int/classifications/icf/en.
22 www.18weeks.nhs.uk/Asset.ashx?path=/AHPs/InformationManagementHandbook
    030408.pdf.
23 www.nahcc.org.au/reports.htm.
24 www.chsd.uow.edu.au/aroc.
25 www.udsmr.org/fim2_about.php.
26 http://secure.cihi.ca/cihiweb/dispPage.jsp?cw_page=casemix_e.
27 www.cms.hhs.gov/TherapyServices/downloads/P4PFinalReport06-01-06.pdf.
28 www.nhsscotland.com/eHealth%20Strategy%202008-11%20final.pdf.

Chapter 9

Data 'sanity': reducing variation

Davis Ballestracci

Introduction

Whether or not you understand statistics, you are already using statistics! The key skill for everyday work is not necessarily mathematical, but the ability to 'think' statistically, which means responding to 'variation' appropriately in order to ask better questions. The famous quality guru W. Edwards Deming said, 'If I had to reduce my message for management to just a few words, I'd say it all had to do with reducing variation'.[1]

Some of you may have had to endure 'Statistics from Hell' courses, in which case, forget everything you learned; and many of you would say, 'Don't worry...we already have!' They are virtually worthless and perpetuate the myth that statistics can be used to 'massage' data and prove anything.

Data 'sanity': statistical thinking applied to everyday data

People generally do not perceive that they need statistics; their need is first and foremost to solve problems. Many of you have encountered the terms or attended courses such as total quality management (TQM), continuous quality improvement, benchmarking, re-engineering, total customer satisfaction, and, most recently, Six Sigma and Lean. There also seems to be a new and increasing tendency for performance goals to be imposed from external sources via 'tough' standards. These efforts are all heavily based in data, but results tend to be disappointing due to poor basic data skills:

- results are presented in aggregated row and column formats complete with variances and rankings
- perceived trends are acted upon to reward and punish
- labels such as 'above average' and 'below average' get attached to individuals or institutions
- stakeholders are outraged by certain results and impose even tougher standards.

These are very well meaning strategies that are simple, obvious...and wrong! They will mislead analysis and interpretation and insidiously 'cloud' decisions every day in virtually every work environment.

The realities are:

- taking action to improve a situation is tantamount to using statistics
- traditional statistics have severely limited value in real world settings
- understanding of variation is more important than using specific techniques
- statistical thinking gives a knowledge base from which to ask the right questions
- unforeseen problems are caused by the exclusive use of arbitrary numerical goals, 'stretch' goals, and tougher standards for driving improvement
- using heavily aggregated tables of numbers, variances from budgets, or bar graph formats as tools for taking meaningful management action are often futile and inappropriate
- there is poor awareness of the true meaning of 'trend', 'above average' and 'below average'.

Despite its age, *Fundamentals of Fourth Generation Management*[2] may be the best overall quality book available. (Everyone going through the legalised torture of Six Sigma belt training should read it to understand what the role of statistics is *really* all about.)

A key concept: process-oriented thinking

The statistics needed for quality improvement are based in the context of *process*. What is a process? All work is a process! Processes are sequences of tasks aimed at accomplishing a particular outcome by manipulating inputs to produce a particular type of output. Everyone involved in the process has a role of supplier, processor or customer. A group of related processes is called a system.

Box 9.1 Process-oriented thinking.

Process-oriented thinking is built on the following premises:
1 Understanding that:
   - *all* work is accomplished through a series of one or more processes, each of which is potentially measurable
   - all processes exhibit *variation*, which inhibits their predictability
   - if a process does not go right, that is undesirable variation
   - processes 'speak' to us through data
   - one's current processes are *perfectly designed* to get the results they are already getting…even if they are getting results they 'should not' be getting!
2 Process inputs falling into the six general categories each of which is a potential source of variation:
   - people
   - methods
   - machines
   - materials
   - measurements – data
   - environment.

3 Reducing *inappropriate* and *unintended* variation by:
- eliminating work procedures that do not add value, that is only add cost with no payback to customers
- ensuring that all workers are performing at the best inherent level of the process's capability with their given inputs
- reacting appropriately to variation because there are two types; treating one as the other will actually make things worse.

4 Improving quality = improving processes (more consistent prediction).

The use of data is also a process

The use of data is really made up of four processes – measurement, collection, analysis, and interpretation – each having people, methods, machines, materials, measurements (data inputs via raw numbers), and environment as inputs, Figure 9.1 Any one of these six inputs can be a source of variation for *any* one of these four processes – they lurk to contaminate your data process and mislead you as to what is going on in the actual system you are trying to improve!

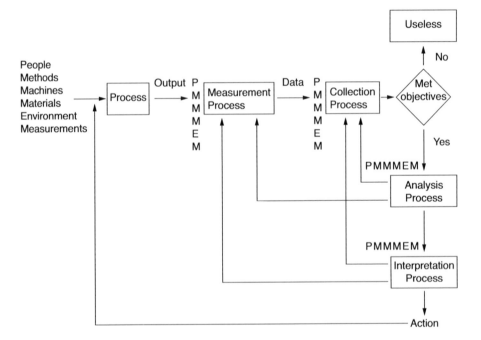

Figure 9.1 Inputs, outputs and data.

Measurement

Any process produces outputs that are potentially measurable. If one chooses, one can obtain a number – a piece of data – characterising the situation through a process of measurement, called an operational definition. If the objectives are not explicitly clear or people have varying perceptions of what is being measured, the six sources of variation will compromise the quality of this measurement process. Deming was so fond of saying, 'There is no true value of anything!'[1] (Those who follow American presidential elections, remember the year 2000. All they had to do was count the votes in Florida. The election was over. How hard could that be…need I say more?)

For example:

1 how many beds does a hospital have?
2 how many patient deaths occurred last year?
3 define 'stopped smoking.'

A key issue: Do the people collecting the data know why they are collecting it and how to collect? If not, human variation will contaminate the data and render any subsequent analysis invalid.

For quality improvement purposes, crude measures of the right things are better than precise measures of the wrong things – as long as it is 'consistently inconsistent' and defined in a way so that all will get the same number, you will benefit from the elegant simplicity of the statistical techniques inherent in quality improvement.

Collection

These individual measurements must then be accumulated into some type of data set, so they next pass to a collection process. If the objectives are clear, the designed collection process should be relatively well defined because the analysis is known ahead of time, the appropriateness of an analysis depends on how the data were collected. If the objectives are not clear, the six sources of variation will once again act to compromise the process. Actually, from the author's experience, it is virtually guaranteed that the six sources will compromise the collection process anyway! Worse yet, many times a data set is an amalgam of continuously recorded administrative procedures (C.R.A.P.)

An objective of quality improvement usually means that more frequent samples need to be collected on an ongoing basis at various times rather than accumulating a large random summary sample.

Analysis

The analysis should be known before one piece of data has been collected.

If the objectives are passive and reactive, eventually someone will extract the data and use a computer to 'get the stats'. This, of course, is an analysis process – albeit not necessarily a good one – that also has the six sources of inputs as potential sources of variation. Or, maybe more commonly, someone extracts the data and hands out tables of raw data presented as computer-generated summary analyses at a meeting. This becomes the analysis process, which is affected by the variation in perceptions and abilities of people at the meeting.

Data not collected specifically for the current objective can generally be tortured to confess to someone else's hidden agenda.[3] Another example of data misuse is the confusion alluded to in the following example given by the famous statistician Walter Shewhart:

You go to your tailor for a suit of clothes and the first thing that he does is to make some measurements; you go to your physician because you are ill and the first thing he does is to make some measurements. The objects of making measurements in these two cases are different. They typify the two general objects of making measurements. They are:

a) to obtain quantitative information
b) to obtain a causal explanation of observed phenomena.[4]

Using data collected for the objective of quantitative information to make causal inferences is usually asking for trouble.

Interpretation

Statistics is not a set of techniques to 'massage' data, but to interpret, appropriately, the variation with which you are faced in a situation, which can be one of two types and that treating one as the other actually makes things worse.

Ultimately, all analysis boils down to interpreting the variation in the measurements. So, the interpretation process – with the same six sources of inputs – results in an action that is then fed back in to the original process.

Think of many meetings, in essence, analysis and interpretation processes; with tabular data, bar graphs and trend lines being compared to arbitrary goals, resulting in interventions. Could human variation in perception also manifest through the six input sources to affect the quality of *each* of the four data processes and subsequent decisions? How many meetings are reacting to variation in the data processes and not necessarily the process attempting to be improved?

When data is looked at as a process in its role of quality improvement, statistics is not the science of analysing data, but becomes the art and science of collecting and analysing data, simply and efficiently.

The eight crucial question of the data process are set out in Box 9.2.

Box 9.2 Eight crucial questions of the 'data process'.

1   Why collect the data?
2   What methods will be used for the analysis?
3   What data will be collected?
4   How will the data be measured?
5   How often will the data be collected?
6   Where will the data be collected?
7   Who will collect the data?
8   What training is needed for the data collectors?

Given the nature of process-oriented thinking, one of the biggest changes in thinking will be to realise the benefit of studying a process by collecting more frequent samples over time, which will cause the need to redefine many current pristine organisational operational definitions to become 'good enough'.

A high level summary of improvement: six sources of problems with a process

The first edition of *The TEAM Handbook* [5] contains what might be considered to be the best high level summary of improvement. To intentionally labour a point: It is all about *process*. The following road map is the best overall summary of improvement I have seen. Any process needing improvement should be approached in the order given. All too often, some data is collected (jumping right to Step 6) and is contaminated by variation caused by (unintentionally) ignoring Steps 1–5:

1 inadequate knowledge of how a process works
2 inadequate knowledge of how a process should work
3 errors and mistakes in executing the procedures
4 current practices that fail to recognise the need for preventive measures
5 unnecessary steps, inventory buffers, wasteful measures/data
6 variation in inputs and outputs.

At the time of writing, 'Lean' seems to be the prevalent quality improvement methodology. So, let us put it in the context of the above, coupled with statistical thinking.

Key elements of 'Lean' are process-mapping and error-proofing (Steps 1 and 4) and an obsession with waste (Step 5). Statistics applies to Steps 2, 3 and 6 to expose the underlying variation and reduce the inappropriate and unintended variation. This will involve using statistical techniques to test theories, assess interventions and hold gains. Improving quality means improving processes to make them as consistently predictable as possible.

More data 'sanity': statistics and reality

Research versus improvement

Many clinicians will argue that the process-oriented approach is invalid because it does not follow established procedures of clinical research. However, in research, all input variations are tightly controlled such that observed differences in the 'control' and 'treatment' groups can be attributed to the 'methods' input and no other. The protocol is also excruciatingly detailed about how measurements will be defined, collected, analysed and interpreted so as to reduce variation in the data process – and it is all defined before one patient is randomised. Pro-actively controlling this variation is inherent in the process and costly, which is why research is expensive.

Hence, research statistics is a specialised subset of process-oriented statistics! It makes the assumption and has the luxury of ignoring the everyday factors lurking to compromise results in busy uncontrolled practice environments. This is the context of statistics generally taught in most courses and makes the naive assumption that one can continuously sample from a stable population to estimate parameters. Good research inherently creates such a stable process, but then what happens?

Unknown and unknowable

There are usually no difficulties carrying out the objectives of a research study other than how to choose the sample; however, when a research result is published and implemented into practice environments, a number of subsequent practical problems still remain.

For example, how does one collect data, say, in a random sample of patients? Consider a chosen group of patients with hypertension included in a randomised controlled study that attends a particular clinic. Either a random method or some complicated method involving random numbers is used to determine who is to get which treatment. But the resulting sample is for the purposes of the clinical trial and not necessarily a random sample of the patients who will be treated in the future at that same clinic.

Still less are they a random sample of the patients who will be treated in any other clinic. In fact the patients who will be treated in the future will depend on choices that have not yet been made! Those choices will depend on the results of the study currently being done and on studies by other people that may be carried out in the future.

So, in an everyday practice environment, there is patient-to-patient variation over and above that of a clinical trial, which is only concerned with sampling variation. This second source is due to the fact that one is predicting what will happen at some time in the future – to some group that is different from the original sample. This uncertainty is *'unknown and unknowable'*. It is rarely known how any produced results will be used, so all one can do is to warn the potential user of the range of uncertainties that might affect different actions.

This is rarely done. Furthermore, how is it expressed? But the uncertainties of this kind will in most circumstances be an order of magnitude greater than the uncertainty, due merely to sampling, making it very dangerous to pretend to be more certain than warranted. Such false certainty many times leads to wrong choices, but the result, in most statistics courses, has been a theory in which the unmeasured uncertainty has just been ignored.

A treatment declared as beneficial: so…what changes?

So, after a significant result is published, researchers lose control over how clinicians use it. There will be variation in how people interpret it and apply it and lack of rigour in how data is collected to evaluate it. This human variation virtually guarantees that they will not necessarily achieve the same results as reported. This variation, usually either inappropriate or unintended, could be present in any or all of the six inputs of five processes – actual and data measurement, collection, analysis, and interpretation!

For example, an antibiotic is found to be useful in the treatment of some infection. Suppose that all testing was done in one hospital in New York in 2010; however, someone may want to use the antibiotic in Africa in 2013. It is quite possible that the best antibiotic in New York is not the same as the best in a refugee camp in Zaire. In New York the strains of bacteria may be different: and the problems of transport and storage really are different. If the antibiotic is freshly made and stored in efficient refrigerators, it may be excellent. It may not work at all if transported to a camp with poor storage facilities. Even if the same antibiotic works in both places, how long will it go on working? This will depend on how carefully it is used and how quickly resistant strains of bacteria build up. The effectiveness of a drug may also depend on the age of the patient, or previous treatment, or the stage of the disease. Ideally it is desirable to have one treatment that works well in all foreseeable circumstances, but this may not be possible.

So, in understanding any variation between the research results and actual results, it becomes necessary to expose the variation between individual use and the research use of the protocol and reduce any inappropriate and unintended variation.

Further clarification: enumerative statistics versus analytic statistics

There are actually three kinds of statistics, and they can be summarised as follows:

1 **descriptive**: what can be said about this *individual* patient?'
2 **enumerative**: what can be said about this *specific group* of patients?'
3 **analytic**: what can be said about the *process* that produced the result in this group of patients?'

An enumerative study always focuses on the actual state of something at one point in the past; no more, no less. For example, one can literally summarise the results of all the participants in any clinical trial once it is completed and because of the way the sample is chosen, consider these patients a 'random sample' of the patients who were potentially available.

An analytic study usually focuses on predicting the results of action in the future – in circumstances we cannot fully know. It is this predictive way of thinking that is fundamental to quality improvement.

However, the process under consideration is different in the clinical trial vis-à-vis the everyday environment. The clinical trial process is concerned only with the effect of the drug and needs to produce a relatively consistent group of patients. The rigour of the protocol ensures a stable group of patients that can be treated in an enumerative fashion via estimation. We want 'the process that produced the result in this group of patients' to reflect variation only due to the presence of the drug. In the context of the future, we want assurance that any group of patients chosen by the same protocol would be similar – no more, no less.

Once the drug is released, it is only part of the subsequent process – the diagnosis process and its interaction with the prescribing process is what is 'producing the result in this group of patients' on whom data is collected. Furthermore, if the drug is found to be viable, this will now introduce a manufacturing process and the types of statistics now answer the questions:

• what can be said about this specific pill?
• what can be said about this specific batch of pills?
• what can be said about the process that produced this batch of pills?

Ideally the manufacturing process must produce as consistent a product as possible. This has the same six sources of input and the same four data processes.

Quality improvement relates to consistency of manufacturing through reducing process variation.

Statistics in a quality improvement perspective

It can be seen that statistics is not merely the science of analysing data, but the art and science of collecting and analysing data. Given any improvement situation – including daily work – it is necessary to:

1 choose and define the problem in a process and systems context
2 design and manage a series of simple, efficient data collections to expose undesirable variation
3 use comprehensible methods presentable and understandable across all layers of the organisation, virtually all graphical avoiding raw data or bar graphs – with the specific exception of a Pareto analysis – to expose further the inappropriate and unintended variation
4 numerically assess the current state of an undesirable situation, further expose inappropriate and unintended variation, assess the effects of interventions
5 hold the gains of any improvements made, generally requiring a much simpler data collection.

The very basics of process-oriented statistics

The best statistical analysis will encourage the art of asking better questions in response to variations in data. The following discussion will debunk the myth that statistics can be used to massage data and prove anything and demonstrate the counterintuitive simplicity and power of merely 'plotting the dots', simple time plots of process outputs. These alone usually yield far more profound questions than the most complicated – alleged – statistical analysis. The manufacturing process is used to demonstrate some basic techniques. These same techniques could be applied to patients as well as 'pills'!

Old habits die hard...hang in there and read on!

Supposing that you have been getting increasing complaints about the quality of a drug on a particular specification. You have three manufacturing facilities and get the summary data for the last 30 batches each has produced. The specification is 50 + 6; summarised in Table 9.1.

Table 9.1 'Statistical' comparison of three plants' manufacturing performance.

	N	Mean	SE Mean	StDev	Minimum	Median	Maximum
Plant 1	30	50.937	0.514	2.815	45.1	50.50	55.7
Plant 2	30	50.527	0.524	2.870	44.7	50.60	57.1
Plant 3	30	50.847	0.573	3.138	44.8	50.05	56.9

Luckily, your local statistical 'guru', a Six Sigma black belt, has come to your rescue and written a report, which is handed out. Several significant findings are shared:

1 Pictures are very important. A comparative histogram was done to compare the distributions of the plants' values of the specification value. There seem to be no differences.

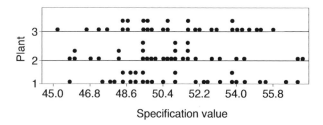

Figure 9.2 Comparative histogram.

2 The three data sets were then statistically tested for the assumption of Normality. The results (not shown) were that we can assume each to be Normally distributed (p-values of 0.502, 0.372, and 0.248, respectively, all of which are > 0.05); however, we have to be cautious – just because the data pass the test for normality does not necessarily mean that the data are Normally distributed...only that, under the null hypothesis, the data cannot be proven to be non-Normal.
3 Since the data can be assumed to be Normally distributed, the analysis of variance (ANOVA) can be undertaken and the 95% confidence intervals generated.

One-way Analysis of Variance (ANOVA)

Source	DF	SS	MS	F	P
Plant	2	2.79	1.39	0.16	0.852
Error	87	754.28	8.67		
Total	89	757.07			

S = 2.944

Individual 95% CIs For Mean Based on Pooled StDev

Level	N	Mean	StDev	
1	30	50.937	2.815	(------------------*------------------)
2	30	50.527	2.870	(------------------*------------------)
3	30	50.847	3.138	(------------------*------------------)

```
                    ---+-----------+-----------+-----------+-------
                    49.70       50.40       51.10       51.80
```

Pooled StDev = 2.944

Figure 9.3 One way analysis of variance.

4 The p-Value of 0.852 is greater than 0.05. Therefore, we can reasonably conclude that there are no statistically significant differences among the manufacturing facilities as further confirmed by the overlapping 95% confidence intervals. Most of these batches were in specification, so there needs

to be systemic improvement of the overall manufacturing process to reduce variation and there will need to be consideration of tightening the final release specification.

Let us see...have we used all the potential jargon?

Mean...Median...Standard Deviation...Trimmed Mean...Normality...Histogram...p-value...Analysis of Variance (ANOVA)...95% Confidence Interval... Null Hypothesis...Statistical Significance...Standard Error of the Mean...F-test... Degrees of Freedom...

Oh, by the way...did you know that this analysis is totally worthless?

But...he certainly sounded like he knew what he was talking about!

There are three questions that should become a part of every quality professional's vocabulary whenever faced with a set of data for the first time.

1 How were these data defined and collected and were they collected specifically for the current purpose?
2 Were the processes that produced these data stable?
3 Were the analyses appropriate given the way the data were collected and stability state of the systems?

How were these data collected? Table 9.1 represents a descriptive statistical summary of the final lab test on that specification for each manufacturing facility of the last 30 batches. Because of good manufacturing practices and laboratory quality control, the labs have been shown to produce consistent results. If possible, individual results can be traced to production dates of individual batches.

Were the systems that produced these data stable? This might be a new question for you. As previously mentioned, everything is a process. All processes occur over time. Hence, all data have a time order element to them allowing one to assess the stability of the system producing the data. Otherwise, many statistical tools can become useless and put one at risk for taking inappropriate actions. Therefore, it is always a good idea as an initial analysis to plot the data in its naturally occurring time order. This was not done.

Were the analyses appropriate, given the way the data were collected and stability state of the systems? But, you ask, the data passed the Normal distribution test. Isn't that all you need to know?

And your local 'guru' also concluded that there were no statistically significant differences among the manufacturing facilities, which led to a recommendation assuming that the problem was the entire manufacturing process regardless of plant and too loose a specification.

As previously stated, the batch production order could be recreated, resulting in the three simple time plots for the individual plants.

No difference? Note that just by 'plotting the dots', you have far more insight and are able to ask more incisive questions whose answers will lead to more productive system improvements.

Compare this to typical outputs encountered like bar graphs, summary tables, and the 'sophisticated' statistical analyses. What questions do you ask from those? Would they even be helpful? You are all smart people – you will, with the best of intentions, come up with theories and actions that could unwittingly harm your system. Or, worse yet, you might do nothing because there are no statistical differences' among the systems. Or, you might decide, 'We need more data'.

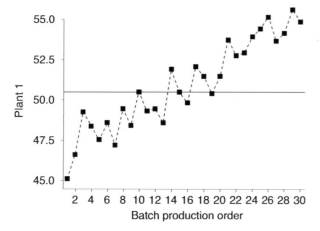

Figure 9.4 Run chart of Plant One.

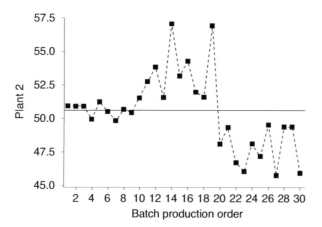

Figure 9.5 Run chart of Plant Two.

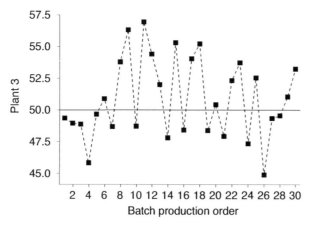

Figure 9.6 Run chart of Plant Three.

Regarding the computer generated 'statistics', what do the 'averages' of Plant One and Plant Two mean? Here's the answer: 'If I stick my right foot in a bucket of boiling water and my left foot in a bucket of ice water, on the average, I'm pretty comfortable.' It is inappropriate to calculate averages, standard deviations, and so on, on unstable processes.

Also, note that you have not calculated one statistic, yet you have just done a powerful statistical analysis!

And note that the conclusion reached was that there was need to overhaul the manufacturing process. However, in looking at Plant Two, one sees two distinct shifts in the data and much less variation than the other two plants (by about half). What if one could study Plant Two's process, determine the reason for the shifts, and control the process to 'target' rather than 'in specification', and implement these improvement in all three manufacturing facilities? Do you think this would result in fewer complaints and a higher quality product? The knowledge for improvement already existed, but needed to be discovered. Is not this an easier solution than a total redesign of the manufacturing process and dithering with specifications – which has nothing to do with the actual manufacture of the drug?

To summarise: *plot the dots!*

The statistics you need for improvement are far easier than you ever could have imagined. However, this philosophy will initially be quite counterintuitive to most of you and very counterintuitive to the people you work with.

If nothing else, it will at least make your jobs easier by freeing up a lot of time by recognising when to walk out of time-wasting meetings! It will also help you gain the cultural respect you deserve as quality professionals because your data collections and analyses will be simpler and more efficient...and more effective! The respect will also be magnified because you will be able to stop inappropriate responses to variation that would make people's jobs more complicated without adding any value to the service.

Plotting the dots – common and special causes

Almost all quality experts agree that merely plotting a process's output over time is one of the most simple, elegant and awesome tools for gaining deep understanding of any situation. Before one can plot, one must ask questions, clarify objectives, contemplate action and review current use of the data. Questioning from this statistical thinking perspective leads immediately to unexpected deeper understanding of the process. This results in establishing baselines for key processes and then allows honest dialogue to determine meaningful goals and action.

A more typical process is to impose arbitrary numerical goals that are retrofitted onto the process and enforced by exhortation that treats any deviation of process performance from the goal as unique and needing explanation – known as a special cause strategy. In paraphrasing the question looking at specific undesirable events into the context of observing a process over time:

> Is this an isolated excessive deviation –'special cause' – or, when compared
> to the previous measurement of the same situation, does it merely reflect
> the effects of ongoing actions of process inputs that have always been

present and cannot be predicted ahead of time – common cause? Would the exact same number necessarily be expected the next time it is measured? If not, then how much difference from the current or previous number is 'too much'?

It is very important to realise that just because an occurrence can be explained – after the fact – does not mean that it was unique. Thinking in terms of process, there are inputs causing variation that are always present and conspire in random ways to affect your process's output; however, they conspire to produce a predictable range of possible outputs. Many explanations merely point out things that have been waiting to happen...and will happen again at some random time in the future! Also, your process prefers some of these 'bogeys' to others. So, how can you collect data to find these deeper solutions to reduce the range of variation encountered by customers – common cause strategy?

So, if a process fluctuates within a relatively fixed range of variation, it is said to exhibit **common cause variation** and can be considered stable and predictable; although one may not necessarily like the results (In Figure 9.6, Plant Three's output exhibited common cause). If there is evidence of variation *over and above* what seems to be inherent, the process is said to exhibit **special cause variation** (In Figure 9.4, Plant One exhibited a 'trend' and, as discussed, Plant Two had two distinct 'shifts' in its process). This usually occurs in one of two ways. Either isolated single data points that are totally out of character in the context of the other data points, or distinct shifts in the process level due to outside interventions – intentional or unintentional – that have now become part of the everyday process inputs.

The most common error in improvement efforts is to treat common cause (inherent) variation as if it were special cause (unique) variation. This is known as tampering and will generally add more complexity to a process without any value. In other words, despite the best of intentions, the improvement effort has actually made things worse.

And note that the summary statistics treated special cause as if it were common cause. Even though the inherent variation of Plant Two was half of the other two, the calculated standard deviation of the 30 batches showed it to be equivalent to the other two. As for the summary of Process 1, how do you summarise it after looking at the plot?

The quality improvement goal

You have been invited to a free pizza lunch in celebration of meeting a quality improvement goal. Two years ago, your organisation had forty five batches of expensive medication rejected at final inspection and set a goal the past year of reducing this by at least 25%. The December data is in, and the yearly total was: 32 batches rejected – a 28.9% decrease! You think of all the hard work in the monthly quality meeting where each individual rejected batch is analysed to find root causes, then dispositioned. Then there are the months where you have zero batches rejected and the reasons for this are discussed and implemented. It all paid off...or did it?

Various graphs were used to prove that the goal had been met.

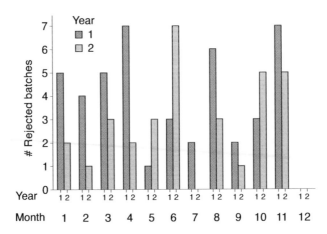

Figure 9.7 Year over year comparison of research batches.

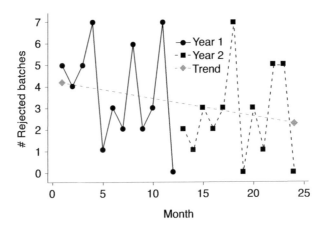

Figure 9.8 Time plot of research batches with trend line.

Figure 9.7, the obligatory bar graph display, shows that adverse incidents in eight months of the second year were lower than those in the previous year – obviously an improvement!

However, as Figure 9.8 so obviously shows, the improvement was much better than originally thought! The local statistical 'guru' did a trend analysis – available in most data packages – which showed a 46.2% decrease! The 'guru' also predicts 20 or rejected batches for the next year.

Regardless, even among people who agree either 'Yes' or 'No', there could still be as many different ways of coming to this conclusion as there are people reading this, which would result in differing proposed actions and a lot of formal meeting time. What is needed is a common approach for quickly and appropriately interpreting the variation through statistical theory.

Run charts

Imagine this data as 24 observations from a process. The chart in Figure 9.9 is a run chart; a time-ordered plot of the data with the overall data median drawn in

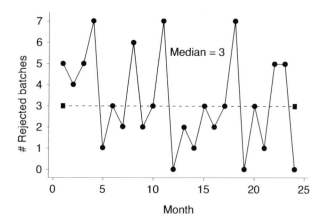

Figure 9.9 Run chart of research batches.

as a reference. The median is the empirical 'midpoint' of a data set, irrespective of time order. Half of the data values are literally higher than the median value and half of the data values are lower. In the present case, the median is 3 (you could sort these 24 observations from lowest to highest and the median would be the average of the 12th and 13th observations in the sorted sequence – both of which happen to be 3).

The initial run chart of a situation always assumes no change was made. A deceptively powerful set of three rules based in statistical theory can be applied to a chart like this to see whether your 'special cause' (you did intervene for the specific purpose of creating a change in the average, didn't you?) did indeed affect the level of the process.

So, the question in this case becomes, 'Is the process that produced the twelve data points of the second year the same as the process that produced the data points of the first year?' There are three statistical tests that can be applied, two of which will be discussed (the third is beyond the scope of this text, yet is still quite simple, and this process is discussed in additional papers by the author).[6, 7]

The first test looks for 'trends', in this case, a downward trend. Defined statistically, a trend is a sequence of seven consecutive points all going in the same direction up or down – in other words, six consecutive increases or six consecutive decreases. This pattern is not observed in this data.

The next test is the 'run of length eight' test. In other words, in the plotted run chart, does one observe a cluster of eight consecutive points either all above the median or all below the median? The theory here is that the process had fewer accidents. If this were true, then one would observe a cluster of eight consecutive points either above the median in the first year and/or a cluster of eight consecutive points below the median in the second year. We see neither.

Thus, despite the alleged achievement of what was seen as an aggressive goal, there is no statistical evidence of it having been met. It just goes to show you: Given two different numbers, one will be bigger!

Thus, given two numbers – 45 and 32 – one was smaller and it also happened to coincidentally meet an aggressive goal. The 'year-over-year' and 'trend' analyses were inappropriate and very misleading.

And it suddenly hits you: The result of all the hard work in the monthly quality meetings has been no improvement over two years and a lot of unneeded new policies!

In fact, if you continue to use this strategy – treating common cause as if it were special cause – you will observe between 20 and 57 accidents the following year!

So…does 'common cause' mean we have to live with it?

No, not at all. In the case of this data, people were treating data from a stable process exhibiting common causes of variation as if there were special causes of variation. Any observed differences were due totally to chance. Looking at individual numbers or summaries and calling any differences 'real' is a no yield strategy, as is looking at accidents individually. Once again, treating common cause as if it were special cause equates to tampering. Statistics on the number of rejected batches does not prevent future rejected batches.

A *common cause strategy* looks for underlying patterns producing the data – a statistical 'slicing and dicing', if you will, to try to expose process inputs that could be accounting for a significant source of the process's variation.

In the case of the rejected batch data, ask: 'Is there a commonality among all the months with higher numbers of rejections, or the low event months, or the months where there were zero rejections? Are some types of rejected batches unique to one of the three manufacturing facilities? Do some reasons for rejected batches occur in *all* three facilities? Does one facility exhibit a disproportionate total of rejected batches because its quality policy enforcement process is sloppy overall? These questions address process patterns that are exerting their influence consistently as inputs to the safety process. Neither the monthly data points nor individual rejected batches should be treated uniquely in isolation. It is only by looking at the aggregated factors contributing to all 77 rejected batches where opportunities in the underlying process inputs will be exposed.

Think of a 'rejected batch' as: an undesirable situation that was unsuccessfully avoided!

It is so common approach to have incident reviews every month and go over *every single* incident individually – in essence, 'scraping it like a piece of burnt toast' – and making a recommendation after each review. Can you see that this treats each incident as if it were a special cause?

Smart people have no trouble finding reasons if they look hard enough; after the fact. There is a high risk of treating spurious correlation as cause-and-effect, which only adds unneeded complexity to the current process, but *no value*.

This also has implications for the current issue of sentinel event analysis without asking the question:

> Was this an individually isolated event (special cause) or is the process such that it has been waiting to happen because the process inputs all randomly aligned to make it happen (common cause) – which means that it could happen again?'

Summary

A quality improvement context invalidates many assumptions perpetuated by traditional research-oriented statistical thinking, hence rendering commonly used analyses inappropriate. Quality improvement is radically different from clinical research! In addition, the stigma resulting from past – often compulsory – statistics courses often presents a formidable cultural barrier to the much needed simple, efficient data collection and analysis methods which are key to improving existing healthcare processes in real time. Proper implementation of statistical thinking has implications for and far beyond clinical outcomes.

It is important to realise that data analysis goes far beyond the routine statistical 'crunching' of numbers and useless displays such as tables of raw data, bar graphs and trend lines. The greatest contribution to an organisation is getting people to understand and use a process-oriented context in analysing situations as well as principles of good, simple, efficient data collection, analysis, and display. Ideally, it will also help gain the confidence and cooperation of organisations during stressful transitions and external assessments.

Whether or not people understand statistics, they are already using statistics and with the best of intentions. It is therefore vital to put a stop to many of the current well meaning but ultimately damaging ad hoc uses of statistics.

As a final summary, Box 9.3 shows the key lessons to keep in mind as you start looking at your organisation or services through a lens of statistical thinking.

Box 9.3 Key lessons.

- Make sure that any data being used were collected *specifically* for the current purpose
- Understand *how* the numbers were calculated and how the data were *collected*
- Make sure any analysis is *appropriate* for the way the data were collected:
  - tables of raw numbers, summary 'stats', and bar graph presentations are virtually worthless
  - the 'normal' distribution is highly overrated and very rarely used in improvement
  - 'traditional' calculation of the standard deviation will typically yield an inflated estimate
- 'Plotting the dots' of an indicator over time is a powerful but simple method for studying a process
- Arbitrary numerical goals by themselves improve nothing – *your processes are currently perfectly designed to get the results they are already getting…and will continue to get*
- Reacting to individual data points and individual 'incidents' in a 'stable' (common cause) system is, many times, a *no yield* strategy
- A stable system can be 'dissected' statistically to look for hidden opportunities

---

References

1   Neave HR. *The Deming Dimension*. Knoxville, TN: SPC Press; 1990.
2   Joiner B. *Fourth Generation Management: the new business consciousness*. New York: McGraw-Hill, Inc; 1994.
3   Mills JL. Data torturing. *New Eng J Med*. 1993; **329(16)**: 1196–9.
4   Shewhart W. *The Economic Control of Manufactured Product*. New York: Van Nostrand; 1931.
5   Scholtes P, Joiner B, Streibel B. *The TEAM Handbook*. 2nd spiral ed. Joiner/Oriel Inc; June 1, 1996.
6   Balestracci D. *Data 'Sanity': statistical thinking applied to everyday data*. Special Publication of the American Society for Quality Statistics Division, Summer 1998.
7   Balestracci D, Barlow J. *Quality Improvement: practical applications for medical group practice*. 2nd ed. Englewood, CO: Center for Research in Ambulatory Health Care Administration (CRAHCA); 1996.

Chapter 10

Outcome measurement in clinical practice

Ann P Moore

Introduction

This chapter sets out the topic of 'outcomes' from a health professional's perspective. It is written within the context of high intensity changes in NHS policy within the UK in response to an increasing number of healthcare reforms. These changes also reflect variations in values, attitudes and expectations towards health and healthcare by health workers, patients, carers, health service managers and officers in the DH, as well as Government officials. Never in the history of the NHS have the challenges for those working at the 'coalface' of healthcare delivery been greater than it is today from a number of different perspectives.

In the UK, *The NHS Next Stage Review – Our NHS Our Future,*[1] put quality at the centre of the NHS. More recently however, emphasis has been placed on quality, innovation and productivity. A number of reports and position statements published by the DH have messages which relate to the value and use of outcome measures in relation to quality and productivity. *Framing the Contribution of the AHPs – delivering high quality care*[2] talked about mandating data collection in respect of referrals, and improving quality through the development of quality metrics. Another paper, *Modernising AHP Careers*[3] set out the need for AHPs to demonstrate their unique contribution to patient care. *High Quality Care for All*[4] emphasised the need for quality metrics and raising standards of care, and finally *The NHS Constitution*[5] talked about maintaining high standards of care amongst a range of other requirements. The key messages arising from all these documents were:

- commissioning, in the future, will be based on local health needs
- a case needs to be made for how AHPs and other health professions meet health priorities
- clinical governance and accountability is vital within the NHS
- new AHP roles are given more autonomy but with autonomy will come greater accountability
- in short, AHPs must:
  - identify the need for their services
  - re-design services as appropriate to need
  - lead change in services in order to provide for these needs
  - focus on cost effectiveness

- influence commissioners indicating how they are addressing local needs
- take on new roles within the health service
- be a flexible workforce for example, in recognising issues such as patient held budgets and how the various professions need to market their skills and services to best effect.

The plethora of DH publications has been disturbing, but recently the key messages have been fairly consistent, AHPs need to produce evidence that they are working effectively and efficiently in achieving high quality patient care. Thoughtful, strategic and informed use of outcome measures will inevitably help AHPs in their efforts to support and sustain their valuable contribution to patient care and also in fulfilling the NHS, DH, agendas.

This focus on the need to demonstrate effectiveness of healthcare provision is not new as reference to the documents *A First Class Service: quality in the new NHS*[6] and *The New NHS: modern, dependable*[7] shows. There is, therefore, an increasing demand for health service provision to be evaluated and this is where outcomes come into play.

So what is an outcome measure?

There are many definitions, but the following are probably the most relevant to AHP practice, for example, Øvretveit defined the outcome of a service as 'the end result of its intervention on a client or a population in the short, medium and long terms';[8] Long, Dixon and Hall however, described an outcome measure as showing 'the results of processes...that part of the situation pertaining after the process which can be attributed to the process';[9] Mayo however specifically referring to physical therapy defined an outcome measure as 'a test or scale administered and interpreted by physical therapists that has been shown to measure accurately a particular attribute of interest to patients and therapists and is expected to be influenced by an intervention'.[10]

As increasingly more emphasis is being placed on health practitioners' roles in health promotion and public health, the following definition is also appropriate as in health promotion terms an outcome is 'the end product of a health programme or activity expressed in whatever terms are appropriate for example, changes in people's attitudes or knowledge, changes in health policy, changes in the uptake of services or changes in the rate of illness'.[11]

In terms of therapy most contact with patients consists of three components in varied proportions according to the nature, stage and severity of the patient's problem, these components are:

- passive/active intervention using one or more treatment modalities
- active participation by the patient where possible as a component leading to eventual focussed self management
- education and advice to enable the patient's understanding of their problem, the examination and treatment they are receiving or will receive and their role in their treatment strategy, this will also illuminate the role of the healthcare provider and their likely prognosis in relation to the specific care being offered.

The emphasis on the evaluation of the three features will vary according to the stakeholders' interests.

So who are the stakeholders?

There are a range of stakeholders interested in the outcome and/or the evaluation of the component parts of a typical therapeutic interaction. These stakeholders are:

- patients
- carers
- commissioners
- clinicians
- departmental managers
- the local NHS Trust
- the DH
- society in general.

The interests and priorities of the above stakeholders in terms of outcome measurement will vary according to their particular role, attitudes, values and beliefs. The concept of outcome measurement is quite complex in terms of fulfilling the needs and requirements of a range of stakeholders such as those listed above.

What are the stakeholders interested in?

Stakeholders' interests in outcomes can vary considerably from the effectiveness of a treatment for a particular problem to improvement in the quality of life of the patient concerned, changes in pain levels, reduction in breathlessness, increased functional ability, increased knowledge of the problem and its management and consequences, together with improvement in health and wellbeing, decreased fear and anxiety and finally cost effectiveness of the treatment concerned. These are all potential outcomes of treatment which need to be addressed in some form or another.

Cost effectiveness can be considered at a number of levels from the patient's perspective, for example, does the treatment outcome justify the time taken off work to attend for treatment and the cost of travel and car parking. From the NHS Trust's perspective there can be early, intermediate and long term cost benefits or costs without benefit implications! For example, in the short term patients may have a successful outcome within a given number of treatments for a chronic problem, but in the intermediate term re-admission rates may be the same as for those receiving fewer treatments so in many ways the treatment may overall not be cost effective. Measuring cost effectiveness is a complex and specialist field and beyond the scope of this chapter but all stakeholders need to be aware of the importance now placed on productivity and hence cost effectiveness features in a number of different agendas. Importantly clinicians need to think deeply and laterally about the short, intermediate and longer term effects of treatments and it may be that instead of trying to cut costs by reducing contact times, it may in the longer term be better in some cases, to increase contact times slightly or offer sessions over a longer period of time in order to aid patient self-management or produce an enhanced problem resolution thereby reducing costs for the NHS in the longer term and improving the overall and longer term quality of life for the patient. Whatever is done it needs to be carefully planned, piloted and evaluated with appropriate outcome measures.

The cost of care includes a wide range of expenditure items for example:

- the clinicians' time
- equipment costs
- estates costs, for example, electricity, heating, lighting, staff costs
- administration and reception staff costs
- ambulance costs – if appropriate
- consultant costs
- GP costs
- cost of admission and treatment in-house
- cost of drugs
- patients' time off work to attend out-patient treatment sessions
- cost of carers and child minding
- transport
- parking
- clinicians' CPD training activities
- GP visits and so on.

This list is not exhaustive and expenditure depends on the patient's needs and the services available. Health economists can and are producing quite complex models which can be used to calculate the cost-benefits – or otherwise – of a particular treatment modality or approach and this can be related to the short, medium and long term costs of care, but these models are dependent on appropriate outcome measurements being in place or adopted in order to contextualise cost effectiveness calculations.

Cost effectiveness can be assessed by measuring the cost of outcomes of different treatments which aim to achieve the same treatment goals in a similar/homogenous group of patients and thus is one of the core roles of NICE.

Why are outcome measures important?

The concept of quality is not new but the language related to quality and the initiatives and directives around the quality model change from government to government and DH initiatives. Outcome measurement has for some time been part of a number of quality assurance techniques which include those shown in Box 10.1.

Box 10.1 Quality assurance techniques.

- Implicit standards, such as professional standards
- Explicit standards, for example, local trusts/departmental standards
- Local problem solving techniques, such as reviews of case records
- Process measurement techniques, for example, qualpacs
- Consumer/user orientated techniques, like surveys and interviews
- Comprehensive review systems, such as audits of record keeping
- Case selection techniques, for example, sampling methods
- Outcome measurement, patient focussed and/or clinician focussed preferably of joint importance to both

Adapted from Ellis and Whittington.[12]

In today's climate quality has been defined as having a series of six key domains:[13]

1 effectiveness
2 access and timeliness
3 capacity
4 safety
5 patient centeredness
6 equity.

These domains can be measured in terms of quality and outcome, *see* Table 10.1.

Table 10.1 Measurement of quality and outcome.[14]

Quality domain	Principle	Example of measurement
Effectiveness	Healthcare services should be based, as far as possible, on relevant rigorous science and research evidence	Mortality rates Compliance rates with evidence-based guidelines (quality standards)
Access and timeliness	Healthcare services should be provided at the time they are needed within the appropriate setting	Provision of emergency care Availability of specialist care or rehabilitation
Capacity	Healthcare systems should be sufficiently well resourced to enable delivery of appropriate services	Staffing levels Number of scanners Information technology
Safety	Patients should not be harmed by the care that they receive or exposed to unnecessary risk	Nosocomial (hospital acquired) infections Medication errors Falls
Patient centeredness	Healthcare should be: 1 based on a partnership between practitioners and patients (and where appropriate, their families) 2 delivered with compassion, empathy and responsiveness to the needs, values and preferences of the individual patient	Survey data on: • patient evaluations of care • shared decision-making • patient experiences and interactions with staff
Equity	Healthcare should be provided: 1 on the basis of clinical need, regardless of personal characteristic such as age, gender, race, ethnicity, language, socioeconomic status or geographical location 2 in such a way as to reduce differences in health status and outcomes across various subgroups.	Comparisons of care provided across different sub-populations (for example, older people versus entire population) Mortality rates by socioeconomic status

Bring clarity to quality	Measure quality	Publish quality performance	Recognise and reward quality	Leadership for quality	Safeguard quality	Stay ahead
NICE quality standards	Indicators:	Quality accounts	PCT contracts, including CQUIN payment framework	PBC, service line reporting	COG registration	Learning from 'never events'
NHS evidence	Local, national, international	NHS choices	Normative tariffs	Social Enterprise	Professional registration	COG Special Reviews
	Patient reported outcome measures (PROMS)	Care Quality Commission (CQC) periodic review	Clinical Excellence Awards	Quality observatories		SHA duty to innovate
	Clinical dashboards	International measures	Quality & Outcomes Framework	SHAs – Medical Directors; Clinical Advisory Groups		Innovation funds and prizes
			Accreditation	National Quality Board		Academic Health and Science Centres
				National Clinical Directors		Health Innovation Education Clusters

Figure 10.1 A quality framework to enable quality improvement DH England (2009).[15]

In the UK the common quality themes for the DH are person centeredness – experience – effectiveness and safety. Importantly in the DH Quality Framework, AHPs are stated as adding 'life to years and not just years to life'. The quality framework, shown in Figure 10.1, clearly sets out the position of outcome measures and measurement in the overall NHS Strategy; for more information on the relevant quality agendas for each country within the UK visit the DH websites for England, Northern Ireland, Scotland and Wales.

Set up in 2004 Patient Reported Outcome Measurement Information System (PROMIS)[16] is an initiative which aims to revolutionise the way patient reported outcome tools are selected and employed in clinical research and practice evaluation, it will eventually establish a national resource for accurate and efficient measurement of patient reported systems and other health outcomes; for more details visit the PROMIS website.[16] Much emphasis has been placed in the NHS on the routine collection of patient reported outcome measures (PROMs). A new standard NHS contract for acute services was introduced in April 2008 and included a requirement for services to report from April 2009 on PROMs data. This data is routinely collected from patients undergoing unilateral hip or knee replacements, groin/hernia surgery and varicose vein procedures using PROMs which have been piloted in the NHS. The outcome measures used include a validated and reliability tested outcome measure for example, the Oxford Hip Score, the Oxford Knee Score and the Aberdeen Varicose Vein Score and in all cases the Euroqol (EQ-5D) which is a standardised instrument for use as a measure of health outcome. This outcome tool is applicable to a wide range of conditions and treatments and provides a descriptive profile and a single index value for health status, it is short and simple to use and has been translated into a hundred different languages; for more detail visit the Euroqol website.[17]

It may well be that in the future as more standardised metrics become agreed that more conditions, particularly long term conditions will be targeted for PROM data collection.[18]

So what outcome measures can be used?

There are hundreds of outcome measures for use in healthcare in addition to those listed above which can be uni-dimensional such as, mortality records – clinician recorded – or multi-dimensional questionnaires, for example the SF36 Quality of Life Questionnaire[19] which has a number of different dimensions included in it and which is patient completed.

A list of major outcome measurement categories is listed as it is not possible to review every outcome measure available for use in healthcare practice. These categories give a clear idea about the areas of stakeholders' interests in relation to healthcare practice.

Box 10.2 Outcome categories and examples.

- anxiety scores and measures of psychological wellbeing – symptoms of anxiety and depression scale
- general health indicators – Nottingham Health Profile
- quality of life measures – Quality of Wellbeing Scale

- disability/functional measures – days of work, Barthel Scale
- pain measures – VAS, McGill Pain Questionnaire
- patient satisfaction measures
- severity of illness classification
- measures of mental health
- measures of life satisfaction and morale – self esteem
- measures of social support – Social Support Questionnaire
- disease specific measures – Oswestry Low Back Pain Questionnaire
- multi-dimensional measures
- standardised data recording techniques
- self efficacy measures
- locus of control measures
- empowerment scales

A web search of these will provide a wealth of outcome measures for practical use. The key is in choosing the right outcome measure for the stakeholders, conditions and situations concerned.

It is important before using an outcome measure, to determine how it was originally developed and this can only be done by reading the literature discussing the development, validity and reliability of the outcome measurement tool concerned, for example, if one is looking for an outcome measure that clearly captures the patient's 'voice', then it would seem entirely inappropriate to choose an outcome measure that was not developed using user input, therefore accessing the original papers describing the development of the measure can be crucial. It is also important to know whether an outcome measurement tool has been validated and tested for reliability in the same context that it is intended to be used, for example, a functional scale may have been developed and tested for validity and reliability in a population of neurological patients and have been used successfully with this population, but is the tool applicable, valid and reliable for use with a group of patients with musculoskeletal problems. This is an extreme example but obviously the same issues apply for whatever outcome measurement tool is being used and whatever patient population is being targeted for its use. Differences in appropriateness of an outcome measure can relate to age, linguistic abilities, level of intelligence, cultural context and the stage of treatment/recovery when outcome measurement is needed or thought most appropriate.

What are the problems associated with the measurement of outcomes?

There are several problems encountered when beginning to use outcome measures, firstly, reaching an agreement as to what are appropriate outcome measures to evaluate effectiveness/quality of care in a particular setting/situation. There is little point in one therapist in a department or practice using an outcome measure that no-one else in the clinical area is using. Agreement upon the use of an outcome measure is vital and the more widespread the use is within a clinical setting locally, regionally and nationally the more data relating to clinical effectiveness will become available. The strength of multiple use of an outcome measure is that performance and effectiveness can be more easily compared. Likewise if patient care is occurring within a pathway in a multi-disciplinary setting then it makes sense for all members of the pathway team to agree on a particular outcome measure or set of outcome measures that can be used to reflect the success or otherwise of the pathway approach. The choice of outcome measurement should also involve a user perspective whenever possible. In the future it is likely that the DH will produce a set of recommended outcomes/metrics for use, but it is important that a discussion takes place as to the applicability/usefulness of using the particular outcome measures in the local setting and with the particular client group concerned, this needs careful discussion with the healthcare team. It is important that the outcome measures that are chosen are patient focussed and are also able to provide information which will support and improve practice and the quality of service provision.

Another problem associated with outcome measurement is disentangling the results of healthcare interventions from the effects of other confounding variables. For example, changes in patient's health/work status, the impact of other interventions, other therapies or drug prescription. This again needs careful thought and discussion regarding the timing of outcome measurement and may need some associated qualitative feedback from patients concerned to get a true picture of the actual perceived outcomes.

Demonstrating relationships between measures of the process of care and measures of related outcomes can also be a difficulty. For example, it is quite common in physiotherapy out-patient research relating to low back pain to measure the outcome of care at the end of active treatment, at three months, six months, one year and two years following the completion of treatment, as is customary following surgical interventions. This can create significant problems as often the success of treatment in the long term after a period of three to five treatments depends substantially on the patient's conformance with treatment and the advice given and also their ability to self manage following discharge, and this post discharge period is something that the physiotherapist has very little control over. The dilemma is when should outcomes be measured in this scenario to truly show the benefits of an intervention? Perhaps it should be that physiotherapists should look more at staged discharge or at building in more strategies to gain treatment conformance, whatever is the case, the timing of outcome measurement is crucial and needs to be explored fully in order to reflect the true impact of an intervention.

Finally and most importantly before using outcome measures in any context, health professionals need to be sure that the proposed outcome measure has been tested for reliability – intra, and inter tester reliability – and also for validity, that is, does the measure, measure what it purports to measure? In other words if the outcome measure is completed by the same patient on more than one occasion without intervention, would the findings be the same, and if used by a number of therapists with a homogenous group of patients, again would the results be comparable?

All outcome measures used in clinical practice should have been tested for validity to ensure academic credibility, in other words, has it been established that it measures what it purports to measure? Does it have face validity with the client group concerned, for example, an outcome measure may have been found to be valid for a group of patients in chronic pain who have their family roots in a western society, but will the results be the same if a group of patients in chronic pain whose cultural roots are from a different part of the world, for example, Africa or the Middle East, are assessed using the same 'tool'?

Before using any outcome measure, it is wise to read about its reliability and validity testing in the literature relating to the 'tool' to assess the rigour of the testing procedures previously undertaken and thus gain insight into the measure's scientific credibility. In addition many 'tools' are designed for patient completion, but it is interesting and illuminating to find out whether the 'tool' was developed with user input as previously stated, if not, it is questionable whether it is a viable and responsive patient reported outcome measure.

It is important to ensure that outcome measures used, truly reflect the management/treatment approach and determine whether the measure to be used reflects patients' and clinicians' needs or is it only fulfilling the needs of another stakeholder?

Summary

The issues relating to outcome measures are:

- are they reliable?
- are they sensitive enough for the clinical scenario in question?
- are they valid? That is do they have face, construct, convergent and divergent validity?
- will they be applied at an appropriate time?
- are they culturally sensitive and acceptable?
- have they been translated appropriately?
- is the outcome measure feasible to be used in the required context?
- is the 'tool' internally consistent?
- is it responsive?

In conclusion the right outcome measures, used in the right way, with the right client group, at the right time, can provide evidence of clinical effectiveness and can contribute to cost effectiveness measurements. To fulfil the quality agenda outcome measurement use cannot be recommended more highly.

References

1 Department of Health. *The NHS Next Stage Review. Our NHS Our future.* London: Department of Health; 2008.
2 Department of Health. *Framing the Contribution of the Allied Health Professions – delivering high quality care.* London: Department of Health; 2008.
3 Department of Health and Skills for Health. *Modernising AHP Careers.* London: Department of Health; 2008.
4 Department of Health. *High Quality Care for All.* London: Department of Health; 2008.
5 Department of Health. *The NHS Constitution.* London: Department of Health; 2009.
6 NHSE. *A First Class Service: quality in the new NHS.* London: Department of Health; 1997.
7 NHSE. *The New NHS: modern, dependable.* London: Department of Health; 1998.
8 Øvretveit J. *Health Service Quality.* Oxford: Blackwell Science; 1992.

9 Long A, Dixon P, Hall R, *et al*. The outcomes agenda: contribution of the UK clearing house on health outcomes. *Qual Healthcare*. 1993; **2(1)**: 49–52.

10 Mayo N. Outcome measures or measuring outcome. *Physiotherapy Canada*. 1994; **46(3)**: 145–6.

11 Ewles L, Simnet I. *Promoting Health: a practical guide*. Edinburgh: Baillière and Tindall; 1993.

12 Ellis R, Whittington D. *Quality Assurance in Healthcare*. London: Edward Arnold; 1993.

13 Institute of Medicine. *Crossing the Quality Chasm: a new health system for the 21st century*. Washington, DC: National Academy Press; 2001.

14 Sutherland K, Coyle N. *Quality in Healthcare in England, Wales, Scotland and Northern Ireland: an intra-UK chartbook*. London: The Health Foundation; 2009.

15 Hughes L. *Creating an Interprofessional Workforce: an education and training framework for health and social care in England*. Conference presentation; 2009.

16 DH England. *PROMIS 2009*: www.niroadmap.nih.gov.

17 Euroqol: www.euroqol.org.

18 Reform: www.reform.co.uk.

19 Ware J Jr, Gandek B. Overview of the SF-36 Health Survey and the International Quality of Life Assessment (IQOLA) Project. *J Clin Epidemiol*. 1998; **51(11)**: 903–12.

Further reading

Suggestions for further reading for a database of approximately 200 outcome measures please visit the Chartered Society of Physiotherapy's website: www.csp.org.uk-outcome measures.

Other recommendations include:

- Bowling A. *Research Methods in Health: investigating health and health services*. 3rd ed. Buckingham: Open University Press; 2009.
- Bowling A. *Measuring Health: a review of quality of life measurement scales*. 3rd ed. Maidenhead: Open University Press; 2005.
- Bowling A. *Measuring Disease: a review of disease specific quality of life measurement scales*. 2nd ed. Maidenhead: Open University Press; 2001.
- Bowling A. *Ageing Well: quality of life in old age (growing older)*. Maidenhead: Open University Press; 2005.

Chapter 11

Benchmarking AHP services

Fiona Jenkins and Robert Jones

Benchmarking your service

Benchmarking is an invaluable means of enhancing understanding of your service's performance achieved through making comparisons with other organisations. It demonstrates how your service is performing in relation to similar AHP services and will also indicate whether the full potential of the workforce and other resources is being fully realised. If, as AHP managers, we have no idea what the standards for a wide range of parameters are, we cannot compare to establish the relationship between our organisation and others. Benchmarking is often used as part of service review and for quality improvement initiatives. The technique is a widely used management 'tool' which had its origins in manufacturing industry and is now used in public services including healthcare.

Introducing our AHP benchmarking tool

We have developed this AHP benchmarking tool, which can be used by managers to help set standards and monitor whether or not these are being met in terms of workforce, resources, activity, availability, access and so on. To date there has been no universally accepted 'validated tool' or process available to AHP managers and their teams to use and undertake this work. In view of this and as a result of our own experience in undertaking service reviews evaluation and consultancy, we recognised that a basic benchmarking process, which is evidence based, would be helpful to AHP managers and wider healthcare organisations.

Initially the 'tool' included a wide range of specialties but following piloting and advice received from heads of AHP services and clinicians, we decreased the number of categories included to facilitate ease of completion and opportunity for comparisons to be made. Our benchmarking 'tool' is designed to be objective and a straightforward process, which can either be used to review your own service in isolation, or to make comparisons with aspects of other services, or other services in their entirety. We hope the 'tool' will support and be helpful to AHP managers undertaking benchmarking exercises.

How to use the tool

Firstly, we set out below data collection forms which we have designed for collecting the data. This is followed by a set of briefing notes which explains how the process should be completed. Our benchmarking 'tool' is one of several AHP management 'tools' developed by us which can be accessed and completed interactively on our website.[1] The 'tool' can be completed anonymously if preferred. The website[1] provides explanatory notes on how to access and use the 'tool' and how to participate in the benchmarking process.

The benchmarking 'toolkit'

The tool has five sections.

1 Your organisation.
2 Your professional group.
3 In-patient services.
4 Out-patient services.
5 Community services.

Briefing notes

The purpose of these briefing notes is to ensure – as far as possible – a consistent and accurate methodology for collecting the data between the provider services participating in benchmarking exercises. Organisations taking part may be widely dispersed across the region, country, or between countries and there are differing practices and definitions in use in different places. Therefore uniformity of approach will help to ensure that the data collected enables valid comparisons and consistent interpretation.

It is possible to select only a few categories for benchmarking, or to include the whole service. The more generic categories that are chosen to describe the service, the more likely it will be to find a comparator to benchmark with. Therefore, consider very carefully the categories you select to benchmark. We recognise, for example, that some areas have elderly care wards and in others areas elderly care is part of General Medicine – we have amalgamated this and have one category, General Medicine.

We also recognise that different professions have different sub-specialisms, for example, gastroenterology is likely to be a high input for dietitians, but physiotherapists may include this in-patient activity as part of General Medicine.

Confidentiality is guaranteed; if your service/organisation wishes to remain anonymous please indicate on the form. The data collection spreadsheet is divided into five sections.

Please fill in the non-shaded boxes.

Table 11.1 Spreadsheet 1: your organisation.

Date:

Provider Name:

Professional groups being benchmarked:

1. .... WTE HPC Reg. Staff .... WTE Non Reg. Clinical Staff .... WTE A&C .... Grand Total WTE all staff ....
2. .... WTE HPC Reg. Staff .... WTE Non Reg. Clinical Staff .... WTE A&C .... Grand Total WTE all staff ....
3. .... WTE HPC Reg. Staff .... WTE Non Reg. Clinical Staff .... WTE A&C .... Grand Total WTE all staff ....
4. .... WTE HPC Reg. Staff .... WTE Non Reg. Clinical Staff .... WTE A&C .... Grand Total WTE all staff ....
5. .... WTE HPC Reg. Staff .... WTE Non Reg. Clinical Staff .... WTE A&C .... Grand Total WTE all staff ....
6. .... WTE HPC Reg. Staff .... WTE Non Reg. Clinical Staff .... WTE A&C .... Grand Total WTE all staff ....

Contact details for the person completing the form (optional)

Name:

Position:

email address:

Provider Type (please tick):

1. Acute Trust
2. Foundation Trust
3. Care Trust
4. PCT Provider
5. Mental Health Trust
6. Combined Acute and Community
7. Tertiary
8. Other please specify:

Catchment Population:

Total number of beds in organisation:

Budget for services being benchmarked (list professional groups)

1. .... Total Budget = £ .... Pay Budget = £ .... Non - Pay Budget = £ ....
2. .... Total Budget = £ .... Pay Budget = £ .... Non - Pay Budget = £ ....
3. .... Total Budget = £ .... Pay Budget = £ .... Non - Pay Budget = £ ....
4. .... Total Budget = £ .... Pay Budget = £ .... Non - Pay Budget = £ ....
5. .... Total Budget = £ .... Pay Budget = £ .... Non - Pay Budget = £ ....
6. .... Total Budget = £ .... Pay Budget = £ .... Non - Pay Budget = £ ....

Grand Totals: .... £ .... £ .... £

Do you want to keep your organisation's name to be kept anonymous? Yes / No (Please identify)

Table 11.2 Spreadsheet 2: your professional group.

Your Professional Group

	WTE Registered Staff									WTE Non Registered Staff						Total WTE staff in this group
	Band 5	Band 6	Band 7	Band 8a	Band 8b	Band 8c	Band 8d	Band 9	Director	Band 2	Band 3	Band 4	Band 5	Band 6	Band 7	
Total WTE Managerial Staff HPC Registered																
Total WTE Clinical HPC Registered Staff for your Professional Group - excluding consultants																
Total WTE AHP Consultants																
Total WTE - Assistants and support staff																
Total WTE Admin & Clerical staff																
Staff from your professional group you provide to other organisations																

Table 11.3 Spreadsheet 3: in-patient services.

Your Professional Group:

Clinical Specialities. Select specialties relevant to your profession - see briefing notes.	Beds per specialty	WTE Registered Staff								WTE Non Registered Staff				Total all staff for specialty	Activity		7 day service Yes/No	Validated clinical outcome measures used? Yes*/No
		Band 5	Band 6	Band 7	Band 8a	Band 8b	Band 8c	Band 8d	Band 9	Band 2	Band 3	Band 4	Band 5		New patients last year	Total contacts last year		
ENT (SALT only)																		
Gastro-enterology (Dietetics only)																		
General Medicine (including elderly care)																		
General Surgery																		
HDU																		
Head and Neck (Dietetics and SALT only)																		
ITU																		
Emergency admissions																		
Mental Health																		
Neurology																		
Obstetrics & Gynaecology																		
Oncology																		
Paediatrics																		
Palliative care																		
SCBU																		
Stroke unit																		
Trauma and Orthopaedic																		
Other 1. Please specify																		
Other 2. Please specify																		
Other 3. Please specify																		
Other 4. Please specify																		
Other 5. Please specify																		

*Please list validated outcome measures used.

Table 11.4 Spreadsheet 4: out-patient services.

Your Professional Group:

Specialties. Select specialties relevant to your profession - see briefing notes	WTE Registered Staff							WTE Non Registered Staff					Total all staff for specialty	Is group treatment included in this specialty? Yes/No	Activity				Validated clinical outcome measures used? Yes*/No
	Band 5	Band 6	Band 7	Band 8a	Band 8b	Band 8c	Band 8d	Band 9	Band 2	Band 3	Band 4	Band 5			Average no. new patients/week per WTE	New patients last year	Total contacts last year	DNA %	
A&E																			
Cardiac Rehab																			
Communication (SALT only)																			
Diabetes (Dietetics and Podiatry only)																			
Dysfluency (SALT only)																			
Fracture Clinic																			
Gait clinics																			
Gastro-enterology (Dietetics only)																			
Hand therapy																			
Head and Neck (Dietetics and SALT only)																			
Hydrotherapy (physio only)																			
Musculoskeletal																			
Neurology (excluding stroke)																			
Nutritional support (Dietetics only)																			
Occupational Health																			
Orthotics																			
Paediatrics																			
Pain management																			
Palliative care																			
Pulmonary Rehab																			
Rheumatology																			
Stroke																			
Voice (SALT only)																			
Wheelchairs and seating																			
Women's/Men's health																			
Other 1. Please specify																			
Other 2. Please specify																			
Other 3. Please specify																			

*Please list validated outcome measures used.

Table 11.5 Spreadsheet 5: community services.

Your Professional Group:

Specialities. Select specialities relevant to your profession - see briefing notes.	WTE Registered Staff								WTE Non Registered Staff				Total all staff for specialty	Activity				
	Band 5	Band 6	Band 7	Band 8a	Band 8b	Band 8c	Band 8d	Band 9	Band 2	Band 3	Band 4	Band 5		Is group treatment included in this specialty? Yes/No	New patients last year	Total contacts last year	7 day service Yes/No	validated clinical outcome measures used? DNA % Yes*/No
Community hospital rehabilitation ward																		
Domiciliary adult																		
Domiciliary paediatric																		
Intermediate Care																		
Learning Disabilities																		
Mental Health																		
Neuro rehab (excluding stroke)																		
Paediatric																		
Social Services																		
Stroke																		
Other 1. Please specify																		
Other 2. Please specify																		
Other 3. Please specify																		
Other 4. Please specify																		
Other 5. Please specify																		

*Please list validated outcome measures used.

Section 1 your organisation — general information

Only one Section 1 form needs filling in per organisation.

- Date: the date the form is completed.
- Provider name: the name of your organisation.
- Professional groups being benchmarked: please list the professions for benchmarking and then insert the WTE HPC Reg. Staff...WTE Non Reg. Clinical Staff...WTE A&C...Grand Total WTE all staff...
- Contact details for the person completing the form: generally the most senior AHP manager in the service. Please give name and e-mail contact, but this may be withheld if you wish.
- Provider type: e.g. Acute Trust, PCT Provider Arm, Care Trust, Foundation Trust, Tertiary provider.
- Catchment population for your organisation: please state the population in thousands.
- Total number of beds in the organisation: list the current declared bed stock.
- Budget for services being benchmarked: first list the services being benchmarked, then include total budget, pay budget and non-pay budget for all of the professional groups combined and finally add up the columns to give the grand totals.
- Indicate whether you want your organisation's name to be kept anonymous: highlight Yes or No.

NB. Each individual profession will need to complete sections 2–5 inclusive as appropriate.

Section 2 your professional group and staffing

- Total WTE managerial staff: please fill in the boxes that are not shaded as appropriate. For staff with mixed managerial and clinical roles, please include here the approximate WTE of their time assigned to management duties.
- Total WTE clinical staff for your professional group (excluding consultants): this includes every member of staff you employ, working within your organisation.
- Total WTE AHP consultants.
- Total WTE assistant and support staff.
- Total WTE administration and clerical staff.
- Staff from your professional group you provide to other organisations: this would include the staff that you employ and that you may have service level agreements to provide to another organisation, e.g. rotational staff, hospices, etc.
- Total staff: please add up rows to give your total staff by band for staff group.

Section 3 in-patient services

An in-patient service is defined as:

One where patients (clients) occupy a bed as part of their episode of care. This may be in acute or community settings and in health or social care.

The list of specialities is not exhaustive, but it is hoped that most therapy services will be able to group their total in-patient activity under several of the categories listed. It is not intended for every speciality to be used by every professional group.

Where highly specialist or tertiary services are provided please list them in the 'Other' category – though this may make it more difficult to benchmark.

- Your professional group: name the professional group you are reporting information for.
- Beds per specialty: for the specialties you are proving data for, please indicate the current number of beds, in the unshaded boxes only.
- WTE registered staff: i.e. staff registered with the HPC.
- WTE non registered staff: i.e. assistants and clinical support staff do not include clerical staff in this section.
- Total staff: please add up rows to give your total staff for the specialty.
- New patients last year: total number of new patients for the last financial year.
- Total contacts last year: total face to face contacts for the last financial year.
- Seven day service Yes/No: this includes routine working, even if only for part of the day and not an 'on-call' service.
- Validated clinical outcome measures used: please identify at the bottom of the sheet the names of the validated outcome measures used.
- Clinical specialties: for each of these broadly defined clinical specialties enter the relevant data in each column. Some clinical specialties listed will not require detailed benchmark scrutiny for every professional group, e.g. gastroenterology is likely to be pertinent to dietetic services, whereas physiotherapy may group this service as part of General Medical services. Similarly it is unlikely that podiatry services will input to ITU regularly. It is anticipated that data will be provided for a wide range of specialties for each profession.
- Other please specify: if your in-patient service is very different from one in the list, e.g. tertiary service, cardio-thoracic, neuro-surgery please identify it and provide data.
- Day surgery: provide data for therapy input to day surgery services, i.e. where there is no overnight stay.
- Total staff: please add up columns to give your total staff by band.

Section 4 out-patient services

An out-patient is someone who attends a hospital or clinic for treatment that does not require an overnight stay.

This section is to gather information on patients who meet this definition. This could include both adult and children's services, and may be in primary or secondary care and normally in a healthcare setting.

The list of specialities is not exhaustive, and is intended to give a reasonable level of specialisation for each profession, but also recognises that to list every therapy sub-speciality would be an exhaustive process. It is not intended for every speciality to be used by every professional group.

Where highly specialist or tertiary services are provided please list them in the 'Other' category – this may make it more difficult to benchmark, so only use when really necessary.

- Your professional group: name the professional group you are reporting information for.
- WTE registered staff: i.e. staff registered with the HPC.
- WTE non registered staff: i.e. assistants and clinical support staff do not include clerical staff in this section.
- Total staff: please add up rows to give your total staff for the specialty.
- Group treatment: answer Yes or No for each specialty.
- Average number new patients/week per WTE: where staff are set an target number of new patients per week please enter this number for each speciality that this applies to.
- New patients last year: total number of new patients for the last financial year.
- Total contacts last year: total face to face contacts for the last financial year.
- DNA %: this includes all DNA and UTA for first and follow up appointments as a percentage of all appointments.
- Validated clinical outcome measures used: please identify at the bottom of the sheet the names of the validated outcome measures used.
- Out-patient specialties: for each of these broadly defined specialties enter the relevant data in each column. Some specialties listed will not be relevant to all professional groups, e.g. dysfluency is likely to be only a speech and language therapy specialty, whereas wheelchair and seating clinics may be pertinent for both physiotherapy and occupational therapy. It is anticipated that data will be provided for a wide range of specialties for each profession, but not each and every one.
- Other please specify: if your out-patient service is different from one in the list please identify it and provide data, this may make it more difficult to benchmark, so only use when really necessary.

Section 5 community services

Community services are those therapy services that are provided away from hospital premises and are neither in-patient services, nor out-patients'. Examples would include services provided to education and a range of community based facilities such as GP surgeries, community clinics and children's centres.

- Your professional group: name the professional group you are reporting information for.
- WTE registered staff: i.e. staff registered with the HPC.
- WTE non registered staff: i.e. assistants and clinical support staff do not include clerical staff in this section.
- Total staff: please add up rows to give your total staff for the specialty.
- Group treatment: answer Yes or No for each specialty.
- New patients last year: total number of new patients for the last financial year.
- Total contacts last year: total face to face contacts for the last financial year.
- Seven day service Yes/No: this includes routine working, even if only for part of the day and not an 'on-call' service.
- DNA %: this includes all DNA and UTA for first and follow up appointments as a percentage of all appointments.
- Validated clinical outcome measures used: please identify at the bottom of the sheet the names of the validated outcome measures used.

- Community types: for each of these broadly defined types enter the relevant data in each column. Some listed will not be relevant to all professional groups. It is anticipated that data will be provided for a wide range of specialties for each profession, but not necessarily every one.
- Other please specify: if your community service is different from one in the list please identify it and provide data, this may make it more difficult to benchmark, so only use when really necessary.

Reference

1   www.jjconsulting.org.uk.

Chapter 12

Management quality and operational excellence

Stephen E Chick, Arnd Huchzermeier and Christoph Loch

This chapter focusses on management quality. A focus on management quality is consistent with Edwards'[1] observation that badly managed organisations fail patients, frustrate staff, deliver poor quality care and cannot adapt to the rapidly changing environment in which they operate. They further note that reports from the Bristol Inquiry[2] and the Climbié Inquiry[3] describe how poor management practice can be at least as lethal as poor clinical practice and that good managers can create an environment that supports clinicians and high quality care. These concerns are not isolated to the UK alone.

What is management quality? What does it mean for healthcare? To answer the first question, INSEAD – the top business school in France – initiated an Industrial Excellence Award (IEA) in 1995 to study how managerial choices lead to outstanding performance in the industrial context. The IEA expanded in 1997 to Germany with academic partner WHU – Otto Beisheim School of Management. The study built a conceptual framework and has been validated by an empirical assessment of high-performance business units from France and Germany. More recently, a number of service firms, including those in the IT and health service sectors, approached us to generalise the questionnaire to a broader context.

This chapter summarises the conceptual model and key learning points from the first decade of the study. We emphasise management quality, rather than technological quality or professional qualifications in isolation; attributes of management which, when performed well, lead to greater effectiveness of an organisation. In the healthcare sector, that means more people that are healthier in a timely and less costly way. Management quality in healthcare is particularly relevant today. Increased specialisation and knowledge, as well as the increasing complexity of patient pathways and technologies in the face of scrutinised budgets, mean that constrained resources must be used more efficiently and effectively. Management quality is one mental framework for approaching trade-offs that leaders and managers in healthcare delivery organisations can use to provide better value for patients.

Introduction

The healthcare sector has changed tremendously through recent decades. Hotly discussed issues include technological advances, biomedical innovations, information infrastructure, standards and accreditation, continuous improvement 'tools', healthcare financing, evidence-based medicine and value-based competition, tension between management and medical roles, tension between national policy and the realities of every-day delivery and continuity in care. Healthcare systems are tremendously complex to manage.

What are the attributes of outstanding management in the healthcare provision? What does an outstanding hospital or community health system look like? Sometimes it is useful to think by analogy. In this case, we would like to make an analogy to the industrial sector. In the industrial sector, technology and information and people issues can also be very complex to lead and to manage. While these systems often have complex management challenges, it is often possible to identify characteristics of high-performance facilities as well as some fundamental measures of process performance. Those key levers and measurements are indicative of the performance and improvement in a few key business processes. Strong performance in several of those processes can lead to outstanding performance for creating value.

The section on management quality improving value creation summarises the structure of the conceptual model of the IEA. That model was first described in the first IEA book[4] and our more recent book describes our continued learning from this long-term project.[5] The IEA study was designed to answer the following questions:

- what is operational excellence in the factory and in the supply chain?
- how can strategy actually be implemented successfully at an operational level?
- how is an excellent operation managed?
- what is the experience of people working in it?
- what does a manager pay attention to?

The IEA study is a framework that is informed by theory from several disciplines and is validated by a large scale empirical study.

While the language of such a study may differ in some respects from that of healthcare management in general, or from that of hospital management in particular, a number of central concepts remain the same. Organisations must create value by organising their processes in an effective and adaptive way and by enabling their employees to perform these processes intelligently and consistently. Value in healthcare has been defined as the health outcome per unit of currency spent.[6] Value for the healthcare chain can also be defined as; the delivery of sustainable, cost-effective value for healthy populations in a 'hassle-free' way.

A number of key processes are required to deliver value. The premise of this chapter is that effective management of the processes that deliver value can improve the cost, quality and effectiveness of healthcare provision. We examine this premise by first reviewing the IEA study, then discussing some ways that the model may apply to healthcare delivery.

Management quality improves value creation

The success of an industrial organisation often gets equated with profitability and short-term share prices, on the basis of the 'shareholder value' paradigm. However, even in an industrial context, clear evidence from strategic management studies indicates the success of an organisation, as perceived by all stakeholders – for example, employees, management, shareholders, other constituencies – is much broader even in an industrial context. An evaluation of success must include not only wealth but also growth, which in turn influences job creation – rather than job destruction – and a sense of a positive role that the organisation plays in a community.[7,8] This broader picture is certainly relevant in healthcare.

Figure 12.1 displays a competitiveness diamond that summarises strategic approaches implemented by the excellent organisations that we have encountered in the IEA. The four external corners of the 'diamond' characterise strategic positions and the inside summarises the execution capabilities. Strategic positioning includes answering questions such as:

- what is the basic value proposition to the population being served?
- what is the population being served?
- what is unique about the value that is provided, relative to the value that other providers offer?
- how are resources and know-how brought together in order to deliver that value?
- how is the target population made aware of that value, and how is the operation sustained financially?

Answers to questions like these are readily articulated in effective organisations.

Healthcare has traditionally employed a less broad range of strategic positions than in other industries. General hospitals that provide a range of services to a broad demographic range can be found everywhere. Increasingly we see innovative healthcare models, such as focussed specialty clinics at both the low and high end of the cost and service spectrum and a greater distinction among

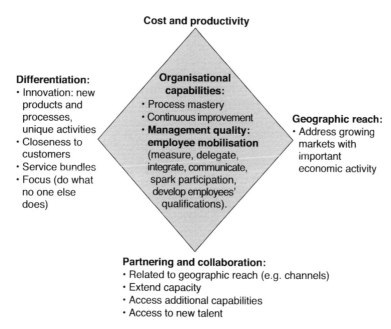

Figure 12.1 The competitiveness diamond.

small providers that goes beyond the traditional focus on local geographic populations as a differentiator.

A greater range of strategic positions allows for a focus that can inspire improvement. For example, an organisation might focus on specific disease groups, on severity and urgency, or on long term conditions management around a core disease. Improvement may include health effectiveness, lower costs, or better services to targeted patient segments that value them, all of which can raise both customer satisfaction as well as the ability of the organisation to be financially healthy. A healthy organisation is able to invest in further improvements, which can turn into a 'virtuous' cycle of success if sustained. The issue of developing a strategic position could be a book by itself. The focus of this chapter is more on the inside of the 'competitiveness diamond' and the successful execution of a strategy.

Management quality model

No strategy, no matter how brilliant, leads to value unless the organisation has the capabilities and discipline to execute it. The real secret of success lies in execution, which often requires multiple, mutually supportive capabilities and this network of capabilities represents the hard-to-copy strength of the organisation. Specifically, the organisational capabilities comprise mastery of key business processes and management quality in executing them.

Execution happens at the level of at least three core business processes.

1 The Strategy Deployment process – the formulation and implementation of strategy.
2 The Supply Chain process – the delivery of products and services from suppliers through the 'sales channel'. Here one might include indirect demand generators, such as GPs who might make a choice to refer patients to one hospital versus another, based on experiences they have had with these hospitals in the past.
3 Product and Process Development – the creation of new offerings and operating capabilities. Performance and improvement across the key business processes, and thus for the entire organisation, are driven by management quality.

The strategy deployment process is the way an organisation organises both top-down and bottom-up communication. How are strategic objectives and focus areas for improvement shared? How are observations for improvement from front-line staff shared throughout the organisation? The supply chain process can refer to the management of consumable flows, but also to the flows of patients through the healthcare system. The new product development process includes the development and adoption of new products and services, whereas the new process development encompasses new ways of delivering those products and services, including methods and procedures. In the healthcare systems of many countries, an important core element to add is the people development process. This governs how medical and non-medical staff are recruited, trained, developed and retained.

The IEA model examines how effective managers use operational 'levers' to improve mastery for key processes such as those above, in order to achieve high

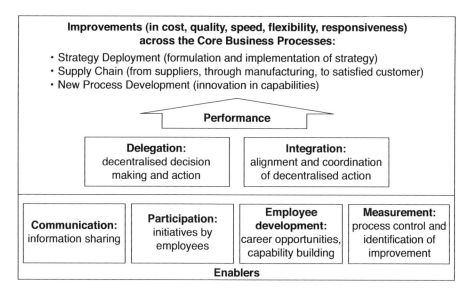

Figure 12.2 Dimensions of management quality.

performance and sustainable value for the organisation and its customers. We define the 'levers' of management quality through the six dimensions described in Figure 12.2.

The first two dimensions, delegation and integration, refer to the classic organisational concepts of decentralised action on the one hand and coordinating the decentralised action on the other hand. Today more than in the past, organisations are often characterised by complex and capital-intensive technology and the need for faster response to changes in the competitive environment. They can no longer, therefore, be run in a traditional command-and-control mode. Management must increasingly delegate decision-making power to the various levels where the detailed knowledge of the manufacturing and service delivery processes resides – delegation is sometimes called 'empowerment'. For example, several winning plants had introduced fully autonomous lines – factories within factories – with decision power over quality, planning, staffing and material flows. As one manager in a consumer products plant put it:

> We are going to the limit of the ability of our workers. I hold many one-on-one meetings with the technicians in charge of the project. They give a status report and I ask them if they need my help, the follow up is close. The combination of monitoring and helping not only reduces errors but also motivates the employees and makes them progress.

The same idea can apply to specialised 'lines' of patients going through a certain type of treatment.

Decentralised action necessitates integration in order to ensure the alignment of common goals within the organisation and across the business processes. Horizontal integration connects the plant with suppliers and customers along the supply chain. Many of the well-managed factories had full access to the customer's production planning system. Several were designated centres of technical expertise for the customer, or lead developers for important components of the customer's products – with customer and competitor engineers on the team. One company developed such a track record and mutual trust that the customer delegated important project management functions for product facelifts to the plant.

> We do our best for the customer, so that everything runs one 100%. That's our goal because we are part of the customer, commented one manager.

The same idea might be applicable for hospitals who seek information about the transferring doctors with whom they work, possibly helping them to prioritise patients, or even supporting them with activities that they have difficulty performing.

Collaborative problem-solving with suppliers for mutual benefit is now also common. For healthcare, this means overcoming issues surrounding some historical mistrust regarding interactions between non-profit and for-profit organisations. For example, some medical systems suppliers are now helping hospitals to improve processes around expensive equipment – such as diagnostic imaging systems – which improves productivity and thus reduces costs while improving the equipment's effectiveness in improving health-critical diagnoses.

Vertical integration applies to the strategy deployment process, including consistent sub-goals for all organisational sub-units. In the best plants, every worker knew the key performance priorities of the plant and could tell us what his or her contribution to these overarching goals was, in terms of quality, cost, volume, delivery times, or similar operational measures. Often, performance indicators and customer quality feedback were posted at the line, and the workers actually used the indicators to manage their daily work. Moreover, these cascaded goals were not simply announced from the top, but developed annually at every level by the manager with their 'direct reports'. The team would start with the deliverables to the next higher level, and every group leader or manager would offer what they were intending to do to reach the goals. If the aggregate result fell short, the team would collectively engage in problem solving until together they had a workable plan to achieve the targets. If investments were needed to achieve the goal, this would at least be seriously considered. Communication goes both up and down from management that sets direction to and from the employees on the front line.

Temporal integration of the plant refers to collaboration with new product development. It has become standard in the best manufacturing organisations that production is represented in product development teams from the beginning. Manufacturing lines are regularly performing prototype runs, which cost capacity in the short run, but help the plant to give input and to learn in the longer run. A superb example is the semi-conductor facility of Thomson, which has become so proficient in testing new equipment and processes that this plant 'ramps them up' and gives them away to other plants once they have been stabilised. Every single production worker is capable of running systematic experiments to find errors and improve yields. Over half of their time is spent on testing and process improvements and yet the plant is highly productive.

Medical equipment producers have begun to apply these lessons by involving hospital staff in the design of machines, in order to ensure the best possible usability and effectiveness. The same lessons hold for the design of operating theatres, birthing rooms and patient wards to facilitate ease of handling and comfort.

Delegation and integration must be supported by four 'enablers'.

1 Communication – is necessary to both establish an open culture and to co-ordinate. That is, to equip empowered employees with the necessary understanding in order to make decisions that are consistent with the overall goals of the plant. This goes beyond posting indicators on boards. It includes an open-door policy, regular information about the overall strategy and situation of the plant, employee satisfaction surveys and open discussion of the work atmosphere. This implies a trustful and constructive collaboration with unions and worker councils – 'you have the worker council you deserve,' observed one plant manager. Information for front line workers must be made concrete and operational rather than conceptual and abstract, but they are nevertheless interested in and capable of understanding the plant challenges and priorities. Hospital studies have shown that openness and trust increases the employees' willingness to contribute their ideas and to enact procedures.[9]

2 Participation – refers to motivating employees to contribute initiatives that go beyond their narrow job descriptions. One plant manager lamented that 'employees who responsibly manage a €50 000 budget in their sports club at home 'turn off their brains' when they enter the locker-room at work'. We observed worker-led machine and process re-design where both the initiative and the project management came from machine operators, who were only supported by an engineer. In the best plants suggestions do not get paid, but workers feel the masters of their own fate and change the face of their workplace because they want to, not because they are paid for a suggestion. In several plants, management put a group of technicians at the workers' disposal, and the workers decided what changes to make to the processes. Hospital processes are, of course, regimented because patient lives are at stake. However, often the staff have deep knowledge of procedural improvements that might improve efficiency and patient comfort at the same time without jeopardising health, knowledge that the doctors do not have. And yet, no change happens because of a strict hierarchy.

3 Employee development – employee initiatives must be supported by knowledge and skills. Employee development refers to continuous training as well as the existence of career paths for employees to advance to broader tasks and responsibility. One consumer goods plant in Germany had the strategy of doubling their output again – after having doubled already – without a head count increase. This happened through automation, with the twist that the workers were not de-skilled, but 'grew' with the increasing technical sophistication of the process. When hiring workers, the plant looked for people with the potential to personally develop higher knowledge, responsibility and breadth of activities. In the best plants, we saw many examples of shift or shop managers who had started as machine operators and worked their way up, with training and support from the plant, to positions of significant managerial responsibility.

4 Measurement – is the systematic tracking of qualitative and quantitative measures of process performance and its 'drivers', providing feedback and the understanding of where to best focus improvements. At Honeywell in Germany for example, workers have on-line access to all process indicators and plan work, maintenance and improvement efforts autonomously based on

them. Mastery of statistical process control is by now quite widely spread for the purpose of process productivity, but Solvay in Laval, France, pushed the method further. When they perceived a small number of tendonitis cases on the line, they applied their problem solving skills to finding the root causes of the injuries, and to eliminate the problem – caused by the ergonomic character of some assembly operations. As a result, tendonitis cases completely disappeared. This improved, above all, workplace quality and as a non-anticipated side-effect, the effort paid for itself within under a year because of reduced sick leave in the plant.

Some healthcare professionals may think that performance indicators (PIs) are not necessary because it is all about saving lives – and the associated physical measurements, such as pulse, blood pressure, body fluid composition and so on – or a nuisance because they are regulated from 'on high'. However, this is erroneous, as many other indicators are useful in giving healthcare staff an understanding of the operational status that determines the quality of service provision. For example: waiting times, time from door to clinical decision, times in intensive care, or as out-patients, quality measures such as post operative problems or repeat hospital visits, equipment use, supply stocks and availabilities. With a better understanding of wider aspects of the operational performance, staff may be able to make better decisions.

Observations about management quality

Over 250 firms in France and Germany have filled out our 10–12 page questionnaire and submitted it to be considered for the Top Factory award. The entrants are typically plants or business units that believe themselves to be effective. An even larger number of firms download the questionnaire in order to do internal 'benchmarking', even if they do not enter. Of the firms that enter each year, the top ten or so receive site visits for validation and clarification of the responses. Of those, the winners and runners-up receive recognition from being awarded a management quality award from academic judges and are also described by articles that are written by media partners, Usine Nouvelle in France, and WirtschaftsWoche in Germany.

> **Editors' note**
>
> See Loch[4] for statistical analysis and Loch[5] for many examples of management quality.

Qualitatively, we observed a number of features:

- the difference from mediocre to world class is management and people, not technology. There is a shift from 'management knows, workers execute' to 'management directs, workers know, manage and improve'
- the old principle 'engineering creates, manufacturing makes, and marketing sells' is obsolete. There is increased interaction at all levels with clients and suppliers

- the principles of 'lean' are widespread – elimination of waste – including the time waiting between activities that actually create value, focussed factories, modular and adaptable processes
- operational excellence is not static, but constantly changing. After three or four years, plants are often largely changed, with new processes and products
- goals are formulated for every department, even support groups, and performance is posted at the line. People at all levels know how what they do influences the business unit's ability to create value
- suggestions do not just get paid with money – important ingredients are recognition and team rewards
- 'open door' policy from management. Everyone in the plant knows what is going on
- operators grow with automation – their knowledge and qualifications grow. There are well defined and utilised career paths
- workers run new processes and new machines on line during production. There is sophisticated proprietary technology
- management quality is applied as a package – it is not enough to pick up one or two 'tools' and to apply them separately. All key processes are improved
- top firms improve year-on-year in key measures. They tend not to remain stagnant until they reach outstanding levels – and then they turn to improvement in other areas.

Management quality trends

We have observed three distinct phases of operational excellence in our study of management quality which have direct implications for healthcare. These phases of industrial excellence are as follows.

1 *Lean excellence.* A decade or more ago – depending upon the industry – a clear competitive advantage could be gained by employing 'lean' principles, such as elimination of excess inventory, set-up times and steps in a manufacturing process that did not add value. 'Tools' like the Toyota production system, TQM and Six Sigma were key. Such ideas remain important today.
2 *Supply chain excellence.* About five to eight years ago, it was no longer sufficient to be 'lean' in order to distinguish one from competitors in many industries. Supply chain collaboration for materials delivery, new product development and a greater emphasis on customer solutions became an increasingly important activity to distinguish outstanding forms from the 'also-rans'. Examples of collaboration include: supplier personnel being present at operations within the organisation, and direct visits and feedback sought from both customers and from end customers.
3 *Strategy excellence.* Over the past two or three years, we have seen an increasing need to achieve consistency and alignment between high level strategy, the key resources, the ability to adapt to competitive forces and the goals of different functional areas as a differentiator. Firms where the R&D department is evaluated on high technical proficiency at any cost and any delay, but where sales and manufacturing are evaluated on the speed of providing new products to market, are not aligned. The strategy deployment and improvement process is becoming more relevant.

Implications for the management of healthcare provision

Discussions of the IEA model have taken place with healthcare managers from a range of professional backgrounds, governmental undersecretaries and healthcare economics academics. These have led to a qualitative understanding of how the IEA model can apply to healthcare.

The phases of excellence

Each of the three main phases of excellence can be found in healthcare: lean excellence, supply chain excellence and strategy excellence.

Lean providers of healthcare use time-based management and TQM 'tools', among others, to streamline care within their facilities. They also use quality improvement 'tools' to enable front line staff to monitor the care processes that they implement in order to improve effectiveness within the facility. An example at the Eastbourne Hospital in East Sussex, UK is an improved use of reminder systems that reduced did-not-attends (DNAs) [10] and the streamlining of service provision arrangements and clinical governance in the orthotics service. This and several other patient-focussed initiatives to sustain and improve patient outcomes improved patient satisfaction and essentially eliminated months-long waiting lists. [11]

Supply chain excellence comes from improved integration across boundaries. An example at the Mid Yorkshire Hospital Trust involves a constraint on bed use for a hospital that discharged a number of patients to social services. [12] Initially, beds were filled to capacity. Some root causes included a sub-optimal triage system that referred too many patients through the A&E area, and poor coordination with social services regarding discharge plans. Solutions included an improved triage plan to route patients to a more appropriate local provider (30% of patients did not need to pass through A&E), and appropriate capacity for much of that demand was available elsewhere and an improved nurse-led discharge planning process from recovery wards. The hospital improved communication with social services to identify appropriate discharge times when social services could accept the patient without logistical choices. These activities required coordinating within the A&E and the Intensive Care Unit with external providers in order to achieve improved patient care across organisational boundaries.

The final phase of excellence is particularly challenging – strategy alignment in the organisation. One example of improved alignment in the hospital context comes from Hôtel-Dieu de France, a university hospital in Beirut, Lebanon. [13] Hospitals in Lebanon have needed to react to crisis situations regularly throughout the past decades of conflict. Hôtel-Dieu de France created and refined disaster plans for managing both massive influxes of patients as well as the risk of a severed supply chain for both medical and food supplies. High level goals for the disaster preparedness plan were set, communicated to manager levels and then to the front lines, with input negotiated up and down the hierarchy at each stage. A 'dummy run' enabled front-line staff to see the effects of the plans, and to continuously improve the ability of the hospital to adapt to urgent situations, while informing high level strategy about organisational capabilities to meet the hospital's strategy for emergency planning.

Part of the challenge at a system level of achieving alignment is the conflicting objectives at different levels of the hierarchy.[14] At a high level, for example, NICE in the UK may provide evidence-based guidance for the cost-effectiveness of a given intervention or technology. At an intermediate level, PCTs may focus more on cost than benefits when making trade-off decisions and at the care delivery level, a clinician may be more focussed on benefits than costs. The press may publicise specific negative outcomes rather than the overall cost and benefit picture. This type of misalignment occurs in many ways due to the many potentially conflicting incentives of the many stakeholders in care. The search for win-win solutions between different units in the same organisation, as well as for public-private partnerships, represents an opportunity for improving sustainable value for patients. This may require a greater emphasis on strategic plans to better define the ways that organisations achieve value for patients, and more effective means for mobilising people around improvement goals. One novel approach is the famous 100,000 Lives Campaign of Institute for Healthcare Improvement.[15] Clear goals with specific timelines, sharing of best practice and engagement can lead to amazing improvements in value for patients.

IEA process enablers

The IEA model has several key processes. The supply chain process can be interpreted in at least two important ways in healthcare.

The first is the flow of patients. 'Mapping' patient pathways, understanding demand levels and managing flow is critical. While 'tools' like process mapping and clinical pathway design are very important, an observation is that information flows to enable action are just as critical as effective management of 'bottleneck' resource steps. For example, bed management is a critical resource and yet information flows between surgical staff and bed managers may be inadequate in some areas. Rationing the portering service might seem penny-wise but may cause havoc for patient flows and opportunity cost losses by preventing other more costly resources from undertaking patient care. Managing patient flows also includes understanding population needs from the community and working to place patients on discharge, whether to their homes or social service settings. Discharge management requires communicating with external partners in this sense, and can have important effects for patient flows. Supply chain measures in manufacturing facilities have direct analogs for patient flows – inventory as the number of patients, the ratio of value-added time to non-value added time maps to patient waiting versus patient care, the percentage on-time delivery directly maps to the fraction of patients that meet national targets in the UK NHS, for example.

A second important supply chain area is the flow of facilitating goods through the healthcare value chain. This includes the flows of consumables, such as drugs, reagents, diagnostic materials and gloves. We have seen process 'maps' and lean principles lead to dramatic reductions of inventory in some cases for pharmaceutical stores that both reduce capital employed and losses due to expiration, while still retaining high levels of availability of key resources.

Innovation is critical to the continued improvement of healthcare. This can be done through new process development and new product development. New process development seeks to identify new ways to deliver care, via managing patient pathways and through ideas for technology improvements to facilitate a smoother process, or more informed and satisfied patients. New product development involves the creation and deployment of new and effective devices, drugs, and protocols. It may be more difficult to separate new process development from new product development in the healthcare context, due to the high level of involvement of the patient in the provision of healthcare services – the product is the process in some real sense.

The observation from the IEA that half of improvements in the effectiveness of leading firms are by re-engineering – top down – and half are by front-line employees appears to be valid here. Bottom-up innovations may include a surgeon adapting a procedure based upon experience, or staff making recommendations to reduce or eliminate operational errors. For example, concerns about hospital work systems that are expressed by the front-line staff that deliver care and create a patient's experience.[9] The authors noted that the two most frequent categories are equipment supplies and infrastructural issues. Those operational failures both frustrate suppliers and can lower the quality and speed of care. It was also noted that such failures are not priorities for national level initiatives to improve care and safety. We note that management quality would enable the mobilisation of employees to make changes that avert such errors – it is not possible to legislate for every possible outcome – local initiative is a must. Mobilised employees are critical to such improvements. It is simply not enough to be satisfied with doing things the same old way, only faster, in order to achieve targets that are imposed from high.

Operations strategy deployment includes the management of tensions between high level clinical and management policy and the day-to-day delivery of quality care. Some of those tensions include issues of focus:

- whether to handle all cases or focus on specific areas of excellence
- trade-offs of time use to make improvements versus getting the job done
- apparent inconsistencies between national level policy and guidance versus local control over health delivery with a finite budget
- the focus of a care giver on an individual patient's outcomes versus overall performance for population health value.

These and other potential conflicts are better resolved when there is a common understanding of the goals of an organisation.

Box 12.1 Useful questions to ask and reflect on when approaching conflicts.

1   What is the goal of this organisation? In a national healthcare system, the desired answer is with respect to the given facility in question, not for the healthcare system as a whole. This improves focus on what the individual unit – hospital, clinic – is trying to achieve for the communities that it serves. For example, general goals like 'save lives' are too aggregated to help an organisation to make good choices. The goal should be specific: is there any focus on diseases/applications, or on

patient segments? Is the goal to give good basic care and diagnoses, and transfer complex cases to specialised facilities? Or is the goal to be leading in some areas, capable of solving the most difficult health problems? Or are education and prevention key goals? Goals at this level of specificity help to guide operational choices and to make visible the trade-offs that need to be struck among multiple goals.

2   How are we measuring progress toward that goal? How do those measures improve through time? Different systems are measured in different ways and for different purposes. The NHS, for example, has an extensive system of measurements and scorecards for evaluating performance on a pre-set range of measures. From an IEA perspective, measures are intended to be metrics that are indicative of progress toward the goal – for example, health outcomes improved for a given budget – rather than as ends to themselves. Each care delivery unit should define measures that it finds useful to gauge progress toward real cost-effective value for patients and not be subservient to national targets.

3   Who uses those measures of effectiveness in order to improve performance?

4   What are the key processes that are required to achieve that goal effectively? This can be thought of broadly speaking, including not only patient flows and compliance measurements, but staff recruitment, training and retention, financial flows, information flows, integration across organisation boundaries with other organisations.

5   How are those process improvements enabled, organisationally?

6   Are the high level goals and the low level process measures aligned with each other?

The answers to these questions and the degree to which individuals at multiple levels in the organisation have a common understanding of those answers, have a number of direct and indirect implications for the dimensions of management quality: measure, delegate, integrate, communicate, participation, and employee development. Sustainable, cost-effective value for patients is not just about medicine, patient safety, hitting national targets, operational optimisation, lean and Six Sigma for clinical procedures and patient maps. It is also about aligning products, processes, suppliers, R&D teams, management, strategy, and the strategy deployment process. It is about improvement through time, by effectively coordinating across the supply chain, across core processes, across the hierarchy of the organisation as well as the selection and inclusion of partners. This can be fostered by effective management practice.

References

1   Edwards N, Marshall M, McLellan A, *et al.* Doctors and managers: a problem without a solution? *British Medical Journal.* 2003; **326**: 609–10.

2   Kennedy I. *Learning from Bristol; the report of the Public Inquiry into Children's Heart Surgery at the Bristol Royal Infirmary 1984-1995* Cm5207-1. Stationery Office; 2001: www.bristol-inquiry.org.uk.

3 House of Commons Health Committee. *The Victoria Climbie Inquiry report.* 2003: www.parliament.the-stationery-office.com/pa/cm200203/cmselect/cmhealth/570/ 570.pdf.

4 Loch CH, Van der Heyden L, Van Wassenhove LN, *et al. Industrial Excellence.* Berlin: Springer; 2003.

5 Loch CH, Chick SE, Huchzermeier A. *Management Quality and Competitiveness: lessons from the Industrial Excellence Award.* Berlin: Springer; 2008.

6 Porter ME, Teisberg EO. *Redefining Health Care: creating value-based competition on results.* Boston, MA: Harvard Business School Press; 2006.

7 Charan R, Tichy NM. *Every Business is a Growth Business.* Chichester: Wiley; 1998.

8 Collins J. *Good to Great – why some companies make the leap and others don't.* New York: Harper Collins; 2001.

9 Tucker AL, Singer SJ, Hayes JE, *et al.* Front-line staff perspectives on opportunities for improving the safety and efficiency of hospital work systems. *Health Systems Research.* 2008; **43(5 Pt2)**: 1807–29.

10 Jones R, Jenkins F. *Key Topics in Healthcare Management – understanding the big picture.* Oxford: Radcliffe Publishing; 2007.

11 Cagna AM, D'Aunno T, Gilmartin M. *Robert Jones and the Eastbourne NHS Orthotics Clinic: make or buy?* INSEAD case; 2006: www.ecch.com.

12 D'Aunno T, Barsoux JL, Gilmartin M, *et al. Leading Organisational Change: improving hospital performance.* INSEAD case; 2006: www.ecch.com.

13 Hourani H, Chick SE. *Hôtel-Dieu de France: the deployment and improvement of a disaster relief plan.* INSEAD case; 2009: www.insead.edu/facultyresearch/research/documents/ Caseupdate2008-2009.pdf.

14 Eddema O, Coast J. Use of economic evaluation in local health care decision-making in England: a qualitative investigation. *Health Econ.* 2010, in press.

15 www.ihi.org/IHI/Programs/Campaign.

Chapter 13

Management Quality in the AHPs Evaluation Matrix

Robert Jones and Fiona Jenkins

Introduction

If quality and excellence are to be at the heart of service provision and the goals which AHP managers strive to achieve for their services, it is essential to be able to measure performance. In order to determine whether we are achieving management quality, it is necessary to establish whether there is alignment between performance, strategy, vision and desired outcomes.

In this chapter, we set out our Management Quality Matrix (MQM) which we have designed for the purpose of evaluating a wide range of performance parameters. The Matrix was developed in the context of management quality and strategy drawing on a range of concepts such as performance management, 'Lean', Six Sigma, Balanced Scorecard, 'Dashboards', TQM and Benefits Realisation. We recommend that the use of IM&T is integral to accurate, timely and relevant measurement for Matrix components, although the evaluation can also be undertaken with paper-based information. Measurement is essential to enable meaningful evaluation to take place. We also draw on the management quality, industrial and healthcare excellence work developed at INSEAD.[1, 2, 3] Also incorporated within the design of the Matrix are ideas from the work of contributors to this book and others in this series[4, 5, 6] together with our own accumulated knowledge, experience and research over many years.

The Matrix, which is set out later in this chapter, comprises fourteen standards each incorporating several components broadly reflecting the six dimensions of management quality:

1 communication
2 participation
3 employee development
4 measurement
5 delegation
6 integration.

The Matrix will enable AHP managers not simply to engage in 'box ticking' exercises, but rather to measure using metrics indicative of progress towards value and responsiveness for patients. The evaluation facilitates best possible clinical outcomes, efficiency, effectiveness and optimal resource use, whilst acknowledging and using national targets, but not merely being subservient to these. Targets are not goals in themselves; value for the patient is the goal. An important objective of using the Matrix is the improvement of performance in all fields of activity within service management; it will enable managers to identify the need to design and implement processes and initiate effective change. The evaluation can be used for performance management as a useful measure to ensure understanding of true performance and as a comparison through time for continuous improvement as well as internal benchmarking. As an external benchmarking process it can be used to draw performance comparison between provider organisations. It may also be used for supporting the management process as an ad hoc service review 'tool' and might also be useful to use in conjunction with our Service Review Assessment of AHP management structures.[4]

Developing strategy and measuring performance, requires participation at all levels. For the achievement of success, actions or activities need to be aligned. It may be helpful to ask ourselves a number of key questions:

- is everyone in the team 'pulling' in the same direction?
- does the direction benefit the patient?
- are there base-line measures?
- are we measuring so that we know whether we are improving or not?
- do staff have the training and motivation to provide value and bring about improvement?
- are tensions around fear of change recognised and managed?
- are problems/mistakes treated as opportunities to improve?

Our Matrix is not only an annual measurement assessment; it can be used to support management quality development throughout the year, assessing progress in strategy and operational developments.

It is not our purpose here to discuss management theories in detail, but an overview of some key definitions and concepts are outlined in order to place the Matrix in context.

Metrics

The term 'metrics' relates to standards of measurement through which efficiency, performance, progress, quality of a process, plan or product is assessed. Examples of these measures, or 'metrics', include indicators, targets, and benchmarks of performance.

Key performance indicators (KPIs)

A KPI is a tool for service improvement, focusing upon significant measurements that indicate degree of success or lack of achievement. A KPI is a composite of:

- a measure of the performance against specific goals or objectives
- a target (or targets)
- an action resulting from the measurement.

Business performance management (BPM)

BPM consist a set of management and analytical processes supported by IM&T and paper systems that enables services to define strategic goals and then measure and manage performance. Core BPM processes include, for example: clinical activity and financial performance; operational planning; reporting; modelling; monitoring of key performance indicators; clinical governance; and human resources. BPM involves consolidation of data from various sources, analysis of the data and putting the learning into practice. It enhances processes by creating better feedback loops and can help to identify and eliminate problems.

Lean thinking

'Lean' was developed by Toyota, becoming integral to their industrial engineering processes. The overall objective is to eliminate non-value added waste to reduce process cycle times, improve delivery performance and reduce costs. This approach is adopted with the objective of improving flow; it is about getting the right things to the right places at the right time, in the right quantities.[7] In the context of healthcare, 'Lean' facilitates patient focussed service provision and is intended to help the patient through adding value. It is designed to eliminate the root causes of non value-added activities such as patients waiting between activities during care.

In eliminating waste, quality improves and at the same time overall activity time decreases and consequently costs decrease. A further objective is to improve patient flow or 'smoothness' of work eliminating unevenness in the pathway, not only waste.

> Lean brings into many industries, including healthcare, new concepts, tools and methods that have been effectively utilised to improve process flow. Tools that address workplace organisation, standardisation, visual control and elimination of non value-added steps are applied to improve flow, eliminate waste and exceed patient expectation.[8]

In order to eliminate waste and ensure evenness of process, the phases or steps in it must be examined to make the process visible so that waste or unevenness is highlighted and can be rectified. Questions might include those in Box 13.1.

Box 13.1 Questions to ask to eliminate waste.

1 Are the steps within the process clear or are parts difficult to identify?
2 Are responsibilities clear for each individual and for teams?
3 Who carries overall responsibility for the entire process?
4 Are there unnecessary phases in the process?
5 Are the right facilities or consumables available when required?
6 Are the processes 'joined-up'?
7 Are the measures and targets appropriate and relevant to the process?
8 Do problems continually recur and need 'fixing' or is appropriate time taken out to 'fix' the system for once and all?
9 Are there gaps, duplications or bottle necks in the service?

It may be useful to adopt the well tested management technique of '5 whys' – asking 'why' five times as in root cause analysis.[9]

The following example demonstrates the basic process.

Patients have long waits for treatment (the problem).

1 *Why?* Not enough treatment slots available (first why).
2 *Why?* Mismatch between new and follow up appointment slots (second why).
3 *Why?* Capacity and Demand has not been modelled (third why).
4 *Why?* Booking process not fully understood or process mapped (fourth why).
5 *Why?* Lacking service improvement and innovative skills in the service (fifth why, a root cause).

The NHI Productive Series[10] supports NHS teams to redesign and streamline the way they manage and work. This aims to achieve significant and lasting improvements predominately in the extra time that they give to patients, as well as improving the quality of care delivered whilst reducing costs.

In a recent survey undertaken by NHSI[10] significant areas of time wasting in management were identified, for example:

- on average leaders spend only 7.5% of time on planning, reflecting and thinking
- of the average 54 hour week worked by an NHS manager, 38 hours were spent in meetings
- of the 26 meetings attended only seven started on time
- only 36% of attendees actively participated in the meetings.

Six Sigma

The fundamental purpose of Six Sigma is the implementation of a measurement-based strategy that focuses on process improvement and variation reduction. The technique was developed for quality engineering using statistical techniques to facilitate understanding, measure and reduce process variation with the goal of improving service quality and cost. The methodology adopts the use of structured techniques to reduce defects. Technically, Six Sigma is a disciplined, data driven approach and methodology for eliminating defects '(driving towards six standard deviations between the mean and the nearest specification limit) in any process'.[11] The word 'sigma' is a statistical term that measures how far a particular process deviates from perfection. A crucial idea behind Six Sigma is that the number of defects in a process is measured in order that they can be eliminated in a systematic way aiming to be as close as possible to 'zero defects' in the process.

The concept of Six Sigma is applicable in healthcare. The DMAIC process (Define, Measure, Analyse, Improve and Control – which is consistent with evidence-based healthcare practice – is an improvement system[11] for existing processes falling below specification and looking for incremental improvement.

Box 13.2 Six Sigma DMAIC process.

- *Define* – process improvement goals that are consistent with patient requirements and the enterprise strategy
- *Measure* – key aspects of the current process and collect relevant data

> - *Analyse* – the data to verify cause and effect relationships; determine what the relationships are and attempt to ensure that all factors have been considered
> - *Improve* – or optimise the process based on data analysis
> - *Control* – to ensure that any deviations from target are corrected before they result in defects; set up pilot runs to establish process capability, set up control mechanisms and continually monitor the process

On the other hand, the Six Sigma DMADV (Define, Measure, Analyse, Design, Verify) process is an improvement system used to develop new processes, or services, or pathways, for example.

Total quality management

TQM is also a Japanese inspired concept, it is an approach centred on improved organisational performance and effectiveness. Deming[12, 13] emphasised the importance of visionary leadership and the responsibility of senior management for initiating change. One of Deming's 14 principles was to eliminate slogans as he argued the importance of doing the right things first time. He focussed on the importance of good management including the human side of quality improvement and how employees should be treated. This is an approach centred on quality, based on the participation of an organisation's staff and aiming at long term success. The 'total' in TQM applies to the organisation or service as a whole; it applies to all of the activities also including culture, ethics and attitude.

> TQM is far wider in its application than just assuring product or service quality – it is a way of managing people and business processes to ensure complete customer satisfaction at every stage, internally and externally. TQM, combined with effective leadership, results in an organisation doing the right things right first time.[14]

Pentecost[15] identified key elements of TQM which can be adapted for healthcare services as shown in Box 13.3.

Box 13.3 Key elements of TQM.

1 A total process – involving all management units in the organisation, and led from the top
2 The patient is 'king' with every strategy, process and action directly related to satisfying customers' needs
3 A greater emphasis on rational information collection and analysis
4 Emphasis on a different approach to looking at the costs of poor quality by examining all processes that add to costs
5 A greater involvement of staff, recognising that they are a great untapped resource
6 Team work – involving multi-disciplinary and multi-level working in problem solving and to meet patients' needs
7 The requirements of creative thinking and the ability to think beyond the immediate job or working environment

Other authors add leadership as a key principle as leaders establish unity of purpose, direction and the internal environment of the service creating the environment in which all staff can become involved in achieving the service objectives.

Benefits realisation

This approach is the identification of target benefits, their definition, planning, structuring and realisation resulting from investing in change. Projects, service changes and service re-design are undertaken to deliver benefits for service users. However, the majority of projects and programmes are criticised for failing to achieve the predicted objectives or benefits. There are a number of possible reasons for this including, for example:

- business cases being focused on financial targets rather than being expressed in terms of the benefits that can be understood and implemented
- too much emphasis on outcomes which on their own do not provide specific benefits
- no mechanisms or structures to manage the realisation of benefits.

It is very important to identify clear benefits that relate to unambiguous service objectives and to assign ownership to the people responsible for ensuring and managing their achievement.

> The challenge for organisations is in identifying clear benefits, assigning ownership, determining how they can be measured and then making sure how they can be delivered. Benefit planning, management and realisation sets out to bring structure, accountability and discipline to the delivery of the benefits inherent in projects.[15]

Important aspects of this approach are:

- the way objectives and benefits are expressed and structured
- differentiating between objectives, outcomes, benefits and also financial results
- the whole planning and management of the process.

Clinical dashboard

High quality information is an important element in the facilitation of good performance amongst clinical and management teams and helps to promote that the right services and best care are provided. A 'dashboard' is a 'tool set' of visual displays specifically designed to provide relevant and timely information to inform decision-making. Dashboards provide data captured in a visual and useable format. It may display local information alongside the relevant national metrics.

The development of clinical dashboards was a key recommendation for 'The Next Stage Review'.[16]

Box 13.4 Five major features of clinical dashboards.[17]

1 Provide better information for clinical teams presented in easy to understand formats, with high visual impact

> 2 Utilise multiple sources of existing data
> 3 Provide information relevant across multi-disciplinary teams
> 4 Information provided in 'real' time with no delay for data cleansing
> 5 Allows configuration to local requirements and comparison against national data sets

NHS information sets and initiatives are complimented by clinical dashboards by providing locally required indicators configured to local needs, supporting clinical teams to deliver faster, improved and safer quality of care. Clinical dashboards are widely adapted for management purposes.

Balanced scorecard

Balanced scorecards are strategic planning and management 'tools' used in many types of organisations worldwide, including healthcare, to align business activities to the vision and strategy of the organisation, improve internal and external communications and monitor organisational performance against strategic goals. The balanced scorecard approach was developed by Kaplan and Norton as a performance measurement framework that added strategic, customer focussed and learning measures as non-financial performance measures to traditional financial metrics to give managers a more balanced view of organisational performance.[18] The balanced scorecard provides a framework for the provision of performance measurement and supports managers to identify what should be done and measured. This methodology is designed for the purpose of transforming the service strategic plan into action.

> **Box 13.5 Reasons for implementing the balanced scorecard approach.**
>
> • Increased focus on strategy and results
> • Measuring what matters to improve performance
> • Align organisational strategy with the work people do day to day
> • Focus on the drivers for future performance
> • Improve communication of the service vision and strategy
> • Prioritise projects and initiatives

The balanced scorecard suggests that we view the organisation from four perspectives, and to develop metrics, collect data and analyse it relative to each of these perspectives. [18]

The four perspectives of balanced scorecards are:

1 learning and growth
2 the business process perspective
3 the service user perspective
4 financial perspective.

In healthcare settings, there is a growing consensus that financial indicators alone are not an adequate measure of performance and that a broader view is needed. The balanced scorecard approach is increasingly used in healthcare organisations as a means of improving performance. The NHS has a very difficult task of fulfilling a wide range of different and complex objective due to the scope and diversity of the service; the balanced scorecard can be used to support in formal recognition and measurement of objectives.

AHP Management Quality Evaluation Matrix

Frameworks for strategy must incorporate the vision, objectives and policies of AHP services setting out the purpose, plans and actions for implementation. Without explicit strategy it will be difficult for AHP services to co-ordinate action and measure performance. To achieve the benefits of 'joined up' working it is necessary for people to collaborate and the absence of explicit strategy will result in staff working at cross-purposes. Strategy must be communicated clearly to enable corporate understanding and 'ownership' at all levels. This requires operational activity to be put in place so that performance can be measured and appropriate learning, change and subsequent action be put in place as necessary.

To succeed, AHP services need structured, strategic frameworks to provide starting points for progress and a means for assessment and evaluation. Our Management Quality Evaluation Matrix is based on AHP strategy and is intended to enable AHP managers to be explicit about their service strategies, facilitating measurement of performance in respect of service provision, activity, processes, people, resources and systems.

Our Evaluation Matrix is designed to enable AHP managers to measure performance; if performance is not measured, it is not managed. An important objective is to enable managers to work towards improving the overall effectiveness, efficiency, responsiveness – in short – the overall quality of services. The Evaluation Matrix is used to evaluate performance against standards on a forward-looking basis so that variances are detected and appropriate actions taken. The Matrix incorporates 14 key Standards for managing AHP services, each being sub-divided into components which make up specific management quality sections within it.

Box 13.6 The 14 AHP Management Quality Standards.

 1 Strategy
 2 Activity
 3 Patient and service user experience
 4 Finance
 5 Staff resource effectiveness
 6 Staff management and development
 7 Information and metrics
 8 Leadership and management development
 9 Clinical excellence
10 Communications and marketing
11 Service improvement and re-design
12 Risk management
13 Corporate governance
14 Key performance indicators

The evaluation of each component has been designed to give information that is easy to interpret. A number of methods are used for evaluating components, for example: Yes/No, percentage achievement or requiring data or text. It may be appropriate to include graphs and bar charts in some places. There is space in the Matrix for comments to be recorded. Each Standard requires a summary and action planning by the AHP manager, when reviewing the management quality of their service.

The evaluation gives an overview of the strengths and weaknesses of the service and where there may be opportunity for improvement and development. When completed, it will also contain valuable data on activity and financial performance.

The Matrix can be used for unidisciplinary AHP services or multiple services where these are managed collectively. When assessing multiple AHP services each profession **should be evaluated separately**.

An important objective of the evaluation is to give guidance and to help focus attention on the service. It is not intended that each and every strategy and component be fully achieved at first, although some managers may be successful in the majority of components within each standard. It may be helpful to focus on one standard at a time, gradually developing the matrix over a period.

In this way the matrix can be used to guide management quality development in AHP services. The matrix can also be used as an aid to the management process as a prompt to instigating work and projects on management quality throughout the service and as an easy source for information retrieval to be used on an ongoing basis.

Standard 1 strategy

The service has a documented strategy which is reviewed and updated annually.

Component	Evaluation		Comment
1.1 Organisational strategy; does your organisation have a strategy?	YES	NO	
1.2 Do you have an up-to-date strategy for your service, written in a business plan? • Is this aligned to the organisational strategy?	YES	NO	
1.3 Is there a 'value statement' that is shared by staff in your service?	YES	NO	
1.4 Service mission statement/vision; is this agreed and documented and up to date?	YES	NO	
1.5 Is your strategy linked to: • National strategies? • Regional strategies? • Local strategies?	YES	NO	
1.6 Service portfolio – the range of services you provide and have responsibility for; is this documented?	YES	NO	
1.7 Major goals/objectives for your service; are these documented?	YES	NO	

Component	Evaluation		Comment
1.8 Do you have service strategies, for example: • Education and training? • Information management and technology? • Marketing? • Clinical governance? • Patient and public involvement? • Elimination of waste (LEAN)? • Quality? • Service improvement?	YES	NO	
1.9 Is the overall contribution of your service (from the patients' perspective) documented?	YES	NO	
1.10 Do you undertake an annual service review, and document findings?	YES	NO	
1.11 Do you have organisational charts for your service illustrating your structure, governance and management team?	YES	NO	
1.12 Do you produce a service annual report outlining for example: • Key achievements against, e.g. target, benchmarks? • Aspirations for continuing service improvement/development? • Activity analysis? • Finance report? • Key performance indicators and performance? • Quality? • Human resource report? • Marketing strategy? • Clinical governance report?	YES	NO	
Standard summary and action:			

Standard 2 activity

Activity is reviewed and analysed on a monthly and annual basis for performance management, and for projections for the coming year.

Component	Sub-component	Total		Comment
2.1 All staff record activity data on the same day that the activity is performed.		YES	NO	
2.2 Total service throughput last Financial Year-defined by total referrals, new patients and total attendances?	Total Referrals			
	New Patients			
	Total Attendances			
2.3 What was your New to Follow-up ratio last financial year for each service? (name each service)	1.			
	2.			
	3.			
	4.			
	5.			
2.4 Do you analyse your re-referral rate and use this for service planning?		YES	NO	

Component	Sub-component	Total		Comment
2.5 What is your anticipated (planned) total service throughput for the next financial year?	New Patients			
	Total Attendances			
2.6 What are your out-patient Referral To Treatment times for each service? (name each service)	1.			
	2.			
	3.			
	4.			
	5.			
2.7 Are you able to report RTT (Referral to Treatment Time) for all patients referred?		YES	NO	
2.8 What are your Service DNA (Did Not Attend) percentage rates? (name each service)	1.	%		
	2.	%		
	3.	%		
	4.	%		
	5.	%		
2.9 Do you have a Demand and Capacity management plan in place?		YES	NO	
2.10 Do you analyse your staff activity time, to review the time allocation between patient contact time, patient related activity and non patient related activity?		YES	NO	
2.11 What is your service standard response time for in-patient service provision(name each service)	1. 2. 3. 4. 5.			
2.12 Illustrate your Referral Trend to your whole service during last five years. (Insert a graph/bar chart with this information)				
2.13 Illustrate your capacity plan projection for next year. (Insert a graph/bar chart with this information)				
2.14 Illustrate your Did Not Attend trend to your whole service during last five years. (Insert a graph/bar chart with this information)				
Standard summary and action:				

Standard 3 patient and service user experience

Patients' views and experiences are actively sought and incorporated into service re-design.

Component	Evaluation		Comment
3.1 Does your service use patient survey data to benchmark its services to patients?	YES	NO	
3.2 Do you actively encourage views from patients about services provided: • How is this done, e.g. surveys, focus groups?	YES	NO	

Component	Evaluation		Comment
3.3 Do you involve service users in service re-design? • Give examples	YES	NO	
3.4 Are plaudits monitored within your service and action plans put in place as appropriate? Detail how learning is disseminated	YES	NO	
3.5 Are complaints monitored within your service and action plans put in place as appropriate?	YES	NO	
3.6 Do all staff collect patient outcome data?		%	
3.7 Do staff collect and report Patient Reported Outcome Measures (PROMS)	YES	NO	
3.8 Is patient outcome data analysed?		%	
3.9 Do you have a procedure for offering patient chaperones?			
3.10 Do you actively involve patients in informed decision-making about their care?	YES	NO	
3.11 Do you have agreed, evidence-based, protocols and pathways in use?	YES	NO	
3.12 Is there a mechanism in place to ensure compliance with NICE (National Institute for Health and Clinical Excellence) Guidelines?	YES	NO	
3.13 Do you undertake environment audits in patient treatment areas?	YES	NO	
3.14 Does you service have a quality monitoring programme for the production and review of patient information leaflets?	YES	NO	
3.15 Do you have a web site that the public can access information about your services?	YES	NO	
3.16 Do you monitor out-patient waiting times, and put action plans in place as necessary?	YES	NO	
3.17 Do you monitor community waiting times, and put action plans in place as necessary?	YES	NO	
3.18 Do you monitor in-patient waiting times, and put action plans in place as necessary?	YES	NO	
Standard summary and action:			

Standard 4 finance

There is comprehensive monitoring and knowledge of the service finances within your management teams and the service is financially viable.

Component	Evaluation		Comment
4.1 Are you the budget holder for your service and responsible for budget management?	YES	NO	
4.2 Do you have monthly budget statements that you analyse?	YES	NO	
4.3 Do you have monthly meetings with your finance team?	YES	NO	

Component	Evaluation		Comment
4.4 Do you monitor your financial performance on at least a monthly basis?	YES	NO	
4.5 If 'yes' to 4.4 what monitoring method do you use? • Monthly budget monitoring? • Monitoring of pay? • Monitoring of non-pay? • Monitoring of income? • Only variance monitoring?	YES	NO	
4.6 Do you have controls in place regarding authorisation of purchases?	YES	NO	
4.7 What is your annual budget? • Pay costs • Non-pay costs • Income			
4.8 Overspend/under spend position last financial year?			
4.9 Reasons for over/under spend?			
4.10 Do you have income generation projects?	YES	NO	
4.11 What type of contracts do you have? for example: • Block contract? • Cost per case? • Cost per contact? • Cost and volume?			
4.12 What is your income from Service Level Agreements?			
4.13 What is your annual income from external contracts?			
4.14 What is your annual income from voluntary organisations?			
4.15 What is your annual income from hiring out facilities/equipment?			
4.16 Do you have income identified from Payment by Results?			
4.17 Do you have income identified from Practice Based Commissioning?			
4.18 Are your service costs identifiable by • Service line reporting?	YES	NO	
4.19 What are your reference costs and how do these relate to the national picture?			
4.20 What is your Earnings before Interest, Taxes, Depreciation, and Amortisation EBITDA?			
4.21 Do you have an inventory of equipment for your service documented?			
4.22 Do you have materials management programmes in place?			
4.23 Are you required to implement cost improvement programmes and Cash Releasing Efficiency Savings. What programmes do you have in place for meeting these?			
4.24 Does your service have Charitable Trust funds with monitoring in place?			
Standard summary:	**Action:**		

Standard 5 staff resources

There is a comprehensive knowledge and understanding of the staff resources used by the service and they are deployed effectively and reviewed frequently.

Component	Evaluation		Comment
5.1 What is the head count of your AHP staff group?			
5.2 What is the Whole Time Equivalent grade profile of each of your AHP staff groups: • Band 2 • Band 3 • Band 4 • Band 5 • Band 6 • Band 7 • Band 8a • Band 8b • Band 8c • Band 8d • Band 9	WTE WTE WTE WTE WTE WTE WTE WTE WTE WTE WTE		
5.3 What is your ratio of registered to non-registered staff	:		
5.4 What is your service annual staff turnover?	%		
5.5 How do your turnover figures compare with the: • National average for your service • Your organisation average? (you may wish to include a graph)	+/− % +/− %		
5.6 What is your annual percentage absence through: • Sickness • Maternity leave • Study leave • Other authorised paid leave • Unpaid leave How does this compare with your organisation as a whole? • Sickness • Maternity leave • Study leave • Other authorised paid leave • Unpaid leave	% % % % % +/− % % % % %		
5.7 Staff Activity – what is the aggregate percentage staff time spent on: • Patient-related activity • Non patient-related activity	% %		
5.8 Does the expertise in your service attract referrals from beyond your normal catchment?	YES	NO	
5.9 Does the service have sufficient expertise to provide comprehensive in-service education/training?	YES	NO	
5.10 Does the service undertake succession planning?	YES	NO	
5.11 Does every member of staff have an up-to-date job description and Knowledge and Skills Framework (KSF)?	YES	NO	
5.12 Do you review each post when it becomes vacant?	YES	NO	
5.13 Do you have a strategy in place to eliminate waste in staff deployment?	YES	NO	
Standard summary:	**Action:**		

Standard 6 staff management, education and development

Staff are managed, supported and developed to meet clinical, organisational and professional requirements.

Component	Evaluation		Comment
6.1 What is your service staffing establishment in Whole Time Equivalent?		WTE	
6.2 Have you benchmarked your staffing establishment against similar organisations?	YES	NO	
6.3 If you have benchmarked how do you compare? (detail in the comments box)			
6.4 What is the ratio between HPC Registered AHP staff to assistants?	:		
6.5 What is the ratio between HPC Registered AHP staff to clerical staffing?	:		
6.6 What is your service percentage compliance with mandatory training attendance requirements?		%	
6.7 What is your service percentage compliance for undertaking Annual Development Reviews (Appraisal)?		%	
6.8 Is your staff HPC Registration checked annually for compliance?	YES	NO	
6.9 Are the numbers of staff grievances/disciplinary investigations monitored on an on-going basis?	YES	NO	
6.10 Are complaints and plaudits about staff monitored and action plans put in place?	YES	NO	
6.11 Is there a monitoring procedure in place for staff competence?	YES	NO	
6.12 Is there a staff education and training policy in place?	YES	NO	
6.13 Is a record of all staff training and education kept and regularly up-dated?	YES	NO	
6.14 Is there a mechanism in place for clinical supervision? How often does it happen?	YES	NO	
6.15 Do you have a mentorship or coaching scheme in place	YES	NO	
6.16 Does your service have Clinical Specialists?	YES	NO	
6.17 Does your service have Extended Scope Practitioners?	YES	NO	
6.18 Does your service have Consultant AHP posts?	YES	NO	
6.19 Do you have a preceptorship scheme in place for your newly qualified staff?	YES	NO	
6.20 Do you have a study leave policy?	YES	NO	
6.21 Does the service take AHP students? Are there established links with the higher education institution(s)?	YES	NO	
Standard summary:	**Action:**		

Standard 7 information and metrics

The service gathers timely, accurate and relevant data as a by-product of clinical activity. Appropriate metrics are used for clinical and managerial purposes.

Component	Evaluation		Comment
7.1 Does your service have a data collection system which is fit for purpose?	YES	NO	
7.2 Does your service have a computerised data collection system fit for purpose?	YES	NO	
7.3 Do clinicians input data at the same time that treatment takes place (real time)?	YES	NO	
7.4 Is your information system capable of providing accurate, timely, relevant reports?	YES	NO	
7.5 Do you have full data on contact and relevant details relating to patients referred to you, including: • Name • NHS number • Demographic data • Disability • Ethnic origin • Gender • Telephone • Diagnosis • Reason for referral • Referrer • Source of referral • Intervention • Equipment or appliances issued • Referral date • 1st attendance date • Discharge date • Discharge destination • Date of discharge letter • Number of contacts • Clinician • Clinical outcome	YES	NO	
7.6 Are you able to report Referral to Treatment Time for all referrals received?	YES	NO	
7.7 Do you collect and use data for Clinical Audit?	YES	NO	
7.8 Do you collect and use data for staff activity analysis?	YES	NO	
7.9 Do you collect and use data for staff case load analysis?	YES	NO	
7.10 Do you have Information about groups of service users, e.g. Voluntary organisations?	YES	NO	
7.11 Do you collect and analyse patient outcome data for all patients?	%		
7.12 Where there are gaps in metrics, are you developing ways to measure the quality of services?	YES	NO	
7.13 Do your clinical staff input the data?	YES	NO	
7.14 Do your clerical staff input data? – are there gaps or duplication in the data	YES	NO	
7.15 Do you have an agreed and updated protocol for data sharing?	YES	NO	
Standard summary:	**Action:**		

Standard 8 leadership and management development

The service has effective leadership and management arrangements in place at all levels.

Component	Evaluation		Comment
8.1 Does the organisational structure support effective leadership and management?	YES	NO	
8.2 Is leadership and management development included in personal development plans?	YES	NO	
8.3 Is there a leadership/management development programme in place for your staff?	YES	NO	
8.4 What percentage of staff in leadership/management positions have undertaken this training?	%		
8.5 Does your service have access to leadership development programmes at: • Local level? • Regional level? • National level? • International level?	YES	NO	
8.6 Can you identify projects within or on behalf of your organisation which your service had led during the last year? (list)	1. 2. 3. 4. 5.		
8.7 Have you identified projects within your organisation which your service will be leading during the next year? (list)	1. 2. 3. 4. 5.		
8.8 Do you have staff members involved in work at national level with Professional Bodies/Regulators?	YES	NO	
8.9 Do you have identified clinical leads in place to lead and develop in specialist areas?	YES	NO	
8.10 What percentage of staff in management positions have undertaken management training?	%		
8.11 Are you responsible for the recruitment of staff to leadership and management positions within your service?	YES	NO	
8.12 Are you responsible and accountable for performance management of your service?	YES	NO	
8.13 Are you a member of, or have access to, the management committees/Boards within your organisation	YES	NO	
8.14 Do you have networks at: • Local level? • Regional level? • National level? • International level?	YES	NO	
8.15 Do you work with service commissioners?	YES	NO	
Standard summary:	**Action:**		

Standard 9 clinical excellence

The service demonstrates procedures and practices to ensure high quality patient care.

Component	Evaluation		Comment
9.1 Does your service have representation on the organisation's: • Senior clinicians committee? • Clinical Governance committee? • Audit committee? • Research and Development committee? • Patient and Public Involvement committee?	YES	NO	
9.2 Are there regular clinical governance review meetings within your service and appropriate action plans put in place?	YES	NO	
9.3 Are there arrangements in place for clinical audits?	YES	NO	
9.4 Is the requirement to undertake clinical audit included in staff job descriptions?	YES	NO	
9.5 Is there a mechanism for reporting results and implementing the recommendations from clinical audit?	YES	NO	
9.6 Do you have staff undertaking Research and Development projects? If so, list current projects.	1.		
	2.		
	3.		
	4.		
	5.		
9.7 Is there a mechanism for disseminating research findings within your service?	YES	NO	
9.8 Do you have mechanisms in place to ensure the provision of evidence-based practice, for example: • Staff appraisal and personal development plans • In-service education and training • Access to Continued Professional Development • Peer review • Staff access to the internet • Staff access to library facilities/journals • Journal review sessions • Participation in professional networks • Active links with Higher Education Institutions • Staff undertaking higher degrees • Clinical Supervision • Mentoring	YES	NO	
9.9 Is there a staff education and training policy in place?	YES	NO	
9.10 Do you have standards for clinical record keeping?	YES	NO	
9.11 Are your clinical records monitored regularly against a set standard?	YES	NO	
9.12 Do you have procedures in place for obtaining and recording informed patient consent?	YES	NO	
9.13 Do you have mechanisms in place for obtaining patient feedback on service quality?	YES	NO	
9.14 Are lessons learned from feedback incorporated into practice? What is the evidence?	YES	NO	

Component	Evaluation		Comment
9.15 Has your service established procedures for developing and implementing? • Clinical guidelines • NICE guidelines • Care pathways • Guidelines • Protocols	YES	NO	
9.16 Do you provide services that contribute to the public health agenda, regarding self-management and prevention? Such as: • Obesity management • Healthy lifestyles/exercise	YES	NO	
9.17 Have you developed staff with extended scope skills? Such as: • Supplementary prescribing • Injection therapy • Podiatric surgery • Radiographic reading and interpretation • Endoscopic techniques	YES	NO	
9.18 Do you monitor staff use of clinical outcome measures?	YES	NO	
9.19 Do you monitor the ratio of 1st to Follow up appointments for out-patients?	YES	NO	
Standard summary:	**Action:**		

Standard 10 communication and marketing

The service has effective internal and external communication processes and well developed links to ensure service marketing.

Component	Evaluation		Comment
10.1 Is there a communication mechanism within your service to keep staff informed and involved?	YES	NO	
10.2 Do you have: • A communication strategy for your service? • A marketing strategy for your service?	YES	NO	
10.3 Have you undertaken a SWOT analysis for your services and developed an action plan?	YES	NO	
10.4 Have you undertaken a PEST analysis for your service and developed an action plan?	YES	NO	
10.5 Do you have an overview of the population served by your service?	YES	NO	
10.6 Is a summary of the 'target' population(s) (Market Segment) for your service documented?	YES	NO	
10.7 Have you developed a service specification for your service?	YES	NO	

Component	Evaluation		Comment
10.8 Do you have a web site for your service? Including, for example: • Locations • Opening times • Facilities • Key managers' contact details • How to contact the service • Referral to service • Service exclusions • Patient information leaflets • Self referral information • Key policies • Expertise available	YES	NO	
10.9 Have you comprehensive and up-to-date leaflets for service users?	YES	NO	
10.10 Have you comprehensive and up-to-date leaflets for referrers?	YES	NO	
10.11 Do you meet multi-cultural requirements in the form of: • Leaflets in different languages • Leaflets in different media, e.g. large print • Access to interpreters • Access to signers for the deaf	YES	NO	
10.12 Have you review dates for updating policies and leaflets?	YES	NO	
10.13 Have you developed links with local media to inform the public about your service?	YES	NO	
10.14 Do you have links and have you developed information about your service for voluntary organisations?	YES	NO	
10.15 Have you undertaken a competitor analysis including identification of possible competitive advantages your service has over other providers or vice versa?	YES	NO	
10.16 Specify the resources that give your service a competitive advantage: • Core competencies • Key assets • Core or critical processes such as pathways	**Please detail:**		
10.17 What are the major types of uncertainty: • Uncertain demand? • Uncertain staff availability? • Uncertainty of funding streams? • Competitor actions? • Technology/treatment changes?	**Please detail:**		
10.18 Have you undertaken a stakeholder views analysis? • Internal • External	YES	NO	
10.19 Have you undertaken an analysis of predicted technological advances? For example: • changes in treatment techniques • changes in equipment • IM&T support	YES	NO	

Component	Evaluation		Comment
10.20 Have you undertaken an analysis of predicted changes in population and made an assessment of possible future demand?	YES	NO	
10.21 Have you established what future commissioner purchasing intentions are?	YES	NO	
10.22 Have you established projected future demand from within your own organisation?	YES	NO	
10.23 Do you analysed service user feedback including complaints and plaudits?	YES	NO	
10.24 Have you analysed the impact of policy on future service provision? • National • Regional • Your organisation	YES	NO	
10.25 Are mechanisms in place for teams to communicate across functional boundaries?	YES	NO	
10.26 Have you developed business cases for service developments, improvements, re-design, in light of your market assessment and other relevant factors?	YES	NO	
Standard summary:	Action:		

Standard 11 service improvement and re-design

Your service actively undertakes re-design and service improvement.

Component	Evaluation		Comment
11.1 Does your service have representation on your organisation's strategic service improvement group or equivalent?	YES	NO	
11.2 Is service improvement embedded in staff job descriptions?	YES	NO	
11.3 Has your service undertaken re-design projects in last financial year? List:	YES	NO	
1.			
2.			
3.			
4.			
5.			
11.4 Does your service have re-design projects in progress during the current financial year? List:	YES	NO	
1.			
2.			
3.			
4.			
5.			

Component	Evaluation		Comment
11.5 Is your service involved in multidisciplinary service improvement projects? List:	YES	NO	
1.			
2.			
3.			
4.			
5.			
11.6 Have you undertaken 'horizon scanning' of other services (internal/external) to inform your service improvement needs?	YES	NO	
11.7 Has your service been recognised at Local, Regional or National level for innovative service improvement?	YES	NO	
11.8 Do you receive requests from other services to visit your department?	YES	NO	
11.9 Are all levels of staff involved in the service re-design initiatives?	YES	NO	
11.10 Do you have user involvement in service re-design?	YES	NO	
11.11 Do you evaluate service improvement initiatives as part of a continuous cycle of improvement?	YES	NO	
11.12 Do you use process mapping as a service improvement tool?	YES	NO	
11.13 Do you have staff trained with service improvement techniques to undertake service re-design?	YES	NO	
11.14 Do you have staff trained with project management skills to undertake service re-design?	YES	NO	
Standard summary:	**Action:**		

Standard 12 risk management

Risk is measured, evaluated and managed effectively with action plans put in place.

Component	Evaluation		Comment
12.1 Does your service maintain an on-going, up-to-date Risk Register including action logs?	YES	NO	
12.2 Does your service Risk Register input to the organisation's Risk Register?	YES	NO	
12.3 Does your service undertake on-going infection control risk assessments and action logs?	YES	NO	
12.4 Does your service maintain an on-going, up-to-date register of serious untoward incidents and 'near misses', with action plans in place?	YES	NO	
12.5 Is your service included in the organisation's major incident planning?	YES	NO	
12.6 Does your service undertake litigation audits and have action plans?	YES	NO	

Component	Evaluation		Comment
12.7 Is there a mechanism in place for ensuring that National Patient Safety Alerts are communicated throughout the teams and action plans put in place?	YES	NO	
12.8 Is there a mechanism for communicating and acting on National, Regional and Local reports? How are these reports accessed and discussed?	YES	NO	
12.9 Are legal claims monitored and reviewed within your service?	YES	NO	
12.10 Is there a named lead for Risk Management for each location within your service?	YES	NO	
12.11 Are Health and Safety assessments undertaken on an on-going basis?	YES	NO	
12.12 Does your service have a named fire officer?	YES	NO	
12.13 Does your service have a mandatory programme with staff attendance monitored?	YES	NO	
12.14 Is training in Risk Management undertaken by your staff?	YES	NO	
12.15 List the major sources of uncertainty for the service – have you a plan in place to manage each one:	YES	NO	
1.			
2			
3.			
4.			
Standard summary:	**Action:**		

Standard 13 corporate governance

The service is compliant with the rules, processes and laws within which your organisation is required to operate and is regulated.

Component	Evaluation		Comment
13.1 Are you aware of and compliant with the 'Nolan' principles of conduct in public life: • Selflessness • Integrity • Objectivity • Accountability • Openness • Honesty • Leadership	YES	NO	
13.2 Have you read and signed your concordance with the organisation's Standing Financial Instructions?	YES	NO	
13.3 Does your service have an identifiable line of reporting to the organisation's Board?	YES	NO	
13.4 Do all staff have signed contracts of employment at the time of taking up employment?	YES	NO	
13.5 Do all staff have up-to-date job descriptions?	YES	NO	
13.6 Do all staff members in your service have clearly defined lines of accountability?	YES	NO	

Component	Evaluation		Comment
13.7 Does your service have representation on the organisation's strategic committees; for example: • Clinical Governance • Research and Development • Capital Planning • Health and Safety • Risk • Equality	%		
13.8 Do you have a mechanism for recording declarations of interest?	YES	NO	
13.9 Do you have a mechanism in place to ensure staff comply with professional regulation requirements (HPC)?	YES	NO	
13.10 Do you have a monitoring system in place for checking registration status of all your staff?	YES	NO	
13.11 Do you have a list of authorised signatories for your service?, for example: • Time sheets • Travel claims • Equipment and supplies ordering • Charitable Trust funds • Petty cash	YES	NO	
Standard summary:	**Action:**		

Standard 14 top five key performance indicators

The service has identified five top KPIs and monitors progress against them annually.

NB. The KPIs selected will depend upon the service and the strategic priorities. They will therefore vary from service to service and change over time. Identify the top five indicators rating performance.

Component	Evaluation	Comment
14.1		
14.2		
14.3		
14.4		
14.5		
Standard summary	**Action:**	

Management quality overall action plan		
The following template is designed to copy and paste in the actions identified. This will enable you to monitor them collectively.		
Standard number	**Standard action**	**Review date**
1.		
2.		
3.		
4.		
5.		
6.		
7.		
8.		
9.		
10		
11		
12.		
13.		
14.		

Management quality record of standard completion and review dates			
Year: 20.....	Service:		
Standard	**Date completed**	**Review date**	**Sign off Manager name**
1 Strategy			
2 Activity			
3 Patient and Service User Experience			
4 Finance			
5 Staff Resource Effectiveness			
6 Staff Management and Development			
7 Information and Metrics			
8 Leadership and Management Development			
9 Clinical Excellence			
10 Communications and Marketing			
11 Service Improvement and Re-Design			
12 Risk Management			
13 Corporate Governance			
14 Key Performance Indicators			

References

1 Chick S, Huchzermeier C, Loch C. Management quality and operational excellence. In: Jones R, Jenkins F, editors. *Managing Money, Measurement and Marketing for the Allied Health Professions*. Oxford: Radcliffe Publishing; 2010.
2 Loch C, Van der Heyden L, Van Wassenhove L, *et al. Industrial Excellence*. Berlin: Springer; 2003.

3 Loch C, Chick S, Huchzermeier A. *Industrial Excellence Award, Healthcare Questionnaire.* Fontainebleau, INSEAD; 2009.

4 Jones R, Jenkins F. *Managing and Leading in the Allied Health Professions.* Oxford: Radcliffe Publishing; 2006.

5 Jones R, Jenkins F. *Developing the Allied Health Professional.* Oxford: Radcliffe Publishing; 2006.

6 Jones R, Jenkins F. *Key Topics in Healthcare Management – understanding the big picture.* Oxford: Radcliffe Publishing; 2006.

7 Womack J, Jones D. *Lean Thinking: banish waste and create wealth in your corporation, revised and updated.* London: Simon and Schuster; 2003.

8 NHS Institute for Innovation and Improvement. *The Lean Simulation Suitcase.* 2009: www.institute.nhs.uk.

9 Latino R, Latino K. *Root Cause Analysis: improving performance for bottom line results.* Boca Raton, FL: Taylor and Francis; 2006.

10 Six Sigma. 2009: www.isixsigma.com.

11 Deming WE. *Out of the Crisis.* Cambridge, MA: MIT; 1986.

12 Deming WE. *The New Economics for Industry.* Cambridge, MA: MIT; 1993.

13 Department for Business Innovation and Skills. 2009: www.dti.gov.uk/quality/tqm.

14 Pentecost D. Quality management: the human factor. *Euro Particip Mon.* 1991; **2**: 8–10.

15 Office of Government Commerce. 2009: www.ogc.gov.uk/documentation_and templates benefits_realisation_plan_.asp.

16 DH. *High Quality Care for All: NHS Next Stage Review final report.* 2008: www.dh.gov.uk/en/ Publicationsandstatistics/Publications/PublicationsPolicyAndGuidance/DH_085825.

17 Connecting for Health. 2009: www.connectingforhealth.nhs.uk/systemsandservices/ clindash.

18 Balanced Scorecard Institute. 2009: www.balancedscorecard.org/bscresources.

Chapter 14

Evaluating clinical performance in healthcare services with data envelopment analysis

Jon Chilingerian

Introduction

Effort to create more accountable healthcare organisations is an emerging global health trend. High performing organisations hold their healthcare staff accountable for both efficiency and the quality of care. Increasing demands for greater accountability will require leaders who focus more time and attention on 'best practice' performance management. Leaders need new 'tools' to measure and assess, as well as benchmark their organisation's performance.

Health policy makers are searching for ways to improve health system performance. The drive for performance has spawned policies and innovations such as payment by results (PbR), accountable care organisations, world-class commissioning, value-based purchasing, value-cost indices and pay-for-performance. What underlies all of these programmes is the idea of holding AHPs, doctors, nurses and clinical managers accountable for clinical outcomes, patient safety, patient experience, patient satisfaction and clinical efficiency.

Why do policy makers want to create more accountable healthcare organisations? Firstly, there is growing evidence that quality and efficiency vary widely among clinicians.[1, 2, 3, 4, 5] Secondly, while demands for safe and acceptable quality and better access to healthcare once justified investment and cost escalation, current budget restrictions re-focus attention on clinical efficiency and cost effective care goals.

Improving both the quality and efficiency of care provided requires measurement and comparison of clinical performance and operational improvement of services. In an effort to ensure that healthcare is neither being over-utilised nor under-utilised, much attention centres on managerial control systems that provide information to help clinical departments to monitor, profile and compare clinical care and treatment relying on audits and reviews. The question is: are there better ways to measure and evaluate clinical practice patterns?

In this chapter a theory-based mathematical methodology called Data Envelopment Analysis (DEA) is introduced as a 'tool' for healthcare policy makers and managers to measure and evaluate the relative performance of clinicians, clinical services and healthcare organisations. DEA is a powerful performance evaluation methodology capable of identifying top performers in relation to less effective performers. It handles multiple, non-commensurate clinical inputs and outputs, including qualitative factors such as patient satisfaction, for example, clinical services can be measured in monetary units, full time equivalents staff, lengths-of-stay, nursing units, time in the operating room, number of laboratory tests or doctor visits. Although these are physical quantities with different units, DEA can combine them in a consistent way. DEA can be used to measure and evaluate the performance of different clinical decision-making units when the care process involves multiple inputs and outputs.[6] Most importantly, DEA estimates a single, summary measure of relative performance without requiring a priori weights.

DEA compares the relative performance of a set of clinical decision-making units using similar resources to care for patients with similar diagnoses and/or procedures. As a 'tool' to establish accountable care, DEA identifies the top performers and estimates a relative performance score for the rest of the units. More than measuring and evaluating relative performance, the methodology also identifies which top performers offer the most realistic benchmarks for a unit. The method estimates what needs to change to improve performance by pinpointing the clinical inputs that are being used excessively, or projecting how many more patients could be treated if the clinicians operated as well as the top performers. Consequently, the information provides benchmarks to guide performance conversations.

DEA can also be used to uncover variables or managerial practices that explain superior, average or inferior performance.[7] Studies employing DEA explained performance variables such as provider age, specialisation and organisational affiliation[8, 9] styles of practice, service concepts and operating strategies,[10] provider experience[11] and mergers.[12] DEA has also been used to trace technical advances and improvements over time.[7, 13] DEA models are explored here to illustrate how to measure and benchmark the performance of clinical providers and hospital departments.

DEA and its application to estimating the performance of healthcare organisations is discussed. Three healthcare applications are presented, evaluating and benchmarking the relative performance of:

1 69 hip replacement teams
2 50 therapy departments treating stroke, hip replacement and heart shock and failure
3 123 cardiac surgeons performing 29 512 coronary artery by-pass grafts (CABG).

Data on these cases are analysed to demonstrate how DEA can be reconciled with quality of care to obtain a comprehensive evaluation of clinicians' performance.

This chapter concludes with a discussion of limitations of these results and how DEA results can be used to help improve accountability and facilitate an evolution of healthcare organisations toward high quality and efficiency.

DEA methodology

Building on the seminal work of Farrell,[14] Charnes,[15] proposed a general methodology – DEA – to measure and evaluate the performance of any decision-making unit (DMU). A DMU is defined as an individual or organisation that uses resources to produce outputs. DEA was developed in the early 1970s when a doctoral student, Eduardo Rhodes, was trying to evaluate public educational programmes that aid children from vulnerable populations.[16] Today more than 4 000 research articles using DEA have been published in journals or books.[17] A recent review of techniques used to measure healthcare performance recommended DEA as one of the most promising methodologies to evaluate performance and identify best performers.[18]

DEA is a linear programming technique that envelops the input and output data with a non-parametric production frontier based on best practices.[16] When comparing a group of decision- making units, rather than focussing on the average performers, DEA focusses on the units that achieved the best results. Once the top performers are identified, every other decision-making unit is given a relative performance score based on that unit's distance from the top performers. Since accountability requires a set of measures that include resource inputs and outputs that increase value, DEA offers a powerful method for evaluating the relationship between outputs and inputs.

Perhaps the most distinct advantage of DEA over statistical methods – such as multiple regression – is that it does not require the functional form of the technology to be known in advance. Thus, DEA allows for a purely empirical study of clinical practices. Unlike many methods that can examine only one input and one output at a time, DEA can manage the complexity of multiple inputs and multiple outputs simultaneously. The ratio of the combined inputs and outputs is regarded as the performance score. The preceding can be illustrated with an example.

Consider a set of n different hip replacement clinics in a health community or region to be evaluated. Although we do not know the mathematical relationship between outputs and inputs – called the production function – we do know how many patients are treated and how many resources were used to care for those patients. Given this situation, the relative performance of a clinic could be determined mathematically by taking the ratio of the outputs (y) to the inputs (x), as shown in Equation 1.

$$P = \frac{y_1 + y_2 + \ldots + y_r}{x_1 + x_2 + \ldots + x_i} \qquad \text{(Equation 1)}$$

Each clinic uses m clinical resources -or inputs- to care for s number of patients - or outputs. If $X_{ij} > 0$ is the amount of input i used by clinic j, and $Y_{rj} > 0$ is the quantity of hip replacement patients treated at severity level r discharged with good outcomes. To measure performance it is very important that the outputs achieve a 'satisfactory' technical outcome. If outputs do not obtain a good or 'constant quality outcome', top performers may be under utilising resources, and offering inappropriate standards of care. Therefore, efficient care always requires satisfactory technical outcomes, that is, an absence of morbidity and mortality, no readmission or recurrence of the diagnosis within a reasonable time period. Herein lies the problem, because the inputs and the outputs are usually measured differently and represent different, or non-commensurate metrics and dimensions scales, they cannot be simply added up in a scale. By using a set of weights, u_r and v_i, the multiple output-input ratio becomes a single 'virtual' output, and virtual input.

To evaluate the performance of n hip replacement hospital clinics, we formulate n fractional linear programs, one for each of the n hospital clinics in the study. If we want to evaluate the performance of a specific hospital clinic k, (h_{kth} = hospital clinic k), we would compare clinic k with the others in the study file.

The mathematical formulation is summarised below, where the relative efficiency of a specific hospital clinic k (the h_{kth} unit) can be determined only by benchmarking it against all of the other units.

$$\text{Maximize } h_k = \frac{\sum_{r=1}^{s} u_r \, Y_{rk}}{\sum_{i=1}^{m} v_i \, X_{ik}} \qquad \text{(Equation 2)}$$

Subject to:

$$\frac{\sum_{r=1}^{s} u_r \, Y_{rj}}{\sum_{i=1}^{m} v_i \, X_{ij}} \le 1$$

$$\text{for } j = 1...k...n$$

$$u_{rk} \ge 0; r = 1, \ldots , s$$
$$v_{ik} \ge 0; i = 1, \ldots , m \qquad \text{(Equation 3)}$$

This new ratio – now a function of multipliers to be determined – becomes the objective function for each clinic or provider to be evaluated. The DEA approach is appealing when applied to the study of the performance of individual providers, departments, clinics and hospitals for several other reasons. Firstly, DEA can be applied in a context of multiple inputs and multiple outputs. Secondly, by employing actual observations in a post hoc analysis, DEA calculates the maximum single, summary score that evaluates the relative performance, and the sources and amount of performance improvement when compared to a reference set or comparison group. The DEA score used to rate each facility varies between 0 and 1, where 1 = best performance efficient, and 0 through 0.99 = lowest to highest performances.

DEA relies on the Pareto-Koopmans definition of efficiency,[19] a derivation of the social welfare criterion of Pareto optimality. To construct the best practice performance frontier, observed behaviour is evaluated using the following input-output criteria:

- a decision-making unit is a 'best performance' if it is possible to decrease any input without increasing any other input and without decreasing output
- a decision-making unit is not a 'best performance' if it is possible to increase any output without decreasing any other output and without increasing any input.

A decision-making unit will be characterised as relatively high performing only when both criteria are satisfied.[15] An example using a small group of clinics illustrates how DEA can be used to define a best practice clinical production frontier.

How DEA works

Consider a simplistic case where 12 clinics in 12 different hospitals are treating 2 types of patients: high and low severity hip replacement patients. The problem is straightforward – we want to measure and evaluate the relative performance of $n = 12$ hip replacement clinics using the conceptual approach.[14, 15] Each care programme has a different mix of high and low severity patients, all patients completed treatment with good outcomes; however, the total number of patients can be severity-adjusted.

When there are multiple inputs, (that is, different types of clinical resources; days in the hospital, hours of nursing care, physical therapy visits, care processes) and multiple outputs (that is, diagnoses and procedures with different levels of severity), it is desirable to have an overall and summary measure of performance. Although ratios and statistical techniques offer some useful measures, they are incapable of estimating a summarising performance into a meaningful measure.

Each of these clinics offers surgical services, nursing care, rehabilitation/ physical therapy for hip replacement patients with good outcomes. Although these clinics also used indirect and overhead expenses,[20] ignoring this, the cost of the actual bundle of direct clinical resources was calculated, including:

- the cost of the operating theatre
- laboratory tests
- nursing care
- rehabilitation
- medication
- ancillary services.

Figure 14.1 plots one year of hypothetical inputs and outputs for each of the 12 hip replacement clinics. Hospital clinics on the top left side of the figure – that is, closer to the vertical axis and to the left of another clinic – treated more patients with fewer resources. The dotted line passing through clinics C_1 and C_2 represents a 'Best Practice Performance Frontier' BPPF for each of the 12 centres. As shown in Figure 14.1, the care teams treating the patients at clinics C_1 and C_2 used fewer clinical resources and dominate the less efficient clinics: C_3–C_{12} inclusive.

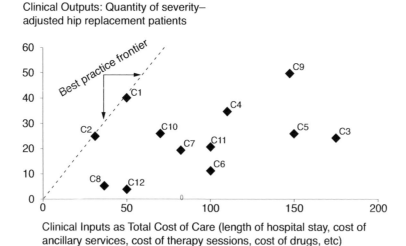

Figure 14.1 Plot of 12 hip replacement clinics with constant returns to scale.

To measure and evaluate performance, DEA ranks and scores all of the clinics by measuring the relative distance of a clinic from the frontier. Facilities on the frontier (C_1, and C_2) will obtain a score of 1.0 (or 100%). Hospital clinics to the right of the dotted line running through C_1 and C_2 are off the frontier and depending on their relative distance from C_1 and C_2, will obtain a score between 0 and 1. For example, C_7 treated fewer hip patients than C_1 and C_2 and used far more clinical resources. Consequently, C_7 is less efficient and its performance is rated approximately 72% when compared with C_2, rated 100%.

The DEA model shown in Figure 14.1 defines a performance frontier in which the average productivity does not depend on the scale of the programme. In other words, if the number of patients is increased by a factor of two, it would need two times or a proportionate increase in the clinical inputs. This is called a constant returns to scale model.

For some healthcare applications, treating more patients might lead to increases or decreases to average productivity. This is called variable – not constant – returns to scale. For example, a clinic learns that by going from 300 to 400 hip replacement patients their weighted y/x average productivity increases. When they do 500 or more cases they have to add more staff and their average productivity decreases. Figure 14.2 reveals how returns to scale – increasing, decreasing and constant – could be interpreted by the intercepts of the segments of the performance frontier.

In Figure 14.2, the dotted line running through clinics C_1, C_2, and C_9 is a BPPF – or a supporting hyperplane – for each of the 12 clinics. The performance score of C_7, a hip replacement clinic that performed more poorly than C_1, C_9 and C_2, can be measured by constructing a line segment from the point f to point e. The output benchmarks for C_7 are hospitals C_1 and C_9. The line segment touches the BPPF at point e. The performance rating of C_7 is equal to the ratio of the length of line segment fg divided by the length of fe (that is, fg / fe). Since the numerator fg is less than the denominator fe, the performance rating of hospital C_7 will be less than 1. Alternatively, input performance can also be evaluated by measuring

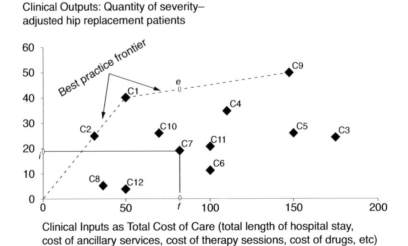

Clinical Outputs: Quantity of severity–adjusted hip replacement patients

Clinical Inputs as Total Cost of Care (total length of hospital stay, cost of ancillary services, cost of therapy sessions, cost of drugs, etc)

Figure 14.2 Plot of 12 hip replacement clinics with variable return to scale.

the scope of resource conservation at point *g* by *ih* / *ig*. It is important to note that while this single input single output example can be solved graphically, multi-input, multi-output problems require a mathematical formulation that can only be solved by using a linear programming model.

To summarise, benchmarking clinical performance requires making significant comparisons of clinicians and healthcare units against their local counterparts inside and outside the organisations in which they practice. With respect to benchmarking performance, DEA has many interesting properties. Firstly, it is a methodology formulated to find best practice rather than central tendencies. By summarising many non-commensurate variables into an overall score, a single summary measure of performance, DEA can 'tame' many multi-dimensional performance problems. Whereas a count of items results in a final reliable value, a measure is merely an approximation, of some true value. DEA, like accounting, looks at how resources were used, what results were accomplished, what happened and tries to determine why. Although one can determine confidence intervals by bootstrapping DEA results, DEA scores are not estimators.

Secondly, since it is non-parametric, the usual statistical requirements such as degrees of freedom, estimators and confidence intervals are relaxed. When using DEA, one needs to identify a comparison group of similar units for benchmarking. To make statistical inferences, requires a large comparison group that is, sample size. An advantage of DEA is the size of a comparison group depends on the number of inputs and outputs. A rule of thumb is size of the comparison group is between two to three times the total number of inputs plus outputs that is, $(2 \times (m + s)$; or $3 \times (m + s)$. For example, with three inputs and two outputs, since $m + s = 5$, $(2 \times 5 = 10)$ and $(3 \times 5 = 15)$, a comparison group of only 10 to 15 units are needed.

Whereas statistical techniques like Ordinary Least Square regression[21] run a single optimisation model, DEA proceeds with a series of optimisations comparing each unit with every other unit in the study file. With the simplex methods and no computational effort, the solution not only measures performance but with the dual problem (every linear programme can be restated into a 'dual' problem with different variables), the methodology uncovers a reference set of comparable units, sources of the problem and projections of a weighted average ways to improve performance.

It is important to note that while this single input single output example can be solved graphically, multi-input, multi-output problems require a mathematical formulation that can only be solved by using a linear programming model.

Using DEA to benchmark clinical performance: three examples

DEA can be used evaluate various categories of efficient performance such as technical, scale, and overall efficiency. Technical inefficiency occurs when a provider uses a relatively excessive quantity of clinical resource inputs when compared with providers practicing with a similar size and mix of patients. Scale inefficiency occurs when a provider is operating at sub-optimal activity level, that is, the unit is not diagnosing and/or treating the most productive quantity of patients of a given case mix. Overall efficiency measures includes both technical and scale efficiency.

DEA can be used to find the minimum set of clinical inputs to produce successfully treated patients. A hospital provider would be considered 100% efficient if they care for patients with fewer days of stay and ancillary services at an efficient scale size. Primary care providers are considered efficient if they care for their patients with fewer visits, tests, therapies, hospital days, medication, and specialist consultations and at an efficient scale.

As stated before, benchmarking clinical performance requires making significant comparisons of clinicians and healthcare units against their local counterparts inside and outside the organisations in which they practice. The preceding section described DEA as a methodology that can be used to measure a healthcare provider's clinical performance by evaluating the relationship between the clinical inputs used to care for patients.

These ideas will be illustrated by three studies of performance:

- 69 hip replacement teams
- 50 therapy departments treating stroke, heart failure, shock and hip replacement patients
- 123 cardiac surgeons performing CABG

Hospital hip replacement teams

Figure 14.3 displays an example of the DEA hospital model for evaluating the performance of hip replacement teams. The clinical inputs and outputs for the productive efficiency dimension displayed are self-explanatory. The hospital's clinical outputs are low and high severity hip replacement patients discharged home with excellent outcomes without re-admission. The two clinical inputs are the total length of stay and the total ancillary services used to care for the patients. Since DEA can handle non-commensurate data, length of stay and the two clinical outputs are simple counts while ancillary services costs are measured in monetary units.

The DEA results are summarised in Table 14.1, which shows the relative clinical efficiency of the 69 hospitals, performing high and low severity hip replacement. The average efficiency score is 86%, and the bottom quartile ranges from 58% to 79%. The DEA model identified 10 of 69 hospitals on the best practice frontier.

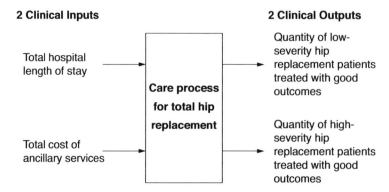

Figure 14.3 Production model for evaluating hip replacement surgery.

Table 14.1 Benchmarking hip replacements with DEA.

Hospital	Score	Hospital	Score	Hospital	Score
H1	92.00%	H23	83.00%	H47	100.00%
H2	80.00%	H24	58.00%	H48	78.00%
H3	100.00%	H25	85.00%	H49	98.00%
H4	92.00%	H26	85.00%	H51	85.00%
H5	81.00%	H27	100.00%	H52	79.00%
H6	75.00%	H28	77.00%	H54	100.00%
H7	74.00%	H29	89.00%	H55	100.00%
H8	66.00%	H30	77.00%	H56	92.00%
H9	77.00%	H31	100.00%	H57	99.00%
H10	100.00%	H32	92.00%	H58	79.00%
H11	87.00%	H33	93.00%	H59	84.00%
H12	100.00%	H34	72.00%	H60	87.00%
H13	87.00%	H35	96.00%	H61	83.00%
H14	90.00%	H36	94.00%	H62	65.00%
H15	80.00%	H37	63.00%	H63	93.00%
H16	99.00%	H38	73.00%	H64	80.00%
H17	76.00%	H39	93.00%	H65	84.00%
H18	100.00%	H42	85.00%	H66	72.00%
H19	84.00%	H43	80.00%	H67	97.00%
H20	84.00%	H44	76.00%	H68	100.00%
H21	78.00%	H45	78.00%	H69	96.00%
H22	81.00%	H46	85.00%		

More than 20 hospitals had scores of less than 80% which reveals a notable opportunity to improve performance, potentially reducing healthcare costs and reducing hundreds of acute hospitals bed days. The average performance for hip replacements was 86% which means that the potential reduction in the use of resources is 14%. In particular, hospital H8 was only rated 66.4% and it did not perform very well. DEA methodology offers interesting insights for using strategic benchmarks and achieving potential for improvement.

Figure 14.4 and Table 14.2 reveal how DEA identifies peer hospitals and the potential for improvement by projecting less effective units onto the frontier. Identification of peers is part of the information that DEA offers and is one of the important features of the methodology. H8's performance is rated 66.4% when compared to the three frontier hospitals H27, H31, and H47. DEA identifies peer hospitals or what could be interpreted as strategic groups – a strategic category of hospitals with a similar patient case mix and practice style. Clinical managers in H8 would focus on what H27, H31 and H47 are doing to achieve their results.

Table 14.2 illustrates another valuable piece of information that DEA offers. A weighted composite of H27, H31 and H47, constructed from the mathematical programming – dual weights – employed in DEA, identifies a potential target to reduce and improve resource use. H8 performed 128 hip replacements and utilised a total of 821 patient days and $3 605 720 in ancillary services. A combination of the actual operation of these three hospitals reveals H8's targets if H8 were as efficient as the other three. The projected improved H8, in

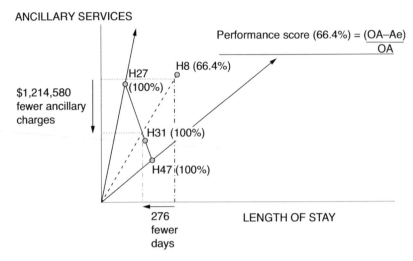

Figure 14.4 DEA projects inefficient hospital onto the frontier: comparing H8 with the reference set H27, H31 and H47.

Table 14.2 DEA identifies hospital H8's potential for improvement: benchmarking against peer hospitals.

	Actual performance (66.4%)	Targets to gain (100%)	Savings
Clinical outputs for H8			
DRG 209 low severity hip replacement	94 patients	94 patients	
DRG 209 high severity hip replacement	34 patients	34 patients	
Clinical inputs for H8			
Total hospital length-of-stay	821 days	545 days	276 days
Total ancillary costs (excluding room and bed)	$3 605 720	$2 391 140	$1 214 580

performing 128 hip replacements, would utilise 545 patient days and $2 391 140 in ancillary services, a reduction of 276 patient days and $1 214 580 in ancillary services. These preliminary findings could be used to sharpen a second stage analysis of the factors associated with improved outcomes and efficient use of resources. H8's clinical managers can use these targets to begin revising operating practices and the innovation process.

Benchmarking cost effective physical, occupational and speech therapy

This example is a one year study of the practice patterns and relative cost per patient of physical therapy, occupational therapy and speech therapy for patients

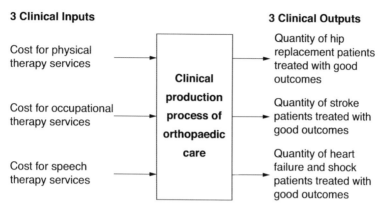

3 Clinical Inputs

Cost for physical therapy services

Cost for occupational therapy services

Cost for speech therapy services

Clinical production process of orthopaedic care

3 Clinical Outputs

Quantity of hip replacement patients treated with good outcomes

Quantity of stroke patients treated with good outcomes

Quantity of heart failure and shock patients treated with good outcomes

Figure 14.5 Primary care model for efficient care: stroke, hip replacement, heart failure and shock.

with stroke, heart failure, shock and hip replacements. A community hospital consortium was interested in the relative efficiency of their respective therapy services. Efficient therapy refers to relationships of multiple clinical inputs to multiple clinical outputs.

The three clinical input measures used were the total cost to the hospital for Therapy services. The three clinical outputs were the quantity of patients with stroke, heart failure and heart shock and hip replacement patients, all with good outcomes, Figure 14.5. The total cost for therapy care for 27 706 patients $16 945 913.

Table 14.3 reveals a wide range of overall efficiencies – between 11% and 100%. Out of 50 healthcare providers, sixteen offered efficient therapy services and had a relative efficiency value of 100% (1.00). As was shown with Figure 14.4, the linear programming formulations projects the inefficient therapy services on the best practices frontier, revealing whether the inefficiencies are with therapies and the potential savings. The average efficiency score is 70%, and the bottom quartile ranges from 11% to 45%. Since the mean efficiency of the services was only 70%, there was a potential to save up to $5 000 000.

Table 14.3 Evaluating efficient patient care for 50 hospital departments: hip replacement, stroke and heart failure and heart shock.

Hospital	Score	Hospital	Score	Hospital	Score	Hospital	Score	Hospital	Score
H1	55.56	H11	76.84	H21	88.14	H31	48.72	H41	17.23
H2	100	H12	45.47	H22	100	H32	26.33	H42	54.92
H3	92.7	H13	100	H23	31.76	H33	56.7	H43	83.05
H4	100	H14	100	H24	100	H34	100	H44	73.56
H5	39.41	H15	100	H25	33.12	H35	55.87	H45	76.97
H6	16.08	H16	100	H26	44.7	H36	11.9	H46	72.38
H7	100	H17	43.82	H27	100	H37	70.16	H47	100
H8	90.23	H18	100	H28	22.97	H38	100	H48	25.52
H9	17.13	H19	90.46	H29	50.71	H39	100	H49	100
H10	77.25	H20	17.77	H30	54	H40	97.76	H50	100

Table 14.4 Evaluating scale efficient patient care for 50 hospital departments: hip replacement, stroke and heart failure and heart shock.

Hospital	Score	Hospital	Score	Hospital	Score	Hospital	Score	Hospital	Score
H1	96%	H11	97%	H21	92%	H31	63%	H41	100%
H2	100%	H12	45%	H22	92%	H32	87%	H42	55%
H3	96%	H13	100%	H23	100%	H33	88%	H43	85%
H4	100%	H14	100%	H24	100%	H34	100%	H44	92%
H5	98%	H15	100%	H25	100%	H35	82%	H45	77%
H6	97%	H16	100%	H26	99%	H36	45%	H46	95%
H7	100%	H17	96%	H27	45%	H37	76%	H47	100%
H8	100%	H18	100%	H28	100%	H38	100%	H48	26%
H9	98%	H19	90%	H29	68%	H39	100%	H49	100%
H10	92%	H20	92%	H30	63%	H40	98%	H50	100%

DEA also can identify whether a therapy programme is operating at an efficient size and scale. Table 14.4 reveals the effect of scale on productive efficiency. Although 20 programmes were 'scale' efficient, 30 programmes were not operating at an optimal scale. Hospital 48 was technically efficient, however, its inefficiencies were entirely due economies of scale. The average efficiency score is 89%, and the bottom quartile ranges from 26% to 87%. Groups interested in accountable care and effective commissioning, like PCTs and healthcare managers could use this type of information for performance conversations, decision support and planning.

Evaluating and benchmarking cardiac surgeons

The final example is a two year study of cardiac surgeons in one large, East Coast State in the US. The database contained 38 577 patients who were given a coronary-artery-by-pass graft and discharged. This study focused on efficiency differences among surgeons producing satisfactory outcomes defined as cases where the patient was discharged home with good outcomes, no readmission, or post-surgery mortality at home. If patients suffered pre-operative cardiogenic shock or renal failure they were taken out of the database. If patients expired or were discharged to a skilled nursing home or other facility they were removed from this study. The availability and use of skilled nursing facilities (SNFs) can vary markedly across regions and lengths of stay in hospitals can be shorter where SNFs are used aggressively. Since length of stay is a key clinical input in the efficiency analyses, elimination of cases where a patient was discharged to a SNF promotes uniformity of cases for efficiency determination.

The result was a database of 26 512 discharges over 2 years who underwent cardiac surgery.

The patient-level data was aggregated to 123 cardiac surgeons who performed 50 or more surgeries in 39 hospitals over a 2 year period. Figure 14.6 shows the DEA model for CABG procedures comprised two inputs (days of stay and ancillary/other charges) and four outputs (low and high severity CABG patients

2 Clinical Inputs   **4 Clinical Outputs**

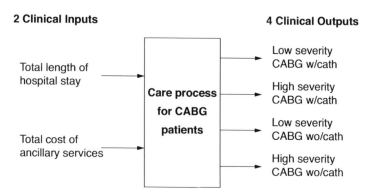

Figure 14.6 Production model for evaluating CABG

with catheterisation, low and high severity CABG patients without catheterisation). The State Authority assigned to each case an admission severity rating which represented an estimate of the patient's clinical stability – probability of in-hospital death – based on the patient's clinical condition at the time of admission. The low severity cases included patients with either few or no abnormal findings upon admission. The high severity patients had significant, severe, and/or critical diagnostic findings upon admission, with a higher likelihood of mortality, perhaps due to a co-morbidity or pre-existing condition.

The Authority use of a logistic regression model was to estimate probability of death as a function of the admission severity measure and several other clinical variables. The independent variables – patient clinical characteristics – included in the logistic regression model were admission severity score, age, age-squared (divided by 1000), cardiogenic shock, concurrent percutaneous transluminal coronary angioplasty, complicated hypertension, dialysis, gender, heart failure, and prior CABG and/or valve surgery.

For both DRGs 106 and 107, all cases were where the estimated probability of death was greater than or equal to 3% ($p \geqslant 0.03$) were classified as high severity which represented 20% of all cases.

A brief example with a small group of surgeons illustrates how DEA can be used to separate practice style from performance. Consider a simplistic case where 10 surgeons each perform 50 CABGs annually on comparable patients. These surgeons used two clinical inputs: diagnostic tests and consultations with other doctor. Figure 14.7 plots one year of hypothetical input and output data for 15 cardiac surgeons.

Cardiac surgeons who are in the bottom left hand corner and to the left of another surgeon used fewer clinical resources to care for similar patients. Figure 14.7 plots a BPPF for each of the 15 surgeons. Although surgeons S_1, S_{11}, S_4, S_{12}, and S_8 dominate S_2, S_3, S_7, S_9, and S_{10} they display different styles of practice.

For example, S_2 and S_9 practice style is similar to S_1 and S_{11} but since they use more resources they are less efficient. S_{15} and S_{10} practice style is like S_{12} and S_8 and they are also less efficient. One style trades off short stay for more expensive tests to get a faster discharge. The other style uses longer hospital stays but many fewer tests and ancillary resources.

Table 14.5 shows performance scores for the 123 cardiac surgeons treating 26 512 patients. The average performance score was 90%, and a bottom quartile

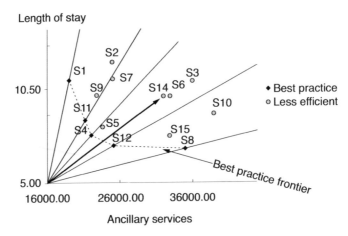

Figure 14.7 Plot of 15 cardiac surgeons undertaking CABG without catheterisation.

range of 63% to 82%. There were 26 out of 123 on the performance frontier. The median score was 0.91% with a standard deviation of 0.086. The minimum score was 0.640, which requires further investigation and explanation. The median score was 91%. Surgeons with DEA scores above the median value were classified as higher efficiency surgeons, while those below the median were classified as lower efficiency surgeons.

To complement the efficiency estimates, this study used CABG mortality rates as a measure of technical outcomes and quality. Mortality rates were not adjusted for patient severity. Overall CABG mortality rates for each surgeon were also obtained by dividing the number of CABG patients with discharge status of expired by the total number of CABG patients – any discharge status. The average mortality rate per surgeon was 3.2% of CABG cases, and the standard deviation was 0.2%. The minimum mortality rate was 0 (1 surgeon), and the maximum mortality rate was 10.2%. The median mortality rate was 2.9%. Surgeons with mortality rates above the median value were classified as high mortality surgeons, while those below the median were classified as low mortality surgeons.

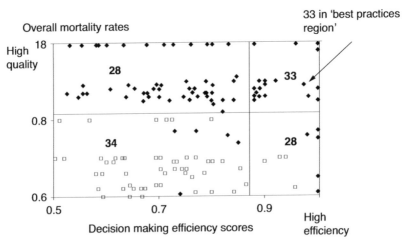

Figure 14.8 Plot of mortality rates and decision-making efficiency.

Table 14.5 Benchmarking of 123 cardiac surgeons.

Hospital	Score	Hospital	Score	Hospital	Score	Hospital	Score	Hospital	Score
S1	74%	S26	92%	S51	97%	S76	83%	S101	100%
S2	84%	S27	84%	S52	100%	S77	100%	S102	87%
S3	88%	S28	91%	S53	68%	S78	100%	S103	96%
S4	83%	S29	87%	S54	97%	S79	91%	S104	70%
S5	94%	S30	97%	S55	96%	S80	100%	S105	82%
S6	92%	S31	79%	S56	100%	S81	100%	S106	81%
S7	100%	S32	100%	S57	100%	S82	100%	S107	99%
S8	77%	S33	74%	S58	81%	S83	93%	S108	81%
S9	78%	S34	74%	S59	79%	S84	100%	S109	89%
S10	96%	S35	80%	S60	75%	S85	99%	S110	90%
S11	75%	S36	91%	S61	100%	S86	96%	S111	100%
S12	89%	S37	90%	S62	91%	S87	78%	S112	100%
S13	100%	S38	78%	S63	89%	S88	64%	S113	83%
S14	94%	S39	100%	S64	100%	S89	90%	S114	100%
S15	95%	S40	94%	S65	93%	S90	100%	S115	93%
S16	89%	S41	89%	S66	100%	S91	81%	S116	89%
S17	79%	S42	96%	S67	94%	S92	95%	S117	92%
S18	93%	S43	88%	S68	94%	S93	87%	S118	100%
S19	100%	S44	97%	S69	85%	S94	79%	S119	100%
S20	85%	S45	88%	S70	83%	S95	87%	S120	92%
S21	77%	S46	93%	S71	88%	S96	87%	S121	94%
S22	100%	S47	82%	S72	93%	S97	87%	S122	93%
S23	76%	S48	89%	S73	81%	S98	93%	S123	100%
S24	100%	S49	96%	S74	85%	S99	87%		
S25	86%	S50	83%	S75	79%	S100	83%		

Figure 14.8 presents the two-dimensional array of surgeon performance, efficiency and effectiveness. Of particular interest are the 33 surgeons located in the top right hand corner. These surgeons displayed high efficiency (average DEA score = 0.966) and low mortality (average mortality rate = 1.6%). By way of comparison, the 34 surgeons located in bottom left corner had an average DEA score of 0.822 and an average mortality rate of 4.6%. The surgeons in the upper right corner were more productive and treated an average of 282 CABG cases over the two-year period, while the surgeons in bottom left-hand corner treated an average of 241 cases. The high quality, high efficiency surgeons could serve as potential role models for efforts to achieve clinical excellence.

Summary and conclusions

With only three examples, DEA found a huge opportunity for performance improvement. The methodology reveals that a substantial amount of money could be saved if hospitals and clinicians adopted the practice style of the top performers who use least clinical resources. From a managerial perspective, DEA could be used to help clinical professionals think about innovative ways to reduce healthcare costs and improve patient value.

By creating a process for improving quality and efficiency, DEA models readily identify opportunities to improve productivity by decreasing clinical inputs, increasing outputs, or some combination of the two. Recommendations will reflect practices employed by the top performers rather than hypothetical proposals based on theoretical efficiency. While DEA is best used as a learning 'tool', it also supports performance evaluations on selected departments, procedures and therapies. As shown in this chapter, evaluations can also be conducted at the level of the individual practitioner.

To summarise, DEA can be used by any type of healthcare organisation to evaluate the practice patterns of any clinician, clinical department or the hospital. The methodology also indicates a variety of ways in which a clinical provider might become more efficient. The linear programming solutions contain multiple options that require discussions about trade-offs in cost, feasibility and practicality. In other words, a strategic thinking process is needed to analyse the situation, set goals and consider the alternatives.

In the past, hospital managers were reluctant to hold physicians, nurses and AHPs accountable for their performance because they were not sure about how to measure quality and decision-making efficiency. Competing views explain the relationship between clinical performance and resource use. One view is that the quality of clinical performance is a monotonically increasing function of the resources and effort invested in a patient. This 'more is better' proposition suggests that more medical care – investing more medical resources – will always improve results. Little evidence supports this contention. Generally more complex and severe illnesses require disproportionately more resources to achieve an equivalent improvement. The principle of diminishing marginal returns seems to apply to healthcare. Seriously ill patients benefit most during the early part of treatment. After some critical point, an additional day in the hospital yields diminishing benefit. Before initiating any change, clinical professionals must assess the potential effects on the quality of care.

There is, however, a secret formula for holding clinicians accountable for their practice behaviour. It has been said by Eisenberg:[1]

> In summary, when feedback is used to alter physician practice patterns, the programmes are most likely to be successful if the data are individualised, if doctors are compared with their peers, and if the information is delivered personally by a physician in a position of clinical leadership...

As the drive for accountable and high performance healthcare progresses, DEA emerges as promising 'tool' that accommodates the 'Eisenberg' requirements by offering individualised feedback based on peer comparisons. Progress towards accountable healthcare requires on-going transparent performance conversations; not only between policy-makers and managers, or managers and physicians, but also with every clinical and AHP who makes a contribution that affects the capacity to perform and the capacity to obtain good outcomes for patients.

A future agenda and new leadership challenge

In the future, clinical health leaders will face two mandates. The first will be simple to understand, yet difficult to fulfil.

1 Offer high quality services at low cost.

The second is related to the first, but may be even more challenging.

2 With increasing demands for accountability, performance that is merely – better than average – or even superior, will soon be inadequate.

Consequently, health and human service organisations of the future will face a mandate to benchmark their performance against the 'best results in observed practice', and they will be paid according to the results they achieve.

Comparative studies of organisations reveal wide variations in innovation and performance among high performing health and service organisations. Over time, these organisations innovate and improve their services by shifting their performance frontiers far ahead of others. Other organisations are then pressured to not only sustain their performance, but also compete and catch up with their rivals.

When confronted with these performance mandates, leaders must then solve a performance puzzle – how is it that some organisations are able to sustain performance on a best practice frontier? And what explains the differences in operational excellence? Many experts believe that rising healthcare costs and inferior quality reflect managerial inefficiency, waste and internal organisational problems.[22, 23, 24] Others argue as much as 90% of the decisions that result in use of medical care are initiated by clinicians.[1] Consequently, the measurement and evaluation of medical practice and clinical decision-making are critical for performance management.[25]

A recent study in the NHS proposed drivers for productivity in healthcare; 'Lean', performance and talent management.[26] Healthcare organisations that established clinical quality and productivity targets; measured and assessed performance, engaged clinicians and communicated performance information with internal and external benchmarks achieved:

- higher patient satisfaction
- lower rates of infection
- fewer readmissions
- higher physician productivity
- shorter lengths of stay
- higher operating margins

The study found that top performing hospitals were continually monitoring internal and external performance indicators and simultaneously communicating results through formal and informal communications. The most important finding was the strong link between hospital performance and two variables:

1 level of physician engagement
2 proportion of clinically trained managers.

The conclusion is that top performers relentlessly tracked their performance and obtained deep involvement of clinicians by recruiting very high proportions of clinically trained managers.[26]

Performance and accounting measures focus on industry ratios and averages, without paying much attention to outliers, or extreme performers. Statistical analyses often ignore outliers, assuming that extreme values represent errors.

Studies of performance suggest, however, that when measured correctly, outliers can represent organisations that have achieved 'excellence' or a 'best practice' consequently, performance outliers could be the most important organisations for future leaders to study and observe.

Increasing demands for greater accountability will require leaders who focus more time and attention on 'best practice' performance management. Leaders will need new 'tools' to measure and assess, as well as benchmark their organisation's performance. Once leaders can measure the relative performance of their organisations, they will be better prepared to build commitment to operational excellence.

Future mandates for quality and productivity will be taken more and more seriously as health and human services organisations face deepening social and economic problems. Meeting the growing imperatives will require a new breed of leader who can mobilise the organisation to create value for patients, service providers and staff, external stakeholders and the organisation. Attending to the behaviour of extreme performers represents a cutting edge approach to performance measurement that traditional statistical approaches have often overlooked. Leaders of the future will be wise to analyse outlier success in order to understand and achieve best practices in their organisations and meet the new mandates for success. Whether DEA will become a leadership 'tool' to support the values and goals of accountable healthcare remains to be seen.

References

1 Eisenberg J. *Doctor's Decisions and the Cost of Care.* Chicago, IL: Health Administration Press; 1986.

2 World Health Organization. *Quality of Care: patient safety.* Report by the Secretariat. A55/13. Fifty-fifth World Health Assembly. Geneva: WHO Press; 2002: www.who.int/gb/ebwa/pdf_files/WHASS/es5513.pdf.

3 Wennberg J, Fisher E, Stukel T, *et al.* Use of hospitals, physician visits, and hospice care during the last six months of life among cohorts loyal to highly respected hospitals in the United States. *BMJ.* 2004; **328**: 607–11.

4 Bernet P, Rosko M, Valdmanis V, *et al.* Productivity efficiencies in Ukrainian polyclinics: lessons for health system transitions from differential responses to market changes. *J Prod Anal.* 2008; **29(2)**: 103–11.

5 US Department of Health and Human Services. *Identifying, Categorizing, and Evaluating Health Care Efficiency Measures.* Rockville, MD: AHRQ Publication; 2008.

6 Banker R, Charnes A, Cooper W. Some models for estimating technical and scale inefficiencies in data envelopment analysis. *Manage Sci.* 1984; **30**: 1078–92.

7 Emrouznejad A. *An Extensive Bibliography of Data Envelopment Analysis (DEA), Volume I: Working Papers.* Unpublished manuscript; 2001.

8 Chilingerian J. *Investigating non-medical factors associated with the technical efficiency of physicians in the provision of hospital services: a pilot study.* Best Paper Proceedings, Annual Meeting of the Academy of Management, Washington, DC; 1989.

9 Chilingerian J. Evaluating physician efficiency in hospitals: a multivariate analysis of best practices. *Eur J Oper Res.* 1995; **80**: 548–74.

10 Chilingerian J, Sherman H. Benchmarking physician practice patterns with DEA: a multi-stage approach for cost containment. *Ann Oper Res.* 1996; **67**: 83–116.

11 Ozcan Y, Watts II J, Wogen S. Provider experience and technical efficiency in the treatment of stroke patients: DEA approach. *J Operat Res Soc.* 1998; **49(6)**: 573–82.

12 Harris II J, Ozgen H, Ozcan Y. Do mergers enhance the performance of hospital efficiency? *J Operat Res Soc.* 2000; **51(7)**: 801–11.

13 Chilingerian J, Glavin M. *A decade of clinical productivity change with Pennsylvania CABG programs.* Unpublished working paper; 2009.

14 Farrell M. The measurement of productive efficiency. *J Royal Stat Soc.* 1957; **120**: 253–81.

15 Charnes A, Cooper W, Rhodes E. Measuring the efficiency of decision-making units, *Eur J Operat Res.* 1978; **3**: 429–44.

16 Cooper W, Seiford L, Zhu J. *Data Envelopment Analysis: theory, methodology and applications.* Toronto: Kluwer Academic Publishers; 2004.

17 Emrouznejad A, Barnett R. Evaluation of research in efficiency and productivity: a survey and analysis of the first 30 years of scholarly literature in DEA. *Socio Econ Plan Sci.* 2008; **42**: 151–7.

18 Agency for Health Care Research and Quality. 2008: www.ahrq.gov.

19 Charnes A, Cooper W, Golany B, *et al.* Foundations of data envelopment analysis for Pareto-Koopmans efficient empirical production functions. *J Econometrics.* 1985; **30(1–2)**: 91–107.

20 Jones R, Jenkins F. Money, money, money: fundamentals of finance. In: Jones R, Jenkins F, editors. *Managing Money, Measurement and Marketing in the Allied Health Professions.* Oxford: Radcliffe Publishing; 2010.

21 Ordinary Least Square: www.ib-net.org/en/Benchmarking-Methodologies/PerformanceBenchmarking-StatisticalTechniques.

22 Porter M, Teisberg E. *Redefining Healthcare.* Boston, MA: Harvard Business School Publishers; 2007.

23 Herzlinger R. *Consumer-Driven Healthcare: implications for providers, payers, and policy-makers.* San Francisco, CA: Jossey-Bass; 2004.

24 Herzlinger R. *Who Killed Healthcare?* New York: McGraw-Hill; 2007.

25 Chilingerian J, Sherman H. Health applications: from hospitals to physicians, from productive efficiency to quality frontiers. In: Cooper W, Seiford M, Zhu J. *Data Envelopment Analysis: theory, methodology and applications.* Toronto: Kluwer Academic Publishers; 2004.

26 Castro P, Dorgan S. Richardson B. A healthier healthcare system for the United Kingdom. *The McKinsey Quarterly.* February 2008.

Chapter 15

Project management for AHPs with real jobs

Janice E Mueller and Ian S Rowe

Overview

Many people struggle with the concept of projects and what a project is. They have a reputation for being big long expensive things that may fail and are generally unpleasant. This chapter sets out some of the reasons people have problems with projects and provides a series of steps designed to help achieve success in projects of any size. It provides an introduction to project management for AHPs outlining the core processes, language and methodology and uses a recognised change management process to explain projects in a logical way, reinforcing these steps with real-life project examples from New Zealand healthcare settings. Finally, the chapter includes a translation table of common project terminology.

Why are projects so difficult?

There is much literature about why projects may not be successful with varied reasons cited. These include a lack of experience, understanding, executive commitment, lack of process, poor planning, doing the wrong project, poor alignment with the organisation's business objectives and failure to recognise the magnitude or complexity of change required.[1, 2, 3, 4] While it is better to learn from projects that succeed rather than the ones that fail, there are only a few real contributors to failure and they are closely linked.

The first major contributor is that people do not know when they should be working in 'project mode' and therefore do not appreciate the impact of the key outcome that projects deliver; which is change. At the end of the project, something important will be done differently from the way it was done previously. For this reason the principles of successful project management are inextricably entwined with the principles of change management.

The second major cause is insufficient practice. Often the first time a project is encountered is in the context of delivering significant change. If the opportunity is taken to first practice on smaller increments of change using project management techniques, there is more chance of success as the scale of change increases.

A project can be anything from a review of a particular clinical policy, through to the implementation of a large new information technology (IT) system, but the basic steps are the same. There is a 'rule of thumb' however; the bigger the project, the more 'fancy tools' and acronyms appear to be required to be successful. It is not the 'tools' or acronyms that make the difference between projects that succeed and those that do not, generally, successful projects have been well planned to achieve the desired outcomes.

What is a project?

Clinicians of all disciplines have an easy way to figure out what is a project and what is not. Clinical work is generally not regarded as project work. For clinicians, working with patients is 'business as usual' (BAU). There are many things that are BAU, for example, treatment, documentation and team meetings. If it is something that is done every day, week or month then it is probably BAU. If an activity is less frequent or does not happen with predictable regularity, or an element of the BAU activity requires change, then treat it as a project and adopt project management techniques.

The key thing to recognise is that the project is likely to change the way the BAU is performed. In summary, when not working on BAU, consider working on a project or having leisure time!

Working on a project is going to change something from the old way to the new and as a specific change can only happen once, every project is different and generally involves many people. This is why it is important to write some key things down. That does not mean a Gantt chart and an issues register are necessarily needed for everything, but it is important to think about things in a systematic way. It means Plan, Execute, Achieve and Review the work.

There are two different stylistic approaches to these four steps. Some would argue that the fastest way to the 'finish line' is to start *Executing* and then repeatedly *Review* the plan on the way. This *Executing for Review* works particularly well when the change is predictable and has been achieved before, but even then there are risks from not having the people affected involved in the process. Alternatively, *Plan to Achieve* sets the scene and direction before *Executing* is started, so there is confidence that the *Execute* tasks are leading closer to the finish line rather than away from it.

Box 15.1 Plan, execute, achieve and review.

Think of a cross country race; should you start running down the first path that looks like it's going in the right direction and then make a decision when you get to the first intersection, or should you get out your map at the start line and figure out the best way to go. *Execute for Review* gives the appearance of progress because you are immediately further away from the start line, but it does not mean you are necessarily closer to the finish.

If it is the first thing you do, then the amount of planning you need to do to achieve the project outcomes becomes apparent. *Plan to Achieve* at the beginning and you may feel that the clock is ticking while you are not *Executing*, however you will find that time spent on the plan reduces the amount of work – and in particular re-work – during the *Execute* phase, and saves a lot of pain and 'soul searching' in the *Review* phase. The plan will

> need to be revised during the *Execute* and *Achieve* phases so the *Plan to Achieve* doesn't need to be perfect before you start to *Execute*. However, you must do enough planning before you start to *Execute* to know that you have the right people doing the right things that are needed to *Achieve*.

Project management and change management

The point of a project is to change something to improve the BAU, so when leading or participating in projects, it is important to develop the 'mindset' of managing the change rather than just managing the project. Kotter commented;

> The most general lesson to be learned from the more successful cases is that the change process goes through a series of phases that, in total, usually require a considerable length of time. Skipping steps creates only the illusion of speed and never produces satisfactory results and making critical mistakes in any of the phases can have a devastating impact, slowing momentum and negating hard-won gains.[5]

He also identified the following steps to achieving successful change:[6]

1 establish a sense of urgency
2 form a powerful guiding coalition
3 create a vision
4 communicate that vision
5 empower others to act on the vision
6 plan for and create short-term wins
7 consolidate improvements and keep the momentum for change moving
8 institutionalise the new approaches.

Table 15.1 links Kotter's steps with the core steps of project management.

Table 15.1 Project management core steps and Kotter's steps of successful change.

Project management steps	Kotter's change management model
Plan the project	Establish a sense of urgency
	Form a powerful guiding coalition
	Create a vision
Execute the project	Communicate that vision
	Empower others to act
	Plan for and create short-term wins
Achieve the desired outcome	Consolidate improvements and keep the momentum for change going
Review the project process and implementation	Institutionalise the new approaches

The authors have used this change management model, applied it and found it to be an extremely valuable 'tool' for achieving successful projects.

> **Editors' note**
>
> In book three of this series, *Key Topics in Healthcare Management – understanding the big picture*, the management of change is explored in detail by the series editors.[7]

Before starting

The first and most important question is 'what do I want to achieve?' It might seem obvious, but getting this wrong is a big problem, yet it happens all too often.

Doing the right project

Surprisingly, this is probably easier in healthcare than in many business environments, because clinical practice has a clear focus – the patient. Most businesses have more challenges around the 'trade-offs' necessary to make the stakeholders feel varying degrees of satisfaction; making the customer happy may not always make the shareholder happy. Generally in healthcare, if the patient is happy then everyone else is satisfied too.

Write down what is planned to be achieved and then think about who this should be shared with. If the project affects patients, co-workers, employers, for example, then it is a good discipline to check if the idea makes sense to them. This is when the first major problem with projects may be encountered; people tend not to like change – especially when it is not their idea – so it is important that conversations start with the benefits of the proposal.

Suppose new chairs are needed for the waiting room. It is better to start a conversation with 'wouldn't it be great if our patients were much happier when we saw them' and get some 'buy in' to the potential benefits rather than to simply request several new chairs 'because they'll make the waiting room look tidier'. Try: 'I find the more relaxed happier patients take five minutes less per consultation than those who are stressed by lack of appropriate seating. So if we improved the seating in the waiting room, I am sure they would be much more comfortable.'

Clearly the benefits first and buy in approach would work better than 'I have found the perfect new chairs for the waiting room'. Staff are inherently problem solvers and are justifiably proud of their ability to come up with a solution, but all too often when presenting change, lead with the solution which has been thought about for some time often with significant emotional attachment. However, because the original recognition of the problem may have been some time ago, they do not convey the sense of urgency for the proposed change. While this may seem a relatively trivial difference in approach, the impact can be extraordinary.

At this stage – assuming the others do not object to the idea – the project has not started, but there are already some of the ingredients to help make the project successful. It is necessary to create a picture about the things that need changing, develop a vision that can be articulated, having first talked to the people who can help achieve it and get 'buy in'. Next declare the need for a project and decide if it's the right time to start.

Box 15.2 Focussing the project – an example.

Ian was appointed as Project Director to a project that was required to implement a software solution; a child immunisation register. The software had been developed by the Ministry of Health (MOH) because the amount of vaccine being deployed only resulted in an immunisation rate of approximately 60%. As a result, vaccine preventable diseases were mutating and children were presenting to GPs with vaccine preventable diseases. The project goal was to implement the software so that the GPs would get reminders about the children they were immunising and the MOH would get information about the GPs who had low immunisation rates.

Rather than just implement the software, the project team reviewed what the project was aiming to achieve. It transpired that the GPs did an excellent job of immunising the children they knew about; the problems occurred when the GPs didn't find out about the children until the first time they were sick. They would then ask if the children's vaccinations were up to date, the answer to this was invariably 'yes' because the caregivers were not experts at knowing which vaccinations their child had received.

The goal of the project was changed to focus on sharing information to increase the immunisation rate. Staff were employed in the hospital to inform the parents of the need for immunisation and when they were due, the parents were also requested to nominate a GP to be responsible for their immunisation and the software was changed from reporting and task management to messaging and information sharing. The GPs then followed up the immunisation and the child's nominated GP was advised even if another provider did the actual immunisation. Doing the right project resulted in an immunisation rate in excess of 90%.

What to do and when to start

Despite being very busy, people have good ideas and sometimes these occur when at their busiest, but it does not always make sense to act on them straight away. For this reason, maintain a Project Register, a list of the good ideas and their benefits is still worthwhile. When things are less busy, start the project. If it never gets less busy bring in extra resources to help make the changes and deliver these benefits. If the list of project ideas is long and the associated benefits are big, find a way to deliver them.

Do not start too many projects at once. Change always takes more effort and time than anticipated. Being well prepared includes thinking of all the things that need to be done and then thinking of all the things that can go wrong and try to allow for them. Think of the Project Register as a 'parking lot' with one entry and two exits (*see* Figure 15.1). All good ideas must go through the entry into the 'parking lot', then as a separate process, the project lead and team should review the Project Register – on a regular basis or whenever a new idea is 'parked'- and choose the best idea to take out through the implementation exit, 'get started'. While reviewing the register, look for ideas that have been around for a long time, or are no longer practical and take them out through the other exit, the one

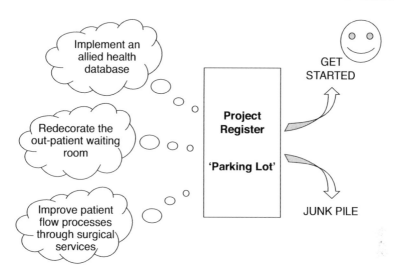

Figure 15.1 The project register.

marked 'junkyard'. It is important to recognise the need for appropriate timing and start with energy, enthusiasm and sufficient capacity to see the project through.

Plan the project

Having worked out what needs to be achieved and found the time to start, a plan is required. This should be written, and could be anything from a simple task list assigned to people, through to a complex Gantt chart with milestones and dependencies. There are two other important things at this stage; establishing a Risk Register and an Issues Register.

The plan

The project plan is a list of tasks that need to be done in order to *Achieve* (see Table 15.2). For small projects this can be a simple list of the things to do that get ticked off as they get done. For larger projects, some tasks depend on primary tasks being completed first. Tracking these dependencies and making sure that things happen in the right order is one of the skills that needs to be accomplished starting with small projects before taking on the big ones, and this is where some of the more expensive 'tools' start to become useful. There is not scope in this chapter to explore all aspects of running large projects, suffice it to say, learn about these 'tools' before embarking on large projects.

Risk register

Projects are often viewed as daunting and a lot of things can go wrong, however many people imagine an even greater number of pitfalls. The risk register is a good place to record potential problems and the control measures. It does not make sense to have tasks in the plan purely on the assumption that everything

Table 15.2 Example plan.

	Task	Who	When	Done
1	Measure waiting room	Peter	Tuesday	(X)
2	Work out number of chairs	Me	Wednesday	(_)
3	Request catalogue	Peter	Today	(X)
4	Review catalogue	Me and John	Thursday	(_)
5	Visit showroom	Me and John	Friday	(_)
	Trial			
6	Get three different chairs on approval	Peter	Next Week	(_)
7	Try for one week	Patients	Next Week	(_)
8	Get feedback	Peter and Reception	Next Week	(_)
9	Select a chair	Me and John	Next Week	(_)
	Buy			
10	Place order	Peter	Week 3	(_)

will go wrong. If these problems arise, having worked out strategies beforehand can be helpful. It is also important to have somewhere to record the risks and worries that people identify. By recording these, they are acknowledged and less likely to be a barrier to change, without necessarily having to deal with them before *Execution* continues. Having the ability to receive a risk point and record it, making it visible, is a key step in empowering and valuing others. Start 'populating' the Risk Register as soon as the project commences (*see* Table 15.3).

Table 15.3 Risk register example.

	Risk	Likelihood (1–3)	Impact (1–3)	Size	Mitigation
1	We cannot fit more chairs in	3	3	9	We will measure the room before looking at chairs
2	We get the wrong chairs	2	3	6	We will try several chairs for a week and get user views
3	We cannot afford the chairs we want	1	3	3	Budget agreed prior to project commencement

Issues register

It is not surprising that some projects do not go smoothly or exactly follow the sequence of tasks envisaged. Some of the things that could go wrong will go wrong and some things that cannot possibly go wrong will also conspire to do so. The Issues Register (*see* Table 15.4) is a way of dealing with these, capturing problems that arise while the project is in progress. When leading a project, it is not the project leader's role to fix everything that does not go to plan, but it is the leader's role to ensure that someone does get them fixed. Have a list of issues, record the things that happen that were not planned and assign responsibility and authority to someone to deal with the issue.

Start the Issues Register when beginning the project, at which point there should be no issues. Make sure everyone knows that if anything does not go according to plan it must be recorded in the Issues Register so that either the Project Manager or Guiding Coalition can do something about it. This helps stop people taking action independently.

Table 15.4 Issues register.

	Issue	Priority 1–3	Action	Who
1	The best chairs are more than our budget	1	Get approval for extra funds	John
2				

Establish a sense of urgency

When making change, establish a sense of urgency, do it now and do it right. If you do not, it is hard to get other people to 'buy in' to change and problems may not be solved immediately. If it is not possible to establish a sense of urgency the project may have come out of the 'parking lot' too soon. Even if there is no sense of urgency about the change itself, remember this task may have to be completed before taking the next one out; you cannot take them all out at once so there needs to be some form of rationing or prioritisation.

> **Box 15.3 A worked example.**
>
> In the early 2000s, a large District Health Board went through a major redevelopment and organisational change programme to improve facilities, merging four separate hospitals into one integrated acute hospital and a separate ambulatory care facility. The goal for the change programme team was to re-design business processes to improve patient flows and re-organise clinical staff to deliver high quality clinical care. The building programme focussed on building a major tertiary hospital and migrating patients, services and staff to the new facility.[1]
>
> The change programme was challenging for the organisation as there had never been the magnitude of change across the organisation previously. When planning commenced for the building of the new hospital, several attempts were made to start the change processes that staff would need to maximise the functions of their new facility, but these were unsuccessful. There was a sense of complacency across the organisation that they were the best at what they did and these skills would take then easily into the new facility, without the need for any significant change.
>
> Two years prior to the planned move date, the organisation finally developed its 'sense of urgency'. Although senior management and the project teams knew they needed to focus on changing their practice models to optimise the function of their planned new facility, when the staff finally saw the new hospital being built, the denial was halted and there was a

> better understanding and motivation that the move and associated change was inevitable. At all levels of the organisation, from the Chief Executive to the nurse on the ward, the 'sense of urgency' took hold. The separate projects within the change programme all 'ramped up' a gear, with staff listening when data and evidence was produced to support the need for change. The organisation finally prepared for the move, 'Without an organisation-wide sense of urgency, it's like trying to build a pyramid on a foundation of empty shoeboxes'.[1]

Form a powerful guiding coalition

Every word in this heading is important.

- *Form* – make a new guiding coalition, do not assume that the group of people who worked on the last successful project are right for this one. There may be other people more affected by the proposed change who need to participate.
- *A* – only one. The 'buck' stops here, there is no confusion over who is in charge or where to go in relation to this change.
- *Powerful* – means full of power within the context of the change. The coalition should either contain at least one member with delegated authority or the coalition itself should be specifically 'blessed' with the power.
- *Guiding* – is different from steering. Remember at the outset it is acknowledged that there is an acceptable good idea with sufficient benefits to proceed. As implementation progresses everyone learns. The coalition is there to guide, give direction and provide resources. The term Steering Committee implies that the people on the committee are in charge of the direction, rather than guiding the exploration of different directions.
- *Coalition* – is an alliance among individuals during which they co-operate in joint action, each in their own self-interest. This alliance may be temporary or for convenience.[1] It is important to distinguish between stakeholders and shareholders. One person can be both, but take care to balance coalition so that the shareholders dominate. The coalition will exist for the period of the change, it de-personalises the impact of the proposal to change. It is no longer about one person's idea. The project becomes about a group of people trying to deliver a benefit and there must be opportunity for those affected by the change to come to the coalition for a constructive discussion on how the benefits are to be realised. It might seem trivial to form this group for minor changes, but even in small projects, thinking about who is affected and getting them working as a team will make a huge difference to the adoption and acceptance of change.

Create a vision

It is imperative that others – particularly those affected by the change, understand and 'buy in' to the project quickly. To do this a vision statement is required. This needs to be something that describes the destination more than the process and it is a picture of the future that is easy to communicate, elicit understanding and interest. Kotter[2] suggested that leaders should be able to communicate the vision in five minutes. If not, they should re-work the vision.

Moore's[4] elevator test helps thinking about how to tell someone about a project in the time it takes to get to your floor in an elevator. The vision should communicate the purpose of the project quickly and clearly. The following format may be helpful:

I am working on (or leading) the................project for..................(briefly describe the target of change, the practice or groups of patients) who want...............(briefly describe one or two major benefits). We are changing...................(describe the major one or two the things that are changing that used to be)...................(old state) to be.................(new state).

Box 15.4 Example of an elevator test vision statement.

I am working on the Kidslink project for the children of South Auckland to reduce the number of children presenting with vaccine preventable diseases. We are sharing birth information from the hospital to primary care so that the GPs know when the babies are born and they can then follow up their immunisations. We are aiming for an immunisation rate of 90% compared to the current rate which is less than 60%. We have found that enabling the GPs to contact the WellChild providers helps them to reach out to the children who have moved.

This vision statement is more likely to receive a positive response from shareholders than, 'I am working on a web based immunisation register written in java' which neither describes the destination nor the benefits.

Communicate the vision

Kotter suggested that leaders should estimate how much communication of the vision is needed and then multiply that effort by a factor of ten. Both stakeholders and shareholders have expectations and these are generally more than the project is able to deliver, despite a great project structure and communication plan. For small projects communicating with both groups can be straightforward. With larger projects communication needs to be more structured to ensure all stakeholders and shareholders receive the right information and can contribute to the project as required.

Who are the stakeholders and shareholders? They are the important people that need to be communicated with to achieve the desired project outcomes. Stakeholders are those who have a 'vested interest' – which may be explicit or implicit – in the project and tend to want to protect the status quo. Shareholders are those who 'invest now' for the future benefits of the project. This does not mean that either group always needs to agree, but that all of the people who are important to the project need to be kept informed and updated about progress, otherwise they may influence the outcomes in potentially adverse ways.

Box 15.5 Handling shareholders and stakeholders.

Stakeholders and shareholders need careful handling – let's say your project is the review of the AHP supervision policy. The first group of stakeholders/shareholders are the people that you can easily identify will be affected by the project outcome: the AHPs themselves, their managers and supervisors; some may be external to the organisation. Other groups will emerge and interested in the project and its outcomes and will also need consideration. The project may potentially have a direct or indirect outcome on them or you need to think of the wider implications of the project for the organisation, will this increase the budget required for training or the need for external supervision? What will the impact be on productivity? Communicating with stakeholders who may have a high level of influence regarding the project outcomes but relatively low levels of interest, will be different from communicating with the AHPs and managers who will be directly affected and influenced by the policy change.

A stakeholder plan (*see* Table 15.5) may be useful. Consider the actual and potential stakeholders and shareholders; identify the benefits and risks from their perspectives; rate these risks and identify appropriate communication strategies to convey the benefits and mitigate risks.

Empower others to act the vision

This is where the strength of the powerful Guiding Coalition comes in. It is often hard for people to accept change. It may be easier to continue doing things the old way. If a sense of urgency is created around a clearly articulated Vision whilst not empowering others to act on the Vision, people will feel conflict, they will know there is a problem and want to do something about it. The powerful Guiding Coalition must seek out and remove the obstacles that could prevent people from acting on the vision and provide guidance so that everyone is working on the same solution. The coalition's approach may be about providing extra resources so that people have the time to work through the change. It may need to remove financial or structural barriers to change; and often it may just give permission to change. The coalition should empower others to act, sets direction, boundaries and guides rather steers.

Project execution

Plan and create short-term wins

Now is the time to start doing 'do' things. There are two major advantages to this approach. The change is introduced gradually, just like starting off on a low dose of medication. It can be tested, monitored for unwanted side effects and adjusted as necessary. If the early change – introducing a few new chairs in the waiting room – works, then increase the intervention; buy more chairs. This approach

Project management for AHPs with real jobs **223**

Table 15.5 Stakeholder plan to review the allied health supervision policy.

Stakeholder	Benefits (Of a successful project)	Risks (If the project is not successful)	Influence (1–5)	Interest (1–5)	Rating (Who requires the most active management?)	Information/management strategy (How will you manage expectations and what do they need to know?)	Responsibility
AHPs	Clear supervision policy	Lack of supervision with potential clinical and personal risks for AHPs	3	5	15	Involve in the policy review Consult on proposed changes Organisation processes to formally communicate/evaluate proposed policy change	Project manager, team members
AHP professional leaders	Clear supervision policy	Potential practice and competence issues Inconsistent organisational behaviour regarding supervision	4	5	20	See above	Project manager, team members
Managers of AHPs	Regularly supervised and competent staff delivering patient care Clear budget and time implications for training	Potential practice and competence issues Training requirements unable to be met	4	3	12	See above	Project manager
Learning and development manager	Will understand training requirements and potential budget/staff impact on trainers	Will not have the resource to implement the policy	3	4	12	See above	Project manager
Director of nursing	Nil	May get nurses asking why they can't have dedicated time for supervision	4	2	18	Regular 1:1 meetings with project manager to consider potential flow on impacts for nurses of the policy, especially where there are multidisciplinary teams	Project manager, project sponsor
Lawyer (medico-legal)	Policy meets privacy and confidentiality requirements	Potential organisational risk exposure	4	2	8	Utilise at key consultation points to ensure policy complies with legislative requirements	Project manager

also 'unlocks' some of the benefits early in the project, creating a sense of success and enthusiasm that reduces the potential adverse impact of future increments of change.

Consolidate improvements and keep momentum for change

- *Keep planning* – as progress is made, tick off the tasks that are completed and consider if new tasks need adding or adjust timelines. Estimating how long things are likely to improve with practice. Generally most projects are better served by spending more time to deliver all the intended benefits, rather than to do things to meet an arbitrary deadline and not deliver. If starting with a sense of urgency and a clear vision, it is often found that instead of losing time or delivering less, people will rally round to work harder to deliver success.
- *Review the risks* – present the risk register at each project meeting, but do not always discuss it. Having the register as a record of what could go wrong and what is being done about it helps people to focus on what they should be doing rather than worrying about what they could be doing. Having the register at the meeting is usually enough to refresh the need to manage these risks.
- *Handle the issues* – the register should be visible to the whole team and reviewed regularly to make sure that the issues are being addressed. Make sure everyone knows that if anything does not go according to plan, it needs to be recorded in the Issues Register so that either the Project Manager or Guiding Coalition can allocate resources and effort to do something about it. This prevents action being taken by individuals at the expense of the tasks they should be doing.
- *Keep communicating* – never assume that people ever fully understand what is expected of them or know what is wanted. Keep the communication flowing throughout the project. Share the important items of the plan, Issues Register and Risk Register with the powerful Guiding Coalition and they will continue to help remove the barriers to change. Communicate with the empowered project team on what has been accomplished, what remains to be done and who is working on the issues, as it will give them the confidence and enthusiasm to work on their own tasks. Celebrate success and publish short term 'wins'. When things are not going to plan make sure they are handled as issues or risks and are communicated to resolve them, rather than allowing people to assume that issues imply failure and a halt to progress.
- *Summary* – managing a project is largely about starting the right project with the right people at the right time. It includes managing lists; the list of tasks that need to be done to achieve the vision – Project Plan – the list of things that could go wrong – Risk Register – and what could be done if they do, and the list of things that have not gone according to plan and who is responsible for fixing them – Issues Register.

Institutionalise the new approaches

One of the most important aspects of projects is knowing how and when to stop. Having started and maintained a sense of urgency it is easier to stop when a team has worked well together to bring about a successful change. The right time to stop is when the benefits are achieved as much as they reasonably can be and the change is part of the BAU. The other time to stop is when the cost of continuing is greater than the benefits that can be achieved, having checked the original vision with the people who are affected by the change. It is better to stop and if necessary start again with a new project, rather than change the vision in the middle.

It is important at this point to disband the Coalition with an appropriate level of ceremony and celebration. When disbanding reflect on the project and what has been learnt, making sure any positive ideas are captured in your Project Register. Then revisit the Project Register, pull the next project out of the 'parking lot', form a new powerful Guiding Coalition with a new sense of urgency and enthusiasm for the next project and get started.

Help! I have been put on a project...what do I do?

One of the problems with some large projects is that often people on the project team are 'project people'. It is important to realise that 'project people' do not have a 'real job', they just do projects. Generally, the more projects they have done, the more they are likely to take project work for granted. This is compounded if there are lots of project people involved because they will start talking in 'project speak' and forget that people who have 'real' BAU jobs may not understand the jargon. Table 15.6 includes an explanation of much of the common project management jargon.

First of all, make sure that you are on the 'right project', and to do that you need to understand what the planned outcome is. There could be a bundle of documents that add up to a 'Plan to Achieve'. Look for the following documents: vision statement; project charter; statement of work and so on, which will need studying. If the *Plan to Achieve* is not obvious from these documents, find another project or suddenly discover a lot of BAU that is more important than the project!

Identify who the project manager is and understand the role(s) assigned. Think about the risk and review the Risk Register, complete tasks on time, contribute to the project team meetings, raise issues when necessary even if you think you can resolve them and celebrate success at the completion of the project. That is all there is to it!

How to structure a large project

Large projects need to be broken down into smaller chunks or work streams in a way that contributes to the overall outcome required of the project. Each work stream must be clearly scoped and defined to be an appropriate size so that:

- the right leaders for each work stream can be identified
- the work can to be done
- the correct skills and resources can be sourced and applied
- all stakeholders clearly know what they are engaging in.

Consider a number of allied health quality improvement projects have been identified in the organisation. Clearly the work in this project cannot be achieved without leadership and project structure to ensure completion on time. The example of a major allied health quality improvement project involving multiple services across a large healthcare organisation is illustrated.

Table 15.6 Common project management jargon.

Term	What it is	What it is not
BAU (business as usual)	What you normally do	Working on a defined project or secondment
Communication plan	List of people you need to communicate with outlining how and when you plan to communicate with them	A plan of what to say, just to whom and when
Gantt chart	A way of presenting and illustrating a project plan	A crystal ball view of how things will actually occur. A way of working out when the last 10% will be done
Issues register	List of things that you didn't expect to encounter and that people are worried about. Everyone on the project needs to be able to raise issues and the project manager is responsible to allocating someone to do something about them	The end of the world
Project administrator	A person who, on larger projects, assists the project manager by looking after the paperwork and routine tasks, leaving the project manager to focus on making the change happen	Administrators who are fixated on just the paperwork
Project brief	A document that should set out what the project plans to achieve	Brief
Project charter	A document that sets out what the project plans to achieve	A trip on a boat!
Project management office	A group of people whose BAU is helping other people run projects. Generally they have experience in multiple projects and can help you with some of the tools	Project police who only tell you when you get it wrong
Project manager	The person who looks after the project plan and worries about who is going to do what and when they are going to finish	Superman!
Project plan	A list of tasks that are arranged and rearranged into a sensible order and assign to people	A crystal ball view of how things will actually occur
Project/programme director	A person who keeps an eye on multiple projects and provides 'direction'. Their role may be to ensure that the multiple projects do not produce conflicting outcomes. The director is usually an experienced project manager who can also advise on project processes that work	Project police!
Project team	People who do the work, with relevant experience and knowledge from the work area	Team of people brought in from elsewhere to do the work
Risk register	List of things that might go wrong and the strategy for managing them	Complete at the outset
Shareholder	A person who is prepared to invest in the changes needed to achieve the benefits	Stakeholder

Subject matter expert	A person with a 'real' job, who is expected to contribute to the project, often without being told what is expected of them	An expert in a different 'field'
Stakeholder	A person who has history, responsibility or any other vested interest in the current way of things	Shareholder
Steering committee	Powerful guiding coalition made up of shareholders who are 'investing' in achieving change	Effective if stakeholders are allowed to dominate over shareholders
Task dependencies	Some tasks must be completed before it makes sense to start the next one	Little tasks that cost lots of money
Terms of reference	A document that should set out what the project plans to achieve	A list of either terms or references
Working group	A meeting of people who have 'real' jobs	People not working on the project

---

Box 15.6 Allied health quality improvement project.

The project included a number of smaller, linked projects that all required specific activity to ensure the overall project goal was achieved. A detailed project structure was used (*see* Figure 15.2) which included four separate work streams.

The project sponsor was the Director of Allied Health, the organisation's most senior AHP position who was accountable to the Chief Executive. The steering group comprised a currently existing group that was representative of staff and managers to avoid unnecessary additional meetings. Group members received training regarding the roles and responsibilities of a steering group. The steering group:
- provided support and guidance to the sponsor
- assisted with decision-making and conflict resolution as required
- assisted with project communication
- took ownership of the project desired outcomes.

Each work stream was led by either a team leader or professional leader. They:
- were accountable for achieving project objectives
- managed the project process within their work stream
- built an effective team, supporting and guiding team members through their work
- ensured communication and change management processes were carried out effectively
- resolved issues and conflict – or escalated as necessary
- reported progress via the steering group to the project sponsor on a regular basis.

The work stream teams were made up of practitioners, discipline-specific professional leaders, managers and union representatives. Practitioners were from key areas across the organisation where the work streams would have impact and they remained on the teams until project completion. They:
- completed specific tasks within the agreed quality parameters and timeframes

- were accountable for the outcomes of their individual work stream
- communicated and consulted with key stakeholders to assist with robust solution finding and change management
- reported progress regularly to their project leader
- escalated project risks to their project leader.

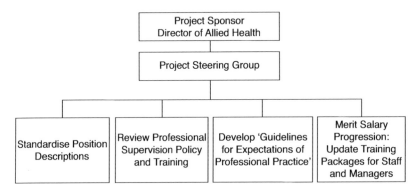

Figure 15.2 Allied Health Quality Improvement Project.

This quality improvement project was complex in that it involved multiple disciplines and teams across the organisation that needed to agree on common policy, processes, recommended guidelines and training requirements. Each work stream had its own inherent complexity and the selection of work stream leaders by the project sponsor from interested individuals was critical to the overall project success.

The work stream leaders needed to be genuinely interested in completing the activity and able to inspire and lead each team to complete all tasks. They needed good leadership, negotiation and collaboration skills to stay focussed, meet deadlines and gain consensus from multiple professions across several practice environments. Each work stream leader needed to obtain support from practitioners, their managers and leaders throughout the process, so that the desired quality improvements could be embedded across the organisation.

Examples of these challenges included:

- how to word a 'position description' so that the purpose statement of the inter-professional team and the resulting key accountabilities made sense and was agreed by all affected disciplines
- how to reflect different discipline-specific requirements for supervision in one organisation-wide policy
- deciding whether training needed to be provided in-house or purchased from external providers
- agreeing the expected level of practice and salary 'step' for all disciplines regarding key common activities such as cultural responsiveness, undergraduate education and undertaking clinical audit
- training practitioners and managers to write appropriate salary progression objectives.

The project outcomes were all achieved, although there was significant time slippage in the supervision policy review work stream, frustrating staff who wanted the policy reviewed and updated promptly. The establishment of training requirements and gaining agreement about funding sources that were affordable for the organisation and still met practitioners' needs took many months of consultation and negotiation. Until this was agreed, the policy could not be finally signed off.

Conclusion

This chapter sets out some of the thinking processes, techniques and 'tools' for successful project outcomes. There is a high level of satisfaction when the benefits from a change that you have 'orchestrated', despite the obstacles and barriers has been successfully achieved. This chapter cannot give you the practice that leads to confidence. Start on small changes that affect few people and follow Kotter's principles of change, *Plan* to *Achieve* before you *Execute* and remember to *Review*, celebrate and learn.

AHPs need to learn the language and discipline of project management, they are already good at team working, particularly inter-professional teams. The ability to work successfully in, and lead teams, is essential skill that will promote success in project environments. AHPs understand how to make teams work and are generally problem solvers and very solution focussed, which can contribute to achieving project goals.

If you are interested in working in a range of organisational projects and 'adding value' as an AHP, then developing technical knowledge and understanding about project management to complement clinical skills will be invaluable. Have confidence in your skills, practice using the 'tools' and techniques whenever possible and above all, have fun.

References

1 Staw B, Ross J. Knowing when to pull the plug. Classic reading. *Harvard Bus Rev.* 1987; March–April: 6564–660.
2 Kotter JP. Leading change: why transformational change efforts fail. *Harvard Bus Rev.* 1995; March–April: 1–20.
3 Obeng E. *The Project Leader's Secret Handbook – all change!* London: Hickman Publishing; 1994.
4 Frigenti E, Comninos D. Reasons for failure and guidelines for success. In: Frigenti E, Comninos D, editors. *The Practice of Project Management: a guide to the business-focused approach.* London: Kogan Page; 2002.
5 Coutts P. Book Review: 'Leading Change'. *Harvard Bus Rev.* 1995; March–April: 1–20: www.coutts.name/Other%20Documents/%25PDF-Kotter.pdf.
6 Potter JP. *Leading Change.* Boston, MA: Harvard Business School Press; 1996.
7 Jones R, Jenkins F. *Key Topics in Healthcare Management – understanding the big picture.* Oxford: Radcliffe Publishing; 2006.
8 Mueller JE, Neads P. Allied health and organization structure: massaging the organisation to facilitate outcomes. *NZ J Physiother.* 1995: **33(2)**: 48–54.
9 McLaughlin MW. *Meet the masterminds: John Kotter on how change is coming*: www.managementconsultingnews.com/interviews/kotter_interview.php.

10 en.wikipedia.org/wiki/Coalition.
11 Moore GA. *Crossing the Chasm*. Rev ed. New York: Harper Business; 1999.
12 Prince 2: www.prince2.com/what-is-prince2.asp.

Further reading

- For those working in the UK NHS, the recommended approach to management of large projects is PRINCE 2.[12]

Chapter 16

Marketing for AHPs

Julian Glover

Introduction

One thing is for sure, you did not become a therapist, radiographer or paramedic to run a business and market your services. After all, business and marketing is for the likes of Virgin and Coca Cola, is it not?

Ten, 20 or 30 years ago, as a health practitioner you trained and qualified in your chosen profession. Patients turned up at your door, you treated them using your skills, they were grateful and went home happy – job done. Despite the fact that they had been told to see you, had little or no medical knowledge of their condition or your skills, and arguably, had limited or misguided expectations of the outcome. Since then, by degrees of stealth, patients have become customers and health provision has become big business. Today, there are products, markets, tariffs and prices just as with any other commercial business. Patients are far more aware of their needs, their rights and what you will do for them and often have high, if not impossible expectations.

As healthcare provision is now big business, so marketing has become an important part of contemporary healthcare services and is one of many traditional business disciplines of which AHPs and other healthcare professionals are expected to have a sound practical working knowledge. They all have to be aware of what their patients want, the costs involved and how to deliver a high quality customer service at a profit – in addition to providing good clinical care.

As marketing is an intrinsic part of business, so branding is an intrinsic part of marketing. Although it is more commonly associated with the high street retailers, branding is a useful 'tool' used by businesses and other organisations, including healthcare, to help deliver good quality products and services to people.

The object of this chapter is to give an overview and some understanding of the core essence of marketing and branding and how they can be related to the healthcare professions, rather than being an in depth tutorial in all aspects of marketing and branding,

So, what is marketing?

When people are asked what marketing is, they usually volunteer a number of words and phrases such as, selling, advertising, promotion and so on. None of these are 'wrong', they all refer correctly to different facets of what is a broad and wide ranging business discipline that touches on every area of an organisation, irrespective of size and sphere of operation. To help understand what marketing is at its simplest level and to understand how marketing works, it is useful to look at the definition given by the Chartered Institute of Marketing.[1]

> The management process responsible for identifying, anticipating and satisfying customer requirements profitably.

As a definition, it is simple and straightforward, and at first sight would appear relevant only to businesses involved in commercial sales transactions to make a financial profit. However, if we break it down and investigate the terminology in more detail we can see that it can be applied equally well to the healthcare profession. If we look at the key words 'customer', 'requirements' and 'profitably', these would superficially appear to relate exclusively to commercial profit making, but in reality they have application in non-commercial and other not-for-profit organisations and beyond.

Customers

The most important word in the Chartered Institute of Marketing[1] definition and for any business, is 'customer'. It is a common enough term, but what exactly is a customer? For commercial businesses it is straightforward – they are the people who purchase their goods and services. They spend money with a business and in exchange, that business gives them something in return – petrol, apples, a photocopier, legal advice, dentistry and so on.

There are two aspects of this to consider; firstly many non-commercial businesses and organisations have customers but are often referred to by another name, and secondly, the exact nature of what constitutes a customer, is not as straightforward as might first appear.

So who are customers? Superficially that is easy. Sainsbury's has customers, BT has customers. A charity shop has customers who are people buying new and second-hand goods. But, if in that charity shop there are people who do not buy anything but put some money in to a collecting tin on the counter, then they are not customers but are donors. However, if they have bought something and then put the change in the tin, then are they donors and customers? This may appear straightforward but it might be a little harder to make the distinction. For example, a customer of the shop buys a second-hand book because they want to read it, but there may well also be a desire to support that charity's aims. Are they then a customer or donor? Making a donation can be thought of as a transaction where the donor exchanges money in return for something – a combination of moral well being and a desire to help the charity towards achieving its aims. This is an exchange or transaction in just the same way as is buying a book.

The concept of a customer can be extended further. Universities exchange students' fees for ideas, education, facilities and so on, and are now very much more aware that students are customers who, in many cases are able to 'shop around' for a university place. Other organisations have already made the leap to using the term customers – many will no doubt remember a time when rail travellers were called passengers.

Similarly the Police service could call the victims of crime its customers. By preventing crime, issuing speeding tickets, by controlling crowds, by investigating fraud, they work for the overall good of the population of their region, or even the country, who can be termed its customers. Considering a transaction as a financial exchange, the transaction is not between the public – unless you count traffic fines! – it is with the Police Authority. It could also be argued that the Police transact with the Home Office and the Government and extrapolated further to include Parliament, the electorate and the tax payer; which leads back in some ways, ultimately back to the general public. Therefore, defining who exactly are the customers of the Police Service can be difficult – is it the victims, the public, local residents, voters, taxpayers or the Home Secretary?

For exactly the same reasons it can be equally difficult for health professionals to identify who are their customers. At the simplest level it is the patient, but if you consider who exactly the transactions or exchanges are with, then it is not quite so simple. For example, a hospital nurse might say it is the patient in the hospital bed, however, a paediatric nurse might say it is the child and their parents, guardians or carers. An elderly care nurse caring for an Alzheimer's patient might not only think of the patient as their customer, but also the patient's children, or their spouse. However, if the customer it is the person actually paying, then is the customer the person who holds the cheque book: the purchaser/commissioner, the insurance company, the health trust or authority, the DH, the Government, the tax payer and so forth?

This leads to a fundamental question, who is the organisation transacting with and with whom is the exchange?

Customers or consumers?

In its simplest form the easiest way to understand this is to examine the difference between a customer and a consumer. A customer is generally regarded as the buyer or purchaser of the product or service, whereas the consumer is the person who uses or consumes the product. Clearly, the distinction between customer and consumer varies enormously. For example, if you purchase and eat a sandwich you are customer and consumer. The choice of bread and filling will – usually – be down to your own personal preferences and your own taste. If you purchase a sandwich on behalf of another person, you are still the customer but they are the consumer and you will – probably – consider that person's requirements and preferences. On other occasions, however, you may have to make those decisions on behalf of the person and anticipate or even dictate their requirements in their absence. People shopping in a supermarket making the purchases are customers and will often be buying not only for themselves, but for others – families, friends, house mates. Each individual customer will have a unique and personal set of purchase criteria and requirements to meet – budget, healthy eating, diet foods, treats, routine purchases for themselves and for others. Thus it can be difficult to distinguish between the customer and consumer.

In the non-commercial sector this distinction also applies. For the Police service, a victim of crime being attended to by the police is perhaps better referred to as a consumer. But, if they pay the taxes that fund the Police service are they also entitled to call themselves a customer? If so, do they have different requirements such as value for money or cost saving measures? What if that victim is a Member of Parliament, or a member of the Police Authority or even the Home Secretary? What about where an offender is a tax payer, Police Authority member or Home Secretary?

This concept can be extended to healthcare. A rugby player paying for a physiotherapy session at a private clinic to treat a sports injury is both customer and consumer. What if he has been referred to an NHS clinic for free – is he the customer or is it the Government? What if he is a student and not a tax payer, or what if he is the Chairman of the Local Health Trust? What if he is a member of a club that pays for such treatment? In a private hospital, a patient may be the customer and consumer, or is the patient the consumer and the customer their insurance company? But if the patient is the customer of the insurance company who ultimately calls the shots?

Faced with this argument, a healthcare professional might argue that the type, level and quality of service provided is determined by the purchaser and is therefore, the customer. They might then feel that they have no need to consider the views or opinions of the consumer or patient!

Another group to consider are those people who take decisions on behalf of others but are neither paying for it – that is a customer – nor using the goods or service purchased – that is a consumer. For example, the purchase of a new train will be influenced and made by accountants, purchasing officers, engineers, and possibly even by drivers. The consumers of the train, the rail passengers will more than likely have no say in the supplier of the train either as fare paying customers or rail travelling consumers. Similarly, in healthcare, this can be likened to a parent requesting an MMR injection for their child, or a daughter or son arranging end of life care for a parent or elderly relative suffering from severe Alzheimer's; neither patient has the capacity or ability to make their own judgements or decisions. In another example, a hospital needs a new X-ray machine. The hospital trust is the customer and the patients are the consumers. But the patient will have had no say in the equipment's specification or supplier, and none in the purchase process. It is the radiographer who actually uses the machine and may even have had an influence on the choice of manufacturer or specification. They are not the customer but are they the consumer?

This shows that identifying who are the customers and consumers, can not only be difficult, but can have important implications as both groups could have very different expectations and requirements and may need to be treated and communicated with in very different ways.

Requirements

Following on from this, the second term in the definition to bear investigation is 'requirements'. It is frequently equated with the more general business term 'products'. Again at the straightforward commercial level, the customers' – or consumers' – requirements will be the products on offer from that organisation. In most cases, products are the goods and services that are a means to an end. These can be anything from coal to a concept. For example, cars are 'goods' that are a means of moving people from A to B. In this sense, a 20-year-old second-hand Skoda performs exactly the same function as a brand new Rolls Royce. But what if it was a 20-year-old Rolls Royce and a brand new Skoda? Although both perform the same basic function, some people are willing pay large amounts of money for a Rolls Royce. They pay not only to be transported from A to B, but for the emotional experience of owning, driving and being seen in a Rolls Royce.

An interesting question to consider in this case would be that if you had the magic power to allow people to travel from A to B in an instant, would all cars then become superfluous? How would this affect Grand Prix racing cars, vintage cars and classic cars? Clearly, in this case, there is more to the good than it being 'just a car'.

A service operates in the same way. A restaurant meal will satisfy the basic objective need of being hungry; but that can be easily achieved by eating a sandwich at home. A restaurant is therefore offering more than just the physical or objective need to satisfy a hunger, it also has to be meeting a more subjective need.

Thus requirements can also be taken as a more subjective need – the expectations or needs of a customer or consumer. The requirements of the donors or customers of a charity will be that charity's efforts to work towards achieving its aims of the alleviation of poverty, injustice or cruelty. The requirement of someone telephoning 999 will be the police, fire or ambulance service's response to a problem. In terms of healthcare, the requirements will vary for patient or carer. They may be the alleviation of medical condition, the long term well being of themselves, another person or a group of people, or support with caring for a person.

Just as patients will have physical and psychological requirements, there are others who also have requirements of the health service. The Government, the PCT and the media will have their own set of needs or requirements; be they meeting targets or the use of the NHS as political capital.

Goods and services

It is useful at this stage to look at what makes up requirements and in particular, the distinction in products between goods or services.

Goods and services are distinguished by four general but linked and overlapping characteristics.

1 Intangibility – a service has no physical presence and cannot be seen, touched, or smelt. Neither can it be possessed. For example, it is not possible to physically touch an insurance policy – you can touch the certificate or schedule but they are only paper and not the service itself! Although a medical examination may be felt, the overall experience and skill of the healthcare professional, their diagnosis, discussion and consultation cannot be touched.
2 Inseparability – a service is consumed as soon as it is produced. For example a haircut is consumed as it is produced. In the same way, an Occupational Therapy session can only happen with the patient present and so is consumed as it is produced.
3 Perishability – a service cannot be stored and only exists at the time as it is consumed. A train journey to Manchester cannot be kept for use later. You might catch a later train, but that is not the original service. A session of physiotherapy cannot be given after the patient has left, nor can it be wrapped up and sent to a patient and the patient cannot carry it home. However, the patient might have exercises to do at home but in this case the service is the assessment and programme and not the exercises themselves and is a different separate service.

4 Heterogeneity – services are usually produced by people and it is impossible to give exactly the same service or experience to different people time after time. There are infinite variations in quality, timing and standards, although they may only be minuscule, which makes each service delivery totally unique. By the same token, one patient cannot receive exactly the same treatment twice and neither can they receive exactly the same service as another patient. Even if the treatments are identical, one patient's experience of that treatment may be totally different from another. Sometimes the differences may be tiny, but they are nonetheless different.

Because a service cannot be held, kept or touched, assessing the quality of a service can be difficult. It is possible to assess objective data such as waiting times, numbers of patients seen or infection rates but it is far more difficult to assess the subjective quality of the service. Perhaps a simple way to understand this is to look at your colleagues. You may be a similar age, have the same job, same qualifications and have a similar background to your colleagues, but if you ask for their favourite piece of music, holiday or TV programme the answers will likely be very different.

People are resourceful and find ways to judge the value or quality of a service. Where directly assessing a service, choice is difficult, people can use physical attributes or properties of the service and its environment, such as cleanliness of a restaurant or the décor of a waiting room. They will also use their own or other people's past experiences such as satisfaction and enjoyment felt before, during or after the service is consumed. For example, remembering what a favourite restaurant is like or asking someone what their dentist is like. In addition, they may also use credence qualities that cannot be assessed until the service is completed. For example, the value of legal advice, the tax saving from financial advice, the ongoing health benefits from an improved diet, the success of some therapy, cannot be judged in advance; users of the service will seek ways to assess the quality of the service, their qualifications, years of experience, or professional memberships.

In some cases, the distinction between goods and services can be very clear; coal is a 'good' whereas legal advice is a 'service'. For most products the distinction can be extremely blurred and very hard to make, most products are a combination of a good and a service. For example, a bus ride will have the service element of transporting a person from A to B, but there will also be tangible elements in the bus itself.

Although a session of music therapy is a pure service, there are tangibles or goods that can be used in conjunction with, and to supplement the service; the instruments, the room's décor, the furniture and how the therapist is dressed. The tangible goods might also provide tangible reminders of that service, such as work sheets, CDs, books, paper and other solid items for a patient to take home. In the same way an airline will provide flight socks, magazines and eye masks as reminders of the flying experience.

Correspondingly, many goods incorporate a service element; a Wii is a tangible good that provides a service that is entertainment and enjoyment. Cars have warranties, free valeting and e-mail service reminders. In many instances the service element will be the only differentiating factor between a supplier and its competitors. A tin of Heinz beans from Tesco is, to all intents and purposes, the same as a tin of Heinz beans from a corner shop, but if Tesco home delivery brings it to your door then there is a service element to the goods provided.

Requirements, therefore, can be seen as more than just a tin of beans or a therapy session. The actual product in terms of a service or a good product delivered to a customer or consumer can be a very complex combination of many different elements. A combination that becomes complicated further when profit is considered.

Profitability

The final word from the definition is 'profitably'. Whereas requirements are the needs of customers and consumers, profits can be seen as the needs of the organisation.

In the commercial world, profit is traditionally associated with financial income, usually excess of income over expenditure and this is how most people view profits. However, the term profit can also have a broader definition which can include returns, benefits or advantages that can be used as a measure of the success of an organisation. For example, for a charity there might be a reduction in the number of people living below the poverty line or for a university, the number of students awarded degrees. For those in the healthcare professions, it could be defined as the number of patients treated successfully, the number seen in a day or in a week, the number referred over a period, a reduction in the numbers of people smoking or overweight, or a drop in the reported number of health acquired infections.

For non-commercial organisations, their requirements and those of their customers may be the same. Using the example of the charity and its donors, both might both measure its success by a reduction in the number of people sleeping 'rough'. Alternatively they might have objectives that differ in other ways. A charity might see its short term success as financial, that will in turn lead to the achievement of its longer term aims. The Health Service might have short term aims in reducing waiting times but have long term objectives in the overall improvement in the health of the nation. Thus, the aims and objectives of a commercial business are not that far removed from a non-commercial business and marketing is just as applicable to organisations such as the NHS.

Competition

One of the fundamental tenets of commercial businesses is competition and this usually means making more money, having more customers or doing more business, than others providing the same or similar services. In theory, commercial businesses engineer their own business to do things better than their competitors by using a combination of price, product quality and distribution. Competition generally comes in one – or a combination – of three forms.

1 Direct – such as someone producing the same good or service as another, for example Ford and Vauxhall or BUPA and PPP.
2 Indirect – where the good or service is not the same but might be used instead, for example rather than joining a gym, a person might take up jogging.

3 Apathy – something is often overlooked but which has resonance with many businesses, but especially with the NHS. Apathy, in this context – and to use a tortuous term – is actively not doing anything. For example, a patient knows they should visit a dentist but they choose not to go. Change4life's[2] biggest competitor is not other health campaigns; it is people not doing anything to change their lifestyle.

The distinction between these three is often blurred and an organisation has to consider each individually as well as in conjunction with each other. For healthcare, the level of competition from these three elements has changed over time in two main ways.

Firstly, the number of other organisations in direct and indirect competition and providing the same or similar services has increased. Private hospitals and health providers might directly compete for primary and secondary healthcare. A private gym or health club might offer physiotherapy. For dieticians, WeightWatchers might claim to offer the same or similar service. Boots, Superdrug and pharmacies are all increasingly providing services to patients that encroach on those offered by AHPs.

Secondly, inactivity or apathy has always been in competition with health professionals, but these days there is a much higher level of information and communication to combat patient inactivity such as a patient failing to turn up for a clinic, a patient who needs help or assistance with a condition actively deciding not to seek professional help despite being advised or informed of its availability such as an obesity clinic or a clinic to help stop smoking.

The Health Service is in exactly the same position as any commercial business in having to look at ways to overcome the competition in order to meet its profit or target. To do this it must create its competitive advantage.

Competitive advantage

To borrow the phrase from Ronseal paints and varnishes, competitive advantage does 'exactly what it says on the tin', they are the advantages you and your organisation have over your competitors. The reality is that creating and sustaining these advantages are not only difficult, but more importantly they have to be seen as advantages by customers and consumers. There are certain factors that need to be considered in creating competitive advantage.

Sustainable and repeatable – the advantage must be there for the long term. A healthy eating clinic offering a bag of free organic vegetables for a month may be a good promotional device but it is not a competitive advantage. Having a portable X-ray machine is an advantage as long as it is permanently available. A service to one patient or group of patients must be available to all patients who might need to receive it.

Unique – a true advantage must be unique to your own organisation. Having a particular skill or qualification is not an advantage if other organisations also have staff similarly skilled or qualified. However, what might be an advantage is to have a significantly larger number of such staff available per patient than a competitor.

Valuable – an advantage is only an advantage if the consumer or customer sees it so and is willing to pay for it. Although this usually means financial value, it can also require some form of investment by the customer, for example, sacrifice of time, physical effort or travel.

Communicable – having a new and expensive piece of radiography equipment may be exciting to you and your colleagues, but patients will probably have no understanding of its significance or benefit and even less interest. The advantage of the new equipment needs to be communicated to the patient so they can perceive that the new machine offers advantages, even if they do not actually understand the science. For example, since 1989, Intel have cleverly created the perception that 'Intel inside' confers some form of benefit to the user, but very few people have any idea exactly what advantage an Intel microchip offers.

It is often the case that creating a clear competitive advantage can be difficult, and an organisation is not able to create or market its own unique advantage. In this case, conducting a simple SWOT analysis to review its strengths and weaknesses, as well as those of its competitors can enable it to build on those strengths, minimise or eradicate its weaknesses and so create a perceivable and communicable advantage to its customers.

The next stage is to pull together these concepts into a clear perception in the mind of the customer and consumer of who you are and what you do – better than anyone else – that can be used as shorthand reference for the organisation and its products. In many ways, this perception is the 'make or break' of a commercial business and for non-commercial businesses it is becoming increasingly important. This perception is wrapped up in the brand and is arguably, the most important element of marketing.

Branding

Competitive advantage must be communicated to customers and consumers who need to quickly recognise and remember these advantages and identify them with a particular supplier or producer.

Brand definition

As with marketing, a simple definition as a starting point is needed. One such definition of what constitutes a brand is that of DeChernatoy and McDonald.[3] This takes the elements of competitive advantage and translates them into what a brand means.

> A successful brand is an identifiable product, service, person or place, augmented in such as way that the buyer or user perceives relevant unique added values which match their needs most closely. Furthermore its success results from being able to sustain these added values in the face of competition.

A second definition from Kapferer,[4] takes a more simplistic approach, but is one that embodies many of the aspects of the NHS:

> A brand is a shared and desirable idea embodied in products, services, places and experiences. The more this idea is shared, the stronger the brand.

The essential point is that although the organisation endeavours to create and manage the brand, it can only be defined by how it is perceived by, for example, the customer or patient. One way perhaps to appreciate this is to make a list of well known supermarkets and think about your perception of each of them. Then ask your colleagues or friends to make a similar list of what their perceptions are. What is important is not only how they may differ, but how that perception takes in more than just the name. The most common mistake people make with a brand is to assume it is only the name, whereas it is everything they know and believe about that brand.

To help understand how brands work and how they can be used by organisations, different aspects of how brands are used or seen can be investigated.

Box 16.1 How brands are used or seen.

Ownership – the oldest definition derives from history. For centuries, livestock farmers have identified their animals by marking them in some way, most commonly by using a branding iron to burn a mark onto the hide of an animal. This marking of ownership continues to this day as goods and service producers identify their products with their name. Cars, baked beans, insurance services are all identified by brand names.

Differentiating device – having created a sustainable competitive advantage, this needs to be conveyed to potential users as belonging to that producer. The customer or consumer sees the name and attaches the characteristics of that product and producer as being different and better than a competitor. For example, British Airways has different characteristics from Ryan Air.

Functional device – the brand tells the potential customer that the product or service will function or perform in an expected way. A Land Rover will be expected to perform off road better than a Mini. An NHS optometrist may well be expected to perform a procedure to higher standard than one in working Specsavers – even though both might both be qualified and skilled in the same way.

Risk reducer – when faced with a choice of product or service, customers and consumers use brand names to gauge the expected quality of a service and reduce the risks involved in purchase. Business travellers often book a Travelodge over an independent hotel because they know exactly what they will get. The risk of being disappointed and having 'hassle' is seen as reduced. A patient might choose an NHS dentist over a private dentist as the perception is that an NHS dentist offers less risk of being charged for treatment that is not required.

Legal device – registering a brand name as a trade mark can give legal protection to a successful product from imitation brands that might try to use the same brand name for their own products. Many household names have had to resort to legal action to prevent other businesses using the same name to promote their own products. EasyJet and McDonald's are both organisations who have taken people to court over the use of the same or similar names.

Strategic asset – a brand can also be a strategic asset that has its own value beyond the cost of production. A typical example is the purchase of Kit Kat by Nestlé for £2.55bn. The price does not reflect the material cost of the equipment and premises to manufacture the bars, but the value of sales and potential profits of the brand, wholly embodied by the name, the taste, look and feel of a Kit Kat.

Symbolic device – people will often use a brand to say something of themselves, it might be as a fashion statement by wearing branded clothes such as Lacoste, or it might be a class issue such as using a Harrods bag for their Tesco's shopping. An individual would prefer to spend a weekend at a Champneys Health Resort than attend an NHS healthy eating clinic, even if the latter may be of far greater benefit.

As ever with marketing, these elements, rather than being independent of each other will overlap. Each individual uses a combination of these aspects of a brand in their choice of product or service. They will have their own unique individual perception and awareness of that brand in their own mind.

Brand awareness

Customers and consumers build up a mental database of information about different brands through a combination of personal and shared experience, hearsay, the media as well as the promotional activities of the brand's producer. This database assists in their decision-making and the main objective of a marketing manager is to generate and develop positive awareness of their brand in the mind of existing and potential customers and consumers. Awareness is characterised initially by brand recognition; a consumer recognises a particular brand on the shelf or in a magazine for example. A customer in a mobile phone shop is faced by a bewildering range of names – Nokia, Sony Ericson, LG, Samsung. In most cases they will opt to purchase the brand they recognise the most and feel is most familiar over a brand that is unknown or unfamiliar. How many people bought an iPhone simply because it was from Apple, without assessing its effectiveness as a phone?

Brand recognition can be further developed into brand recall when the consumer can remember the brand name, albeit when prompted. For example, when asked about diet plans, they may recall WeightWatchers, Slimming World or the Atkins diet. At the next level, brand salience is where the brand is most familiar to consumers. In a simple test, ask colleagues to name one brand of instant coffee. Which brand comes to mind first? Chances are it comes in a jar and is manufactured by a rather large Swiss company! The ultimate ambition for brand and marketing managers is where not only is the brand top of mind, the product or service is the brand of choice and the customer will not accept a substitute, preferring to shop elsewhere. Ironically, it can backfire where a brand becomes synonymous with the product such as Hoover and vacuum cleaners, iPod and MP3 players.

There are two basic issues facing the marketing or brand manager. Firstly, perception can substantially differ with each individual. For example, consider the customer's choice of supermarket for shopping. There will be a range of views on each brand and why people choose to shop where they do. For some the differences might be small, for others, huge. One person will have a different view of the NHS based on their own experiences of hospitals, doctors and clinics.

The second, and one of the biggest problems that brand managers face, is that there can be a substantial difference in the view or perception of the brand between those outside an organisation and those within. For evidence, look no further than Woolworths whose marketers seriously over estimated the value and perception of the brand to the British consumer.

The perception of the NHS from those working within it will differ from those outside. For example, those within have greater technical knowledge and a better – and possibly 'jaundiced' – understanding of the organisation including how it works and its problems than patients. This could mean they may not see or understand where something is an issue or problem for a patient. Similarly, they might not be able to communicate effectively with the patient, leading the patient to misunderstand a diagnosis or treatment. If evidence is needed that this can happen, simply ask the IT department to explain how a computer network works when your PC breaks down!

Branding and non-commercial organisations

Although later into the starter's blocks than commercial business, non commercial organisations have brand identities that have changed and created new perceptions, just as well managed and designed as those of many profit making businesses. The Met Office and the Royal Navy are both organisations that have successfully established a brand and others have even re-branded and reinvented themselves, such as Ofsted.

Charities have known for a long time how powerful the brand can be. An example of the recognition accorded to the power of the brand is Scope's rebranding from the Spastic's Society in 1994. The word 'spastic' had increasingly become a cause of concern to those working and living with the condition. Consequently, the Society wanted to move away from the negative connotations of the word and so after some lengthy discussion and research chose 'Scope' as a name with more optimistic and positive connotations.

How does this work with the NHS and healthcare? As the UK's largest employer and the one single organisation that touches everyone in the UK from before the cradle to the grave, the NHS has been perhaps, one of the slowest to adopt branding. It was not until 1999 that a single brand identity was agreed for the whole of the NHS.

Surprisingly, the NHS does not even appear in the 2009–2010 Superbrands list of 500 UK Superbrands whereas Boots (40), BUPA (138) and even WeightWatchers are listed. Perhaps it is most telling when looking at Superbrands UK Ltd's own definition of a superbrand:[5]

> A superbrand has established the finest reputation in its field. It offers customers significant emotional and/or tangible advantages over its competitors, which (consciously or sub-consciously) customers want and recognise.

But what is the NHS brand's reputation? One of the largest influences on the reputation of a large organisational brand is media coverage. The NHS receives more media coverage than any other organisation in the UK and the problem that it shares with many other non-commercial organisations is that the majority of this coverage is negative. Notwithstanding the use of the NHS as a political 'football', in one year alone there was major news coverage of Swine Flu, C. diff, MRSA, and individual hospitals such as Stafford Hospital and individual patient stories. The NHS public relations machine works hard to counter this negative publicity, by creating positive responses and marketing, by actively taking the initiative on issues such as Swine Flu. The fortunate irony for those working in the NHS is that the media's negative perception is rarely shared by patients.

Creating and maintaining a successful brand is achieved in part by a combination of marketing methods such as product design, distribution, price and how it is promoted. It is also a perception of a brand created by the personal and shared experience of all of its customers, consumers and others – as individuals – and for the NHS whether as a patient, customer or carer. It is the combination of millions of these unique experiences that have contributed to the NHS being possibly the biggest and most popular brand – even if not the most successful – in the UK. The crucial element of all of this is that those experiences are shaped by the people within the NHS.

Managing the brand

On one level, the overall direction of the NHS brand and other related healthcare organisations is no different from commercial business, in that although the brand is designed, engineered and managed by senior management and their marketing teams, it is the detailed 'people' level that frequently has the greatest influence on the experience brand. Responsibility for these details rests with individuals within the organisation, and it is their actions that can make or break a brand. The power of the individual members of staff is often seriously underestimated. To quote Anita Roddick:[6] 'If you think you're too small to have an impact, try going to bed with a mosquito.'

The success of a haircut, the enjoyment of a meal out or the stress of flying are all dependent on the quality of skills and abilities of the individuals involved in delivering the service. It is individual people who shape the experience of consumers and customers. Boots the Chemists is one retailer who prides itself on ensuring individual staff give a high standard of service. When a customer asks where a product is located, the staff member will – should – take them to the shelf, suggest a comparable Boots product if applicable and ask if there is any other help they can give. Whether it is the cleaner, the receptionist, the healthcare assistant or the doctor; all have a role in shaping the perception and therefore success of the brand.

Even when the service is remote from human contact such as on-line banking, it is still dependent on individual people to ensure that every contact between the customer or consumer and the brand is efficient, effective and a positive experience.

Touch points

At their simplest level touch points are the individual contact points between the customer or consumer and the brand. These make the difference at a practical level.

The level and range of these touch points can vary enormously and accordingly will have a varying level of impact. They may be totally infrequent and impersonal; a vending machine, a cash machine or online enquiries. Others may require minimum human interaction; a shop purchase, a ticket check by a conductor or asking directions from a police officer. For a patient undergoing an X-ray or ultrasound scan, contact with the radiographer might be a 'one off' and only involve a few minutes. Others will be more frequent and regular as well as more complex. For a therapist, they might build a long term relationship with their patient and with their carer, but it can still influence the perception. The problem is that even in a short time, a huge amount of damage can be done.

A brand such as Virgin has shown that by concentrating on this level of service and developing an holistic approach to the brand, they can successfully operate into other sectors of business. What this means is that much of the power to market the organisation and positively develop the brand rests with individual actions. These can be managed at the human scale and combined to make the brand experience positive. There are a myriad of ways and means that the individual can create positive touch points that will have a positive impact for the brand.

Creating and managing touch points

The first step is to stop and think of all the ways the brand touches or comes into contact with individuals. A good starting point is to work backwards and forwards from the principal contact. To help understand this, a group of students were asked to consider the different touch points that British Airways had with its customers (*see* Table 16.1).

Table 16.1 Student perceptions of British Airways touch points.

Aircraft condition	Cabin cleanliness	Seat allocation
Seat comfort	Space	Reception on board
Flight crew appearance	Cabin crew appearance	Childcare
Catering and refreshments	Literature	Entertainment
Merchandise	Shopping	In flight delay handling
Problem passengers	Baggage reclaim (or not!)	Communications from BA
Frequent flyer	Advertising	Public relations
Promotions	Ticket selling	Ticket delivery
Airport journey and arrival	Luggage tags	Departure lounge
Check-in	Security	Departure punctuality
Information	Flight crew announcements	Flight quality
Technical problems	Leaving the aircraft	Send off

What is immediately apparent is the huge range and variety of these touch points in terms of how they are set up, managed and operated. Many are under the control of central management such as public relations and advertising and others devoid of superficial human contact by being computerised or automated such as ticket delivery. However, what is important is that the vast majority, are in the direct control, management and responsibility of individuals at a local or ground level. It is not just the check-in staff, flight or cabin crew. They are the professional face of the airline and as such, one would expect high quality service. In other cases it is not the interpersonal skills that are important, it is the actions and responsibilities of people who are not visible or do not communicate directly with the traveller and can be just as – and in some cases perhaps more so! – important to the traveller; aircraft engineers and technicians, aircraft cleaners, baggage handlers, catering staff. Some people may not be employees or even directly linked, but can still affect the airline's brand, for example, air traffic controllers, security staff and parking attendants.

It is important to explore and look at every aspect of service provision. In this example, a high standard of personal appearance is synonymous with cabin crew, but ensuring and helping other staff achieve a high standard can pay a dividend. Other organisations not usually associated with personal appearance have taken this 'on board'. Eddie Stobart – the road haulage and warehousing business – recognised some years ago that the personal appearance of its drivers impacted on the overall image and success of the brand. Consequently, all their drivers have clean and smart uniforms and even the lorries are well turned out. In healthcare there has been endless debate about the merits of staff uniforms, but most patients seem to prefer staff to have uniforms that not only single them out but make it easy to identify their role.

What next

For those working in the NHS and related organisations it should be easy to see how it is a short step to use the example as a starting point and create a similar list for your own sphere of expertise and department. It is possible to look at how the experience of patients and customers can be improved in a number of small but effective ways to improve the brand.

Every aspect of the process and service provision needs to be considered. From first point of referral, time taken to process appointment, advising and reminding of the appointment times, attitude of receptionists, time in waiting room, ambience of waiting rooms, toilet facilities, client handling skills, literature, follow up, explanations of treatment, after-care, self treatment...the list of areas that can affect and be managed at a local level is long indeed.

Each part can be considered and ways found of making small improvements that can have far reaching effects. For example DNAs are a problem in all areas of healthcare. A text message or e-mail to the patient – or the person responsible for ensuring the patient makes the appointment – might improve DNA rates. Some would argue that this is time consuming and laborious. But is it more time consuming than the time wasted waiting for the patient? Is it more laborious than remaking the appointment? If more patients show up and are treated, are overall waiting times reduced, targets met more easily, productivity and profitability increased?

Summary and conclusion

This chapter is not intended as a definitive guide on marketing and branding. It is intended to give an understanding of the importance of marketing and branding and its role in healthcare and how this can influence the brand in a positive way for patients and staff. It is also designed to give a greater appreciation of how branding works and how its development and management can positively affect and benefit the organisation in both commercial business and not for profit and other non commercial businesses.

Whilst marketing and brand management comes from the top, the experience and perception of the organisation and its brand is shaped at the 'grass roots' by individual experience. Control and management of that experience is in the hands of AHPs, their colleagues and their administration staff at all levels.

Why is this so important? Perhaps it is easier to ask another question: what happens if you do not create and own your own brand? Other competing organisations are becoming increasingly aware of how important the brand is to the potential market. To see the importance and power of the brand, look no further than Virgin Healthcare. This is reflected in how the general public are not only becoming increasingly brand aware, but also brand promiscuous. People are more willing than ever to shop around. Brand loyalty is not as strong as it was and businesses are investing large amounts of money to persuade customers to come to them and also to stay with them. Complacency is not longer an option.

References

1   Chartered Institute of Marketing: www.cim.co.uk/home.aspx.
2   Change4life: www.nhs.uk/Change4Life.
3   DeChernatory L, McDonald M. *Creating Powerful Brands*. 2nd ed. Oxford: Butterworth Heinemann; 1998.
4   Kapfer J-N. *The New Strategic Brand Management*. 3rd ed. London: Kogan Page; 2004.
5   Superbrand: www.superbrands.uk.com.
6   Roddick A: http://thinkexist.com/quotes/anita_roddick.

Further reading

* Blythe J. *Essentials of Marketing*. 3rd ed. Harlow: Pearson Education; 2005.
* Rizebos R. *Brand Management – a strategic approach*. Harlow: Pearson Education; 2003.
* Dibb S, Simkin L, Pride WM, *et al. Marketing – concepts and strategies*. 5th European ed. Boston, MA: Houghton Mifflin; 2006.
* Elliot R, Percy L. *Strategic Brand Management*. Oxford: Oxford University Press; 2007.
* www.scope.org.uk/downloads/publications/scopename_change.pdf.
* www.nhsidentity.nhs.uk/about-the-nhs-brand/background-and-aims.

Chapter 17

Effective report writing

Julie Shepherd and Natalie Beswetherick

Introduction

The purpose of this chapter is to discuss why reports are important management 'tools' to aid achievement of service objectives, ensuring written reports are of high quality raising the profile of the service within the organisation.

A well written report presents information succinctly and in a format that is clear and easy to read. Reports need to be evidence-based and present to the reader the desired outcome, what actions need to be taken, or the desired 'direction of travel'. Good communication in a well written report facilitates decision-making and often leads to success. Reports inform the reader about the service and provide an indication of the service quality and future plans. They can be powerful as part of business cases and help to re-define what the organisation wants and the roles that services can play.

A poorly written report may confuse and bore the reader. It may also lead to the conclusion that the writer is a muddled thinker and poor communicator. Good planning and making time to consider how the report will be understood and construed by readers reduces confusion and aids clarity. The process of planning and compiling a report is outlined. An example of a service review report is presented highlighting the parameters to include.

Background

The NHS Plan 2000[1] and NHS Improvement Plan 2004[2] set out the strategy for continuing change within health and social care and a more evidence-based and outcome oriented NHS. Increasing pressure to provide better services against a background of financial stringency and target-setting has challenged traditional practices. Doing things because 'that's the way they've always been done' is no longer a viable option.

Subsequent health policy reforms such as the 'Choice' initiative,[3] the 18 week pathway directive[4] and the 'Next Stage Review',[5] have promoted faster access to patient-centred services. Additional 'levers' for change include for example, the requirement for commissioners to purchase care 'closer to home', whereby services are moved out of hospitals into community settings, with integration between health and social care.[6, 7]

Challenging clinicians to evaluate the outcomes of their practice and to provide cost effective and evidence-based management of patients is often a barrier to change. Clinicians from all disciplines, whose patient care is based on historical practice alone, may become defensive when challenged. They may feel that their practice is being threatened by cost-cutting and other changes rather than what is in the best interests of patients.

Carefully planned projects and concise reports are essential to demonstrate the efficacy of services or the need for change. It may also indicate a focus for investment. As a key part of service improvement, good report writing needs to be embedded in the culture of services. The process of planning, executing and evaluating projects saves time and effort in the longer term.

Reports should:

- be factual, evidence-based and verifiable
- present information that is relevant, interesting and easy to both read and understand
- be underpinned by the 'KISS' principle – keep it short and simple.

Planning the report

There must be clarity around the aims, objectives, scope and purpose. It is worth asking yourself the question; 'Who is the report aimed at, as well as what you want to say?'

Overall objectives must be focussed and SMART – specific, measurable, achievable, realistic and timed. There needs to be clarity about the desired result. Consider the style, formality and focus required taking care to minimise the use of jargon.

Editors' note

The third book of this series, *Key Topics in Healthcare Management – understanding the big picture* (Chapter 2), explores techniques for the management of change including objective setting.[8]

Questions to consider:

- if the report is about a service, does it relate to proposed improvement, development or is it a review of current practice, for example?
- who is the report intended for? Knowledge of the potential audience will help pitch the contents appropriately.

As the NHS develops 'World Class Commissioning',[9] (*see* Chapter 3) report writers must consider the 'big picture' and requirements of service commissioners and the local delivery plan. This will require the report to include quantitative as well as qualitative content. Reports may be circulated to a wide audience, which could include people with detailed knowledge of the subject as well as those new to the topic area.

Service review report planning requires clear aims and objectives and thorough measurement methodology. Collection of baseline data is essential in order to ascertain whether any change has had the desired effect. The template below was developed for this purpose. It has been beneficial in providing a focus for planning, clarifying objectives and also providing a framework for report writing.

Box 17.1 Improvement project plan template.

Project title:
Project leads:
Project team:
Comments
Background to the project:
What needs to be found out?
How is this to be done?
Who should be involved and informed?
    e.g. service users, stakeholders, commissioners.
Data collection:
    to include baseline.
Type of project:
    e.g. service review, re-design, improvement, developmental.
Evidence-base and references:
Action plan with timescales using SMART objectives:

Data must be robust and accurate with consideration given to what might be the most appropriate method of data presentation, for example, bar charts, pie charts, scatter plots, box plots, graphs or tables.

There are a number of publications on the measurement and evaluation of service improvement. 'Evaluating improvement, general improvement skills',[10] outlines: Why, What, When, How and Who should evaluate? 'Measurement for improvement, process and systems thinking',[11] outlines which measures to use and how data should be presented (*see* Chapter 9).

Presentation of the report

There needs to be a clear structure with headings and sub-headings to guide the reader through the document. The report must outline the evidence, how it was collected and verified and its significance. Conclusions are drawn from the evidence leading on to presentation of recommendations.

A framework for presentation might be as follows.

Front page: an eye catching front page, with name of organisation and logo, title, author(s) and date, set out using the organisations' 'house style'. The title needs to be succinct and attractive.

Table of contents: the contents include headings for each section providing a quick reference guide with numbered pages.

Executive summary: this is often one page or shorter, containing précis information to enable clear understanding of the main points in the report. It outlines the subject, background and major recommendations. It is a very important section, and may be the only part that a busy person will read.

Introduction: this relates to the subject and purpose of the report. It provides the background to the report, or the background may be a separate section on its own.

Methodology: this describes the research methodology where applicable, how and what data was collected and in what time-scale. It also describes the evaluative methodology employed.

Results: this section sets out the findings of the area under investigation or review.

Presentation of data: most reports include evaluative data as part of the results section, which must be presented in a way that is easy to read and does not 'switch the reader off'. Graphs, charts and other visual representations are often a better method of providing clarity, than numbers included in blocks of text. Some people may prefer reading data within the text. The KISS principle applies. Data needs to be tailored to focus on key issues. Additional detailed data may be included in appendices at the end of the report.

Tables: a table is a means of arranging data in columns.

Table 17.1 An example of a table.

	Apr	*May*	*Jun*	*Jul*	*Aug*	*Sep*	*Total*
Year 1	48	82	92	67	67	74	430
Year 2	49	61	116	133	151	186	696

Bar charts: a bar chart, also known as a bar graph, is a chart with bars of lengths proportional to the value that they represent.

Pie charts: a pie chart, is a circular chart with segments proportional to the value that they represent.

Graphs: a linear representation depicting the relationship between two or more variables with a discrete or continuous range.

Scatter graph: a scatter graph or scatter plot is a type of display using Cartesian coordinates to display values for two variables for a set of data. The data is displayed as a collection of points, each having the value of one variable determining the position on the horizontal axis and the value of the other variable determining the position on the vertical axis.

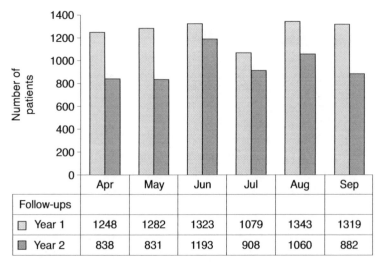

Follow-ups						
	Apr	May	Jun	Jul	Aug	Sep
☐ Year 1	1248	1282	1323	1079	1343	1319
▣ Year 2	838	831	1193	908	1060	882

Figure 17.1 An example of a bar chart.

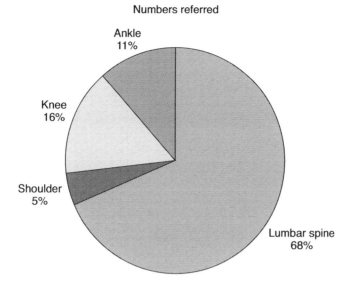

Figure 17.2 An example of a pie chart.

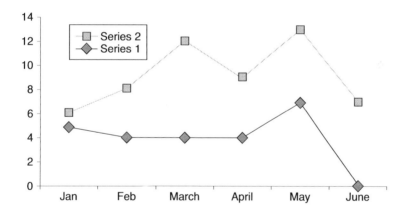

Figure 17.3 An example of a graph.

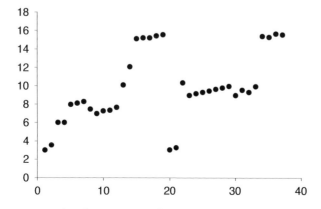

Figure 17.4 An example of a scattergraph.

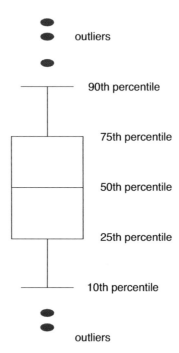

Figure 17.5 An example of a box plot.

Box plot: in descriptive statistics a box plot (also known as a box-and-whisker diagram or plot) is a convenient way of graphically depicting groups of numerical data through their five-number summaries (the smallest observation, lower quartile (Q1), median (Q2), upper quartile (Q3), and largest observation). A box plot may also indicate which observations, if any, might be considered outliers.

Analysis of data: in this section the findings that have been presented in numerical, graphical and text format are discussed.

Financial information: when the report includes proposals or recommendations which have funding implications presentation of financial information and analysis must be included.

Options appraisal: this may be included as a section if relevant to the type of report.

Discussion: it may be useful to introduce a discussion section before conclusions are made.

Conclusions: draws the report to an end, summarising the main points.

Recommendations: sets out the requested actions or outcomes succinctly. Recommendations should:

- flow from the preceding contents
- be clear and specific proposals for action
- set out concise and unambiguous proposals
- be realistic, affordable and not too numerous
- be numbered in priority order.

References: to conform to standard referencing techniques, following the 'house style' of the organisation.

Appendices: these should be numbered and contains supporting information to the main document.

Box 17.2 Report writer's checklist.

1 Is there a clear purpose for writing the report?
2 Is the target audience identified?
3 Is the report structure clear?
4 Are headings consistent and used as signposts?
5 Is there a deadline for submission?
6 Have you set a deadline for completion?
7 Identify a proof reader prior to final drafting
8 An easily readable typeface and consistent font to be used along with line spacing of one and a half
9 Presentation of the report is important; do not try to squeeze text in too small a space. Take care with margins, headers, footers and paragraph spacing
10 Text should be broken up regularly, with charts and diagrams as appropriate
11 Pages, figures and tables must be numbered
12 Check spelling
13 Correct use of grammar
14 Check use of tenses, generally 'third person' for formal reports
15 Avoid convoluted sentences and use of jargon
16 Consistent use of headings, bullet points and sub headings
17 Consider whether the use of colour is desirable and affordable, but expect that some people may copy off in black and white only
18 Check punctuation
19 Consider final presentation of the report, for example, is binding required
20 Is the report suitably formatted for electronic circulation?

Truss,[12] sets out examples of the 'use and abuse' of punctuation and quotes:

There's the famous telegram: 'Not getting any better. Come at once.' Which became: 'Not getting any. Better come at once.'

This light hearted example clearly shows that punctuation can change the meaning of a sentence.

Example of a report in outline

This report demonstrates the efficacy of a new service that resulted in funding being secured from three organisations.

'A review of the occupational health physiotherapy musculoskeletal assessment service.'

Author: ....

Date: ....

Executive summary

Following the success of a physiotherapist working in Occupational Health (OH) in a neighbouring Trust, funding was secured for a six month pilot project. The aim of this was to ascertain the value of a physiotherapist working as an assessor and case manager in the OH departments within the Trust.

A secondment was advertised and a physiotherapist recruited with relevant musculoskeletal skills to undertake two clinics, eight hours per week for the six month pilot. Before to the pilot, musculoskeletal assessments were carried out by OH Doctors and Nurses. The Nurses had no formal training in musculoskeletal assessment. Self referral to physiotherapy was available for staff, however there were still significant numbers of referrals to OH.

The pilot demonstrated a 50% decrease in sickness days for staff presenting with musculoskeletal disorders across the Trust and a decrease in waiting times for assessment from 20.4 to 15.2 days.

The cost of the physiotherapist for the pilot was £3 500. The cost of employing a doctor to do this work would have been significantly higher. There were significant benefits to the members of staff and cost benefits to the employing organisation. The estimated savings of salary and locum 'backfill' for the sickness days saved was £33 538. The results clearly demonstrated that a physiotherapist working as a case manager was an effective addition to the OH team.

It is recommended that the funding for the physiotherapist is provided substantively for the continuation of the service. Further evaluation of the service is required, to assess and monitor its efficacy utilising both qualitative and quantitative outcomes.

Background

Close links exist with other OH departments in the area. A neighbouring OH department employed a physiotherapist providing consultancy with the benefits of improved outcomes and a reduction in staff sickness days. Funding was therefore sought via the Trust Employment Committee and secured by the lead OH physician, to run a six month pilot for a physiotherapist to be seconded to OH. The aim was to decrease staff sickness absence for those presenting with musculoskeletal problems and to assess whether there would be added value resulting from a physiotherapist working as a case-manager in the OH team.

Although staff were able to self refer to the physiotherapy service for physiotherapy assessment and management, the need was identified to employ a musculoskeletal specialist physiotherapist to assess and case-manage patients attending OH. The aim was to expedite staff return to work. The physiotherapist would not offer treatment, but advice and support regarding return to work.

Musculoskeletal referrals accounted for 28% of consultations with OH. Before the employment of the physiotherapist, OH nursing staff managing musculoskeletal patients had received no formal training in musculoskeletal assessment.

The seconded physiotherapist worked for eight hours a week providing two clinics on different sites. The role included:

1 advice for departments such as vascular day surgery and the plaster room, which identified problems regarding ergonomics and manual handling
2 car ergonomic assessments for 'pool' car users
3 work-station ergonomic assessments
4 liaising with manual handling advisors
5 liaising with healthcare professionals and managers regarding appropriate treatment for staff and arrangements for return to work
6 assessment of staff with musculoskeletal problems
7 training sessions for OH nursing and medical staff
8 working with OH staff to develop the physiotherapist's skills in, for example, the management of stress and anxiety.

Methodology

Data was collected retrospectively for staff assessed by OH for the six months prior to the commencement of the physiotherapy pilot. Further data was collected for the six months of the pilot itself.

Data collected:

• waiting time in days, from referral to appointment
• sickness days taken after the OH appointment
• method of return to work, phased or full time
• clinical conditions managed
• profession of assessing clinician.

Results and presentation of data

This data is presented in a graphical format to illustrate trends. Where data was incomplete on records, it was excluded. This equated to nine patients, an overall 8% of total assessments. 105 staff patients were assessed, of these 51 new patients were seen during the pilot period and 54 had been seen in the six months before the pilot began.

Table 17.2 Staff assessed per site.

Profession of staff patient	Site 1	Site 2
Trained nurse	9	7
Healthcare assistant	4	8
Allied health professional	5	2
Estates/portering	3	0
Administration	3	5
Domestic	2	0
Catering	3	0
Total	29	22

There was a different skill mix of staff patients consulting OH attending on the two sites. In addition to these 51 new patients, there were a total of 44 follow up appointments conducted during the pilot. There were 20 'did not attends' for both new and follow up appointments. Two consultation visits to departments in the trust took more than two hours where specific ergonomic and manual handling problems had been identified. There were five and a half clinics not covered due to staff sickness, annual leave and training. Two training sessions were provided by the physiotherapist for other members of the OH team. The physiotherapist also spent approximately six hours at meetings within OH for personal development.

Figure 17.6 highlights that the average post appointment sickness days were reduced from 13.6 to 6.8. It also shows that the average waiting time for a musculoskeletal assessment had decreased from 20.4 days to 15.2 days.

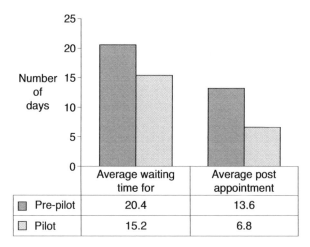

Figure 17.6 Average waiting time for assessment and the number of post appointment sickness days.

No member of staff assessed after the start of the pilot had to wait more than 50 days for an assessment. Prior to the start of the pilot, seven patients had to wait longer than 50 days. Of these, five had been off sick for the whole period of their wait for an appointment.

Figure 17.7 presents the categories of conditions seen in OH musculoskeletal assessments. This concords with the general population who seek healthcare services for musculoskeletal problems.[13] Approximately 58% of the population suffers from low back pain at some time in their lives[14] and it is the most common pain complaint together with headache.[15] The chart shows that the staff group is broadly representative of the general population; however there is a higher incidence of back pain.

Figure 17.8 indicates that 34 patients were assessed by doctors and 20 by nurses in the pre-pilot phase.

Financial information

The cost of employing a doctor would have been significantly higher than that for a physiotherapist. Only a few patients would need to see the doctor for further management. During the pilot only one patient seen by the physiotherapist,

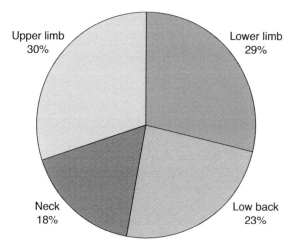

Figure 17.7 Categories of conditions.

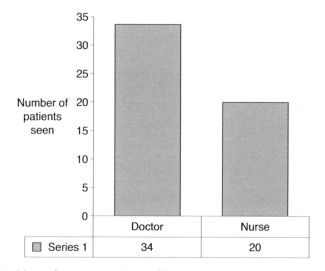

Figure 17.8 Health profession assessing staff patient pre-pilot.

needed further assessment by the OH doctor. In the six month pilot the physiotherapist undertook two clinics a week at a total cost of £3500.

The pilot demonstrated:

- a reduced waiting time of 5.2 days on average
- a reduced sickness absence post appointment of 6.8 days on average
- a total saving of 12 days absence per staff member seen on average
- 51 staff members were seen during the pilot with an estimated average salary of £20 000.

Estimated savings of salary and locum 'backfill' costs for the six months pilot was calculated using average salary costs:

£54.80 × 12 days × 51 staff = £33 538

Conclusion

Previously nurses and doctors were assessing musculoskeletal staff patients. However, during this pilot the physiotherapist assessed and managed the majority of these patients.

The most significant finding was that the average sickness absence days were reduced from 13.6 to 6.8. There was a decrease in the waiting time for musculoskeletal appointments in OH. The decrease in waiting times and earlier return to work correlates with significant cost savings for the Trust.

This pilot demonstrated that there would be cost and efficiency savings and other benefits if the physiotherapy role as a case manager in OH was continued.

Recommendations

It is recommended that:

1 the role of the physiotherapist as a case manager in OH should be made substantive
2 the service continues to be funded as the pilot has demonstrated that physiotherapy input is cost efficient and clinically effective
3 clinical audit should be undertaken on a regular basis to further evaluate the service
4 a feedback survey of both staff and manager views should be undertaken as part of on-going evaluation
5 the physiotherapist continues to work with other OH staff to improve the overall clinical effectiveness of the management of musculoskeletal conditions within the OH service.

Appendices

These would be normally included to provide further background and more detailed information and data supporting the content of the report.

Summary

This chapter sets out important aspects for effective report writing. There are many different types of report from, for example, short A4 length briefing reports, reports on specific elements of service or issues, detailed service reviews, annual reports, reports for the Trust Board, performance or clinical governance reports and many more. Reports may be formal or informal depending on the circumstances, intended or target audience and purpose.

In these days of electronic communication through vast quantities of e-mail the art of good report writing can be worth its 'weight in gold' for success in achieving desired outcomes. Reports must be methodically structured, clearly written with a minimum of jargon with correct use of grammar, punctuation, spelling, appropriate use of graphical, tabulated material and diagrams. The appearance, layout and overall presentation of reports is crucial to making successful cases and arguments getting the 'message across'; 'clean', concise and clear presentation is invaluable.

Editors' note

Top tips

Writing successfully takes practice and is a skill in itself. The following list outlines some tips we have found helpful.

1 The faster and easier your audience receives your key messages the more successful your report will be.
2 Know your audience – beware of jargon and do not over estimate or underestimate their technical understanding of the topic.
3 Signpost your document to facilitate reading, a good content page and headings are essential – do not assume the audience will be as keen to read it as you were to write it.
4 Give attention to the title page, make it stand out.
5 Write a short summary – one or two sentences that give the condensed version of your whole document, this helps you focus.
6 Make sure you ask the reader for the action you are wanting – not just a passive essay.
7 Give the reader a date by which action is required.
8 Write for the reader who 'scans' make sure headings convey the key points.
9 Do not make it too long! It may never get read.
10 Make sure you explain the benefits of your request, make good use of the Appendices.
11 Avoid telling the readers what they already know.
12 Avoid negative text, turn it round to be positive with a solution to the problem.
13 Keep sentences short. Use bullets effectively, but not repeatedly, never more than six bullets.
14 Figures and tables – number them and use strong headings to convey key messages.
15 Avoid pointless words – like basically, actually, undoubtedly. They add nothing to the message and often can be removed without changing the meaning or the tone. You will find sentences survive, succeed and may even flourish without them.
16 Focus the conclusion and recommendations section – have you drawn together all the main ideas without adding in new information?
17 Do not forget references and acknowledgements, use a consistent style.
18 Write a draft report and get someone to read it and give you honest feedback.

Tips for report presentation

Skill 1 – be sure of your objectives
- Have an objective in mind for your presentation and think about the objectives of your audience
- Make sure you know about the group, who they are and what their levels of knowledge/experience is, why the presentation is taking place, what the audience is hoping to gain from it
- Decide what style of presentation is appropriate

Skill 2 – be prepared
- Preparation is key to success in any presentation
- Allow plenty of time for preparation
- Know who the audience are
- Speak to the event organisers before the event
- Know the roles of people in the audience in respect of influence, authority, decision-making
- Know why individuals are at the presentation
- What do you know about the 'agendas' of those attending – why are they there?
- Who supports you, who is potentially against you?
- What objections can you expect and what arguments or strategies have you got to rebut them?
- If more than one of you involved in making the presentation, who will lead on which areas and why?
- Presentation checklist:
  - Phones off
  - Someone on the door to welcome
  - Is there a fire alarm test due!
  - Room layout and seating/tables
  - No barriers – take control of the space
  - Break times if a long presentation
  - Lighting arrangements
  - Timing
  - Stand, lectern where appropriate projector table positioning
  - Test all audio media equipment
  - Have spare handouts where appropriate
  - Rehearse if you can

Skill 3 – have structure
- Keep it simple and straightforward
- Strategies for eliciting:
- Why?
  - Universal truths,
  - Stories and metaphors
  - Rhetorical questions
  - Ask the audience
  - Discussions
  - Recap
- What?
  - What are the key points to be covered?
  - What are the main elements of each point
  - What is the right level of detail for this audience?
  - If selling (or an idea) what are the benefits of what you are proposing/selling?
  - Focus on tangible results and softer intangible benefits
  - Repeat and emphasise key points
- How will it work?
  - Examples

- Using demonstrations, models, graphs, figures
- Getting them to do it – role play where appropriate
- Doing an exercise, apply to real situations with examples
- Getting them to talk about how they could use this – with others in the audience
- Drawing, writing, brainstorming
- Questions
  - Always summarise the benefits
  - Focus on the core benefits
  - Call to action
  - Recommend future actions and agree next steps where appropriate

Skill 4 – take notes with you
- Never rely on the PowerPoint – it may not work!
- Use brief notes of salient points
- Use mind mapping for planning presentations

Skill 5 – use engaging language
- Do not be long winded
- Use straightforward (not over complicated words)
- Create audience involvement
- Use signposts – let people know what's coming
- Be positive
- Talk about benefits
- Avoid vague, wishy washy words
- Avoid useless phrases
- Avoid being overly technical or complex

Skill 6 – use presentation aids appropriately
- No-one likes 'death by PowerPoint'
- PowerPoint should only aid, illustrate, use to spice up, it should never be used as an aide memoir
- Use variety of presentation slides, not just words
- Handouts:
  - Must be 'branded' and must be clear they are presentation material
  - Should leave room for note taking
  - Should expand on the bullet points on the screen, not just reiterate them
  - Can be used actively during the presentation 'now what I want you to do is...'
  - Must be something they will want to keep

Skill 7 – engage your audience
- Speak to some people early on as they arrive if you can
- Smile, make eye contact
- Learn some names if you have chance
- Bring people in – walk around, own the territory
- Use fizzy exercises, ask questions, divide into groups, ask for volunteers, vote on something, give something away, play a game
- Use 'yes' sets
- Ask questions
- Look for energisers

- Watch your body language: symmetrical, upright, palms down, hands moving down and outward from chest level, open, asymmetrical, leaning forward
- Never turn your back to the audience to read from the screen!
- Go there first, whenever possible go to the presentation room first, claim the area, make it your own

Skill 8 – take questions and deal with challenges
- Questions are a sign your audience is 'still there' and interested
- Ask questions yourself
- Listen and demonstrate you are listening through your body language
- Ask individuals to repeat or elaborate
- Ask others their opinions
- Be honest
- Prepare answers to likely questions

Skill 9 – get the edge
- Avoid monotonous pitch
- Consider the emotion behind key messages examples and sentences
- Be slow to drive home key points and benefits
- Use pauses for emphasis
- Seek feedback and listen to feedback non judgmentally
- Enjoy! If you enjoy the presentation, your audience probably will too

Authors' note

The authors would like to thank Lucy Booth and David Taylor from the Physiotherapy Team at Gloucestershire Hospitals NHS Foundation Trust for their contributions to this chapter.

References

1 Department of Health. *The NHS Plan: a plan for investment, a plan for reform*. London: HMSO; 2000.
2 Department of Health. *The NHS Improvement Plan: putting people at the heart of public service*. London: HMSO; 2004.
3 Chartered Society of Physiotherapy. *Making the Business Case. A physiotherapist's guide to commissioning*. London: CSP; 2007.
4 www.18weeks.nhs.uk.
5 Department of Health: www.dh.gov.uk/en/publicationsandstatistics/publications/publicationspolicyandguidance/DH_085825.
6 Department of Health. *Shifting the Balance of Power*. London: HMSO; 2002.
7 Department of Health. *Our Health, Our Care, Our Say: a new direction for community services*. London: HMSO; 2006.
8 Jones R, Jenkins F. *Key Topics in Healthcare Management – understanding the big picture*. Oxford: Radcliffe Publishing; 2007.
9 Department of Health. *Operating Framework: world class commissioning*. London: HMSO; 2007.
10 NHS Institute for Innovation and Improvement. *Improvement Leaders' Guide. Evaluating improvement, general improvement skills*. Warwick: NHSI; 2005.

11 NHS Institute for Innovation and Improvement. *Improvement Leaders' Guide. Measurement for improvement, process and systems thinking.* Warwick: NHSI; 2005.

12 Truss L. *Eats, Shoots and Leaves: the zero tolerance approach to punctuation.* London: Profile Books; 2003.

13 Hackett GI, Bundred P, Hutton JL, *et al.* Management of joint and soft tissue injuries in three general practices: value of on site physiotherapy. *Br J Gen Prac.* 1993; **43**: 61–4.

14 Papageorgiou AC, Croft PR, Ferry S, *et al.* Estimating the prevalence of low back pain in the general population. Evidence from the South Manchester back pain survey. *Spine.* 1995; **20(17)**: 1889–94.

15 Raspe HH. Back pain. In: Silamn AJ, Hochberg MC, editors. *Epidemiology of the Rheumatic Diseases.* Oxford: Oxford University Press; 1993.

Further reading

- Cormack D, Benton D. *Writing for Health Care Professions.* San Francisco, CA: Wiley-Blackwell; 1994.
- Forsyth P. *How to Write Reports and Proposals.* 2nd ed. London: Kogan Page; 2006.
- Harbert E, DiGaetani JL. *Writing for Action: a guide for the health care professional.* Chicago, IL: Irwin Professional Publishing; 1984.
- Inglis J, Lewis R. *How to Write Reports.* London: Collins Educational; 1995.
- Mort S. *Professional Report Writing.* Farnham: Gower Publishing; 1995.
- http://us.deskdemon.com/pages/us/career/business-report-writing.

Chapter 18

Demonstrating worth: marketing and impact measurement – self-referral

Lesley Holdsworth

Modern healthcare delivery is constantly evolving requiring services including those of the AHP to continually re-invent themselves. The greater emphasis on effectiveness and value for money together with the introduction of various models of 'commissioning' have reinforced the need for services to prove their worth.

In this chapter some of the key concepts that determine the success of AHP services particularly in relation to marketing, the 'selling' of the service and, measuring impact demonstrating worth are explored.

What do we mean by marketing?

A definition commonly used states that it is…'the process of planning and executing the conception, pricing, promotion, and distribution of ideas, goods, and services to create exchanges that satisfy individual and organisational goals'.[1]

However, it is also considered that marketing as a concept covers organisational culture and positioning, market research, new product development, advertising and promotion, public and press relations and the sales functions. It is the process by which an organisation decides what it will offer, to whom, when and how.

Over the last decade, there has been a growing recognition within AHP services of the need to embrace and put into place many of the principles of marketing. This has resulted in significant benefits to many in terms of gaining support for developments and confidence in their efficacy and value. Others who have not adopted these principles so readily have not fared so well and struggled with introducing new or re-designed services.

The objective of this chapter is to capture the experience gained over 20 years of service development and in particular, the experience of introducing and evaluating the efficacy of patient self-referral to physiotherapy. These developments have always been in response to a desire to introduce 'improvement', in making services more responsive to patient need and professional development. Key lessons learned in relation to marketing and demonstrating impact are explored and practical tips provided to assist in addressing these issues. Although patient self-referral is focussed on, the issues highlighted are equally applicable to all models of service provision and for all professions.

The growth of autonomous AHP practice

Professional autonomy can be summarised as the freedom to practice independently of external controls. Practicing autonomously not only brings freedom of practice, but also both professional and personal responsibility with increased accountability for the management of patients.

For the last decade, healthcare policy throughout the UK has challenged the NHS to re-design themselves, be more patient-centred, innovative and responsive, focussing the locus of care away from hospital to community settings.[1, 2, 3] As a consequence, traditional roles, with doctors as gatekeepers to other services both in primary and secondary care, have also changed allowing greater autonomy and role extension for a range of professions including the AHPs. Improving access to services has also been a priority of policy. Prior to the 1990s, it was not uncommon for patients to have to wait for anything up to one year to be seen by a secondary care doctor and then experience another significant period of waiting to gain access to the most appropriate service for their problem. Rather than being a phenomenon, this was common in many AHP services throughout the UK.

Within this context, the 1990s saw the development of non-medically led services reported firstly within nursing services followed by patient self-referral to

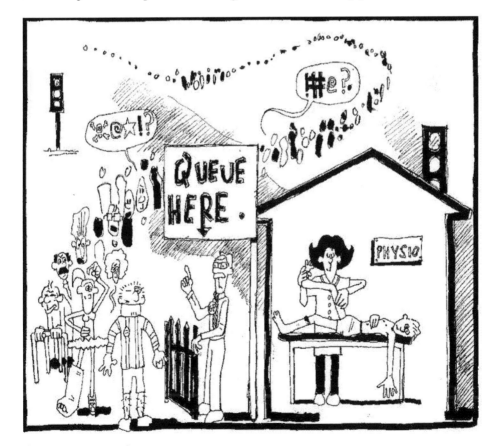

Figure 18.1 Queue here.

AHP services.[4, 5] The concept of patients accessing services without medical referral first is not new. Within physiotherapy for example, patients in the UK have been able to access services directly since 1978. This has often been on a privately funded basis through private practitioners, occupational health therapists and sports specialists. The same level of access, however, did not fully extend to the NHS where doctors continued to act as 'gatekeepers'.

What is meant by patient self-referral?

> A system of access that allows patients to refer themselves to a healthcare provider directly without having to see or be prompted by another healthcare practitioner. This relates to telephone, electronic technology or face to face services.

This definition was endorsed by the Chartered Society of Physiotherapy in 2006[6,7] and by other AHP leads in 2008.

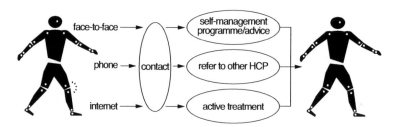

Figure 18.2 Patient contact.

The most recent UK Government health policies have reinforced the need to improve quality, achieve better, fairer access with increased flexibility, improved communication and reduced waiting times. They also emphasise that patient access and flexible provision are important strands of the modern NHS. This, together with a general growth in societal consumerism has greatly influenced how healthcare is provided. Patients are better informed about healthcare options and have greater expectations which they vocally express. It would appear that there is wide public support for easier access and particularly self-referral to a range of healthcare services. Public polls undertaken in 2003 and 2004 by Mori and YouGov reported over 88% of respondents would prefer to refer themselves to physiotherapy than attend their GP first.[6]

The efficacy of patient self-referral to physiotherapy services reported by a Scottish national trial provided the first documented evidence of the feasibility, safety and acceptability of such services to physiotherapy and other AHPs.[7, 8, 9, 10, 11, 12, 13, 14] More recently, in 2006, recognising this evidence and the potential that increased access to AHP services could bring, a DH policy document identified the need for formal consideration of self-referral services, particularly within therapy services in England.[1]

> Self-referral to therapist services has the potential to increase patient satisfaction and save valuable GP time. In order to provide better access to a wider range of services, we will pilot and evaluate self-referral to physiotherapy.[1]

In response, the DH established six pilot sites as well as holding AHP workshops to explore the wider relevance of self-referral. The results of this work were published in 2008[15] further commendation to self-referral was made in 'Framing the Contribution of Allied Health Professionals'.[16] These documents supported the findings from the Scottish work that patient self-referral to AHP services is:

- accessed by patients of all ages, both genders from all sectors of society and all geographical settings
- safe, clinically and cost effective
- supported by patients, staff and managers.

There are many examples a range of AHP services offering patient self-referral whereby patients re-refer themselves back for further treatment as their need dictates.

Private therapy practitioners worldwide have a long and successful track record of providing services to patients who refer themselves. They have developed approaches, processes and systems that ensure that patients are managed professionally, effectively and safely and there is much to learn from the experience of the private sector.

Experience shows that the two key determinants of successful implementation of self-referral are how services are marketed and impact is demonstrated. This is required internally to staff who provide the service as well as externally to:

- traditional referrers such as doctors and AHPs
- commissioners and healthcare managers
- public and patients, who it is hoped will access services in this way.

The pre-marketing phase

Marketing self-referral services

Before contemplating marketing any proposed changes in services, there are a number of 'internal' key considerations to be made and information to gather.

The internal focus

What's in a name? Anyone considering introducing service changes should think about how they call or refer to it. When the author first started introducing patient self-referral physiotherapy services in the mid 1990s, it was initially called 'direct access services' or 'Physiotherapy Direct'. A logical choice of name that quite transparently described what was being offered, that patients had direct access themselves, or did it? In 2003, the decision to stop using this term was made for a number of reasons.

As interest grew in the concept, other services started to emerge throughout the UK. Many called themselves 'Direct Access' services, but on closer examination, these proved to be very different in terms of how patients accessed them. The subsequent emergence of services that were fundamentally different, but referred to by the same name, was confusing to patients, the public and staff. This confounded attempts to compare the impact between sites. GPs, for example, often report that they already have direct access to a range of AHP services and from their perspectives, they do. This lack of clarity also extended to the policy makers who were unclear about what constituted a 'Direct Access' service. If confusing for those who provide or commission services, what must it be like for potential service users? When deciding what to name a service, think about it from the user's perspective. These services are now called 'patient self-referral' removing ambiguity, distinguishing them from the variety of other options available.

Top tips 1

- Ensure that whatever you decide to call your service, the title is a true reflection of what is being provided and consider the issue from a number of perspectives.
- It is important to apply consistent terminology to avoid confusion particularly for patients.
- Test your ideas out with a variety of 'audiences' including potential service users before making a definitive decision.
- Keep key messages simple and clear.

Intelligence gathering

Marketing or selling services successfully requires underpinning with local intelligence which involves gathering key information about the population and your service.

Knowing your population

Can you answer the following questions?

- The size of the population the service covers?
- What proportion of the population lives in urban, semi-rural or rural areas?
- The deprivation indices of each area?
- The gender, age and ethnic mix and if there is variability throughout the area?
- Whether the profile and size of population has changed during the last three years?

Why is this important?

The demand for healthcare provision differs throughout the country and within individual regions. The available evidence, however, relates mainly to medical services. Although there is no cause to believe that this should be any different for AHPs, information about these services is not as robust.

With regard to physiotherapy, the reported national trial of patient self-referral in Scotland identified that there were differences in the average number of referrals in locations that differed in terms of their geography, and to some extent, their levels of deprivation. Other work identified that in some settings, the demand for physiotherapy was directly linked to an increased older population, an issue that will be equally as appropriate to other AHPs.

Having up-to-date information about the local population makes predictions of potential outcomes much more relevant and credible.

Knowing your service

For the same reasons that it is important to know about the local population, it is advisable to have a thorough knowledge of the service.

Box 18.1 Are annual statistics/data available?

Can you answer the following questions?

1 What is the referral rate to your service; do you know how many new patients you see?
2 Can you express this as a proportion per 1000 of the population?
3 Can you provide an analysis of referral rates per individual site?
4 Can you provide a breakdown of exactly where all the new patients came from?
5 Do you know the referral sources – GPs, consultants, other referrers?
6 Do you know what investigations or drugs these new patients were prescribed?
7 Do you have a waiting list? If so, how long is it? Does it vary and if so to what extent?
8 Can you provide a breakdown of the profile of your patients? By age, gender, condition, number of contacts, outcomes.
9 Do you have patient employment and work absence statistics?
10 Do you know how many fail to attend for their first appointment or do not fully complete their treatment episode?
11 Do you know what happens to patients after they are discharged?
12 Do you know how many proceed for consultant referral, surgery, or other options?
13 What is the whole time equivalent staffing per treatment location?
14 Do you know exactly what your staffing establishment is – skill mix – expressed as whole time equivalents by grade?
15 Do you have full understanding of how your staff divide time between direct and non-direct patient care and other work?
16 How much treatment time is available, have you a capacity and demand plan?
17 Do you know how many student placements your service provides?
18 Do you have patient and stakeholder feedback about your service?

It cannot be emphasised strongly enough how important this information is. It will form the backbone of baseline data, which is vital to make any credible judgement of impact into the future.

Top tips 2

- Gather as much information as you can.
- Having some information is better than having no information.
- Consider a short prospective data collection project to assist with accurate baseline data.
- Baseline data is essential for future measurement and evaluation.
- Contact an information analyst in the organisation to support you in verifying the data.

Preparing the workforce

In order to be able to market your service, you need confidence in, and commitment from, staff who will be providing the service. Service development requires change and strong leadership. Patient self-referral requires AHPs to reflect and evaluate their practice critically and identify learning needs throughout the process. Staff providing new services need to be fully supported and involved in the development process. It should not be presumed that all therapists will enthusiastically embrace the concept of change to their practice. Good leadership will facilitate positive team working. With increased responsibility comes increased accountability. Some AHPs may feel wary of assuming a role when the perceived 'safety net' of screening traditionally undertaken by the referring doctor has not taken place. With no 'gate keeper', there is always the chance that potentially complex and inappropriate self-referrals may occur.

On qualification, AHPs are legally and professionally competent to accept patient self-referrals. However, it is essential that staff have the knowledge to recognise the breadth and depth of practice and expertise required. They also need confidence to deal with all aspects of patient management, including recognising when their professional expertise is not the most appropriate. In some instances, self-referring patients may be more demanding or more anxious, which could be challenging for some staff.

It is therefore imperative that time is taken to fully prepare staff prior to introducing any changes in service.

Top tips 3

- Support and encourage your staff.
- Take time to prepare them fully.
- Do not presume that all staff will happily move out of their 'comfort zone'.
- Address issues of accountability, responsibility and authority.
- Communicate at all levels.
- Identify your supporters and 'champions'.

Cautionary point

Staff who lack confidence or have misgivings about the development can not only undermine their own practice but may inadvertently convey these feelings to patients and colleagues with negative consequences.

The external focus

Making 'critical friends' is important during the vital planning stage, it is essential to find out what others think about the concept of introducing the change to the service. Why? You will need their support throughout but this may require cultivating some of these relationships.

Who are 'critical friends'?

Critical friends have the following characteristics in common:

- influence
- an interest in innovation

- are focussed on improving the patient experience
- meeting organisational objectives
- are fairly senior in the organisation.

Before meeting your 'critical friend' to discuss ideas, it is advisable to prepare a business case that clearly sets out items as shown in Box 18.2.

Box 18.2 Some items to include in the business case.

1 The overall rationale including the political and professional context
2 The evidence supporting patient self-referral, quoting key sources, the potential benefits for patient services and the organisation
3 Facts and figures about the local population and service be specific.
4 Include any resource implications identified. Include projections that not only relate to the service but the potential knock-on effects for other, such as potential reduction in investigations and drug prescribing
5 Include intentions with regard to evaluation and reporting
6 Cite sources of support gained already
7 Include the possible relevance and applicability that patient self-referral could have for other AHP services.
8 A carefully thought out and presented plan is normally well received

---

The direct marketing phase

Publicising the service change

Having a good idea about the proposed service change, how this change is communicated or 'marketed' to potential key stakeholders should be considered. For example, there is no point introducing changes to services that rely on patients referring themselves if they do not know they can actually do this. It is often useful to have a publicity and marketing strategy or documented plan of action.

If the intention is to introduce a change to service access and availability that potentially applies to the full local population, there are many options to publicise this. A marketing campaign could include all or some of the following.

Marketing options

1 **Posters.** Advertising service changes using posters allows information to be presented in an informative, eye catching manner. Points to bear in mind are:

- ensure that service users are involved in poster development – do not assume that they will understand your messages – ask them!
- not trying to put every piece of information about 'what you do' on a poster
- specify how the service can be accessed
- include information about professional registration status
- guide potential referrers to more detailed information such as additional leaflets in libraries, community centres, GP surgeries
- include key information as to what type of conditions would be appropriate for your service

- specify what kind of service is being provided, for example, if there are 'drop in' clinics or a telephone advice service
- include opening times and locations
- advise how patients can refer themselves or access the service
- give information about accessing referral forms if they are needed
- decide where the posters will be displayed
- enlist the help of a communications or marketing specialist to ensure your posters get noticed and that they are designed to catch the eye
- ensure resources are available to update and replace your posters as necessary
- ensure language requirements have been addressed.

2 **Leaflets.** Leaflets are a useful way of providing key information in a 'mobile' format. Potential users can take leaflets away with them and the information they contain can be accessed by more than one person, if the information is shared. Leaflet and poster design need to be consistent. Produce clear, simple leaflets which contain the same information as detailed above in the poster section.

Displaying posters and leaflets – the choice of location will depend on the target population. Consider the following:

- GP practices
- health clinics
- therapy departments
- accident and emergency departments
- community centres
- libraries
- leisure centres
- local shops.

Also target specific groups, for example; senior citizen groups, mother and toddler groups, sports groups, local condition specific voluntary groups.

Top tip 4

- Do not forget to inform healthcare staff know, word of mouth is still one of the most powerful publicity 'tools'.
- Place publicity materials in places where people go, think creatively.

An experience to learn from

One area advertised their patient self-referral service in local pubs, hotels and restaurants as well as the range of places identified above – they were surprisingly successful!

3 **Using the media.** Consider placing a feature in the local staff publication. Local press may also run a feature in their home and health or local news section. Local radio including hospital radio will reach a different audience.

4 **The 'world wide web'.** Where do patients find out about which private AHP healthcare practitioners there are in their area? Two of the most popular ways are the internet or telephone directory.

NHS services have not been very creative about publicising themselves. Try 'googling' your profession with 'NHS services' and the local area and see what comes up. The likelihood is that the answer will be 'not a lot!' Can anything be done to publicise your service on the web?

5 **Presentations.** Presentations to groups of healthcare providers, managers, patient groups and others are another way of providing information about changes to services.

Remember to ensure that the language you use in these types of presentations does not include technical or 'jargonised' terms or abbreviations; 'plain English' is needed. [17]

Targeting publicity

When introducing change in services to a section of the population, ensure that publicity is tailored to avoid confusion. This may require targeting patients directly via newsletters, leaflets or personal approaches.

Changing patterns of behaviour particularly longstanding ones does not happen overnight. It can take some time for people to adapt to changes in service delivery, in the case of patient self-referral to a range of healthcare services in the same way they currently do for dentistry.

- Seek the involvement of user groups, community groups and the public when developing publicity strategy. It should appeal to and be clearly understood by the intended population. Remember cultural differences may make messages inaccessible. So seek guidance on adapting parts of the strategy.
- Target the intended population appropriately.
- Remember to inform other healthcare providers.
- Think creatively about where publicity material is placed and renew regularly.

Publicising the service at launch

There is no point in advertising the new service until ready for launch. Premature publicity can cause frustration. Launch the publicity strategy at the same time as introducing the change. Although the response may be slow to start with it will allow for the opportunity to ensure that:

- the publicity is getting to the right 'audience'
- referral mechanisms are rigorous and efficient
- staff are prepared and confident in all aspects of the systems administration
- the approach to data collection and definition are appropriate and unambiguous
- arrangements for monitoring and reporting impact are in place.

Measuring and demonstrating impact

The importance of being able to demonstrate impact cannot be over emphasised. It needs to be carefully considered and proactively planned from the outset. Doing this well is reliant on the approach taken to measuring including the reliability, validity and robustness of the data used.

To survive in today's healthcare sector, services need to be able to demonstrate their clinical and cost effectiveness on an on-going basis. This is particularly so for newly introduced or re-designed services. Not only is this a professional requirement, it is also needed to provide assurance that standards of care are being met, that there are positive benefits for patients and services and that value for money is demonstrated. A rolling programme of impact planning, guideline implementation, clinical audit and patient and staff feedback should be integral to service re-design.

Traditionally, demonstrating impact has not been a strong point for most services. Consistently, AHPs have struggled with demonstrating what impact, if any is made on patient care. This means that in an environment where there is ever increasing competition for scarce resources, the inability to make a credible case severely hampers the ability to attract on-going or additional support.

Major effort needs to be put into planning how the impact of the service change will be monitored and demonstrated. It should include the impact on patients, AHP services, on referral sources and other services and how it meets organisational and national objectives.

Measuring impact

In order to demonstrate impact, measurement is required. Some parameters may be obvious, for example how many patients have self-referred in comparison with the baseline data. Other measures of impact are more complex or subtle but may prove to be very useful in the future.

Many organisations have objectives that are developed and reviewed regularly based on a combination of national, professional and local priorities. Having an Impact Plan allows the objectives of the organisation, service and profession to be 'pooled' into one working document that focusses effort. Bringing objectives together provides an overall view and helps to ensure that all perspectives are covered. It allows the key objectives that are directly relevant to the service and the change to the service specifically to be identified.

In compiling this list, it is advisable to explore all sources of information. Do not forget to think laterally and prospectively, for example, if one of the organisational objectives relates to waiting times to what are currently predominantly medical specialties, think about how introducing patient self-referral, could contribute, these may not have been previously considered. If there are objectives relating to the prescribing of drugs or specialist investigations, think about how the service could potentially offer a more cost and clinically effective alternative.

Top tip 5

- Link the service change to key organisational and service objectives.
- Think laterally, be creative.
- Review and update regularly.
- Exploit the 'expertise' of others.

Information collection

Having worked out what questions need to be asked, the next stage is to ensure that the correct data are being collected. Many services will already be collecting some of the data needed. There may be a requirement to review the overall data set and update it in light of the Impact Plan.

The agreed data set should allow collection of all the data needed for ongoing service monitoring and to demonstrate the impact of the development.

A copy of the data set and data definitions used in the national physiotherapy trial undertaken in Scotland can be found on the self referral web site,[18] although developed primarily for physiotherapy out-patient use, over 90% of the data items are relevant to all AHP services.

Top tips 6

- Establish accurate baseline data.
- Develop an agreed data set and definitions that can.
- Monitor the impact plan.
- Use validated and standardised definitions and scales.
- Ensure that all staff are proficient and 'signed up'.
- Pilot the dataset.

Utilising information to demonstrate impact

Information is knowledge and knowledge is power and powerful.

Two important reasons for having accurate information about any service are:

1 to monitor progress for internal use – identifying where improvements need to be made
2 to report impact to others – providing assurance of effectiveness.

Irrespective of how well a service is planned, if it does not meet the perceived or actual needs of its users, it will not succeed. The involvement of users is service development is recommended from the outset. Invite representatives to contribute to the design by sitting on steering and development groups.

Not only is it important to elicit the views of users but mechanisms should be identified to provide feedback to them so they know their views are both valued and acted on. One way of doing this is to develop a 'user' newsletter that can be handed to new service users to encourage their involvement. Consider setting up a user group as part of ongoing monitoring.

Feedback from staff is equally important at all stages. Make it clear that this is welcome and that their input is valued during all stages of development. Staff and patients will be your greatest critics as well as ambassadors.

Reporting impact results

Who is the 'audience?'

There can be significant benefits for services if they can:

- proactively engage with a wide range of stakeholders including patients. The wider involvement the better as some may not have previously appreciated the contribution the service can make

- demonstrate the impact of the results in terms that are relevant to the intended 'audience'. Remember to make their meet objectives. Providing a report that meets this purpose will be well received.

In addition to targeting information at individuals or teams, consider also adopting a general dissemination approach. Does the organisation have an annual report, newsletter or other means of communicating with staff, patients, other agencies and the public? It is also recommended to explore the implications of publishing the impact report via the world wide web to widen accessibility.

Remember to share good practice and successful implementation with a wide range of networks.

What should be reported?

The content of the report should vary according to the intended audience. This principle also applies to the frequency of reports. Be prepared to make reports on an interim basis, but particularly with regard to staff, so that they are kept informed and involved.

The chief executive of an organisation may be primarily concerned with demonstrating the extent to which the organisation is achieving Government targets. The report will need to emphasise the impact made on waiting times, efficiency of resource use and access. Other 'audiences', patient representative groups and others may be concerned with these issues therefore include outcomes that have meaning and are tangible to all, for example:

- convenience
- decreased work absence
- patient choice
- improved experience.

Ensure that patient centred impact measures and user views are included. This can be incredibly powerful. The majority of reports highlight positively experiences, it is also helpful to identify aspects that were not so well received and how these issues were rectified.

In order to meet the many and demanding challenges of modern healthcare, AHP services need to ensure that they value, consider and appropriately apply business approaches. Marketing and 'selling' your service is well worth the effort. Being able to demonstrate a services' impact is also necessary and when done skilfully reaps considerable benefits. These are the 'tools' that all AHP services need to use in order to gain support for, and confidence in, the services they provide for the benefit of patients.

Box 18.3 Useful websites.

Allied Health Professions: professional body website addresses.
- British Dietetic Association www.bda.uk.com
- Chartered Society of Physiotherapy www.csp.org.uk
- College of Occupational Therapists www.cot.org.uk
- Royal College of Speech and Language Therapists www.rcslt.org.uk
- Society of Chiropodists and Podiatrists www.feetforlife.org.uk

- The Association of Professional Music Therapists www.apmt.org.uk
- The British Association of Art Therapists www.baat.org.uk
- The British Association of Drama Therapists www.badth.org.uk
- The British and Irish Orthoptic Society www.orthoptics.org.uk
- The British Association of Prosthetics and Orthotists www.bapo.org.uk
- The Society and College of Radiograthers www.sor.org.uk
- Physiotherapy self-referral information www.selfreferralphysioinfo.com

Resource/Information Packs produced by each of the professional bodies are a great source for clarifying issues such as scope of practice, legal issues, etc. Most are available via the members' website.

References

1 Department of Health. *Our Health, Our Care, Our Say. A new direction for community services.* London: DH; 2006.

2 Scottish Executive. *Better Health, Better Care.* Edinburgh: Scottish Executive; 2007.

3 Welsh Assembly. *Designed for Life: creating a world class health and social care for Wales in the 21st century.* Cardiff: DH; 2005.

4 Dowling S. Nurses taking on Junior Doctors work: a confusion of accountability. *BMJ.* 1996; **312**: 1211–14.

5 Rayner C. Stuff and nonsense. *Nurs Standard.* 1999; **13(39)**: 22–3.

6 Chartered Society of Physiotherapy Annual Report. London: CSP; 2005.

7 Holdsworth L, Webster V. *Patient Self-referral: a guide for therapists.* Oxford: Radcliffe Publishing; 2006.

8 Ferguson A, Griffin E, Mulcahy C. Patient self-referral to physiotherapy in General Practice. A model for the new NHS? *Physiotherapy.* 1999; **85**: 13–20.

9 Holdsworth L, Webster V, McFadyen AK. Direct access to physiotherapy in primary care: now? – and into the future? *Physiotherapy.* 2004; **90(2)**: 64–72.

10 Holdsworth L, Webster V, McFadyen AK. Self-referral to physiotherapy. Deprivation and geographical setting: is there a relationship? Results of a national trial. *Physiotherapy.* 2006; **92**: 16–25.

11 Holdsworth L, Webster V, McFadyen AK. Are patients who refer themselves to physiotherapy different from those referred by GPs? Results of a national trial. *Physiotherapy.* 2006; **92**: 26–33.

12 Holdsworth L, Webster V, McFadyen AK. What are the costs to NHS Scotland of self-referral to physiotherapy? Results of a national trial. *Physiotherapy.* 2007; **93**: 3–11.

13 Webster V, Holdsworth L, McFadyen AK. Self-referral, access and physiotherapy: patients' knowledge and attitudes: results of a national trial. *Physiotherapy.* 2008; **94**: 141–9.

14 Holdsworth L, Webster V, McFadyen AK. Physiotherapist and General Practitioner views of self-referral and physiotherapy scope of practice: results from a national trial. *Physiotherapy.* 2008; **94**: 236–43.

15 Department of Health. *Self-referral Pilots to Musculoskeletal Physiotherapy and the Implications for Improving Access to Other AHP Services.* London: DH; 2008: www.dh.gov.uk/en/ Publicationsandstatistics/Publications/PublicationsPolicyAndGuidance/DH_089516.

16 Department of Health. *Framing the Contribution of Allied Health Professionals – delivering high-quality healthcare.* London: DH; 2008: www.dh.gov.uk/en/Publicationsandstatistics Publications/PublicationsPolicyAndGuidance/DH_089513.

17 www.plainenglish.co.uk.

18 www.selfreferralphysioinfo.com.

Chapter 19

Improving access to services: a practical approach to understanding demand and capacity to support service re-design

Zak Arif and Elizabeth Roberts

There is a wealth of knowledge available on improvement 'tools', techniques and methods. For example, information produced by the former NHS Modernisation Agency – good practice guides,[1] the NHS Institute for Innovation and Improvement,[2] and the 18 week programme.[3] Whilst the examples in this chapter relate largely to the AHP services the information and approach suggested can also be used or modified for other services.

This chapter provides an insight into practical approaches which can help improve access and performance, without being a definitive 'how to' guide. It provides helpful tips for consideration when embarking on local re-design initiatives.

Re-designing the service

To ensure the success of any re-design project it is crucial that all team members who need to be involved are included. It is important to include service users to obtain their views. There are clear benefits to adopting a team approach:

- ensures 'ownership' and clarification of the issues
- facilitates good communication
- identifies and collectively agrees the possible benefits.

A structured and systematic approach is required to guide the work to ensure that a whole system review is undertaken rather than 'cherry picking' which may miss some of the more difficult issues.

Five steps to successful re-design[4] provides a structured approach to service review and re-design. The time taken to complete re-design from start to finish is variable.

The present state

It is important to 'pinpoint' areas which may be contributing to unnecessary waits. Examine:

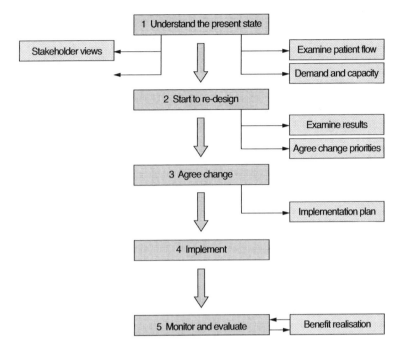

Figure 19.1 Five steps to successful re-design.

- views of staff working within the service to identify those areas which are performing well, but also where delays and poor access exist
- patient flow and how resources are managed throughout the pathway
- demand, waiting time data and how existing capacity is used.

Staff workshops

Workshops may be useful throughout the change process acting as a focus. They may generate work for smaller sub-groups but most importantly provide the momentum required to progress.

The workshop may commence by reviewing service achievements before moving on to explore the more difficult areas. It is easy to focus straight away on problems, which can be demoralising when faced with long waits, with some staff feeling overwhelmed leading to possible disengagement from the process.

It is useful to review the core purpose, to ensure that it is focussed on agreed objectives. Many services have 'drifted' into providing what they do, not in a planned way, but rather responding to various initiatives which contributes to loss of direction.

The next step is to discuss areas which give cause for concern. Workshop leads or facilitators play a vital role in ensuring that there is a healthy balance between time spent exposing areas of potential difficulty and exploring possible alternative solutions. Workshop findings must be recorded and summarised and then circulated to participants, as well as those not able to attend.

Some simple questions act as a prompt for further discussion, as set out in Box 19.1.

Box 19.1 Reviewing service core purpose – useful questions.

1 What is the strategy and purpose of the organisation?
2 Is the service aligned with this strategy?
3 What are the commissioners' purchasing intentions for the services?
4 What do service users and other stakeholders want from the service?
5 What needs to be provided?
6 Is there any service provision that can be stopped?
7 What are the main changes needed to align the service to organisational strategy?
8 What are the potential barriers to changes?
9 What benefits will these changes bring?

There are many useful 'tools' for guiding discussion, a popular one being the tried and tested Strengths, Weaknesses, Opportunities, and Threats. This is a simple tool which provides a straightforward structure which can be used at team or department level.

Editors' note

An in-depth discussion of the process of change management is presented in Chapter two of the third book in this series: *Key Topics in Healthcare Management – understanding the big picture.*[5]

Some reasons for poor access

Access and waiting times have been issues for the NHS since its inception. The 18 week programme[3] launched by the DH in 2006 to reduce waits – from the time of referral to first definitive consultant led treatment – by 2008, saw confidence grow in tackling long waits in England. Collection of waiting time data in a consistent way provides a picture of waiting times nationally and allows services to compare themselves with one another. Measuring service performance enables improvements to be made and together with a focus on quality, safety, user experiences and outcomes will collectively improve quality within services.

There are many reasons for waiting lists, but some of the most common are:

• demand exceeding capacity to treat
• inappropriate demand made by referrers
• lack of clear processes and agreed systems to handle referrals
• staff capacity and skills not used appropriately
• pressure on space and facilities.

Without a complete understanding of the demand for services and the capacity required to meet demand, service re-design will almost inevitably fail to have the outcome intended.

Box 19.2 Fixing the wrong problem.

The number of referrals has increased and the waiting list is growing.

Assumption: we do not have enough capacity to meet demand.

Proposed solution: more clinic sessions and extra staff to meet demand.

The real problem: an analysis of demand and capacity shows that there is sufficient capacity available to meet the needs of the patients being referred to the service and to tackle the waiting list. The main problem is lost time in clinic sessions – for example, due to DNAs, cancellations and poor scheduling. The problem is exacerbated by time lost by staff travelling between clinics because of the way they have been scheduled. Service re-design needs to focus on maximising patient contacts at each clinic and minimising unnecessary travel – the capacity may be there already but being wasted.

It is also essential to understand the flow of patients through the service before commencing service re-design initiatives associated with demand and capacity. A key objective of most service re-designs should be to improve the flow of patients through the system by more effectively matching capacity and demand.

It is easy to make incorrect assumptions about demand and capacity making attempts to tackle them unsuccessful. Some examples of such misconceptions are illustrated in Box 19.3.

Box 19.3 Common pitfalls in tackling demand and capacity.

- You only need to look at demand and capacity once
- If there is a problem with meeting demand, it is because we do not have enough capacity
- You cannot do anything about capacity – it is fixed and beyond control
- You cannot do anything about demand – referrals will just keep increasing
- You concentrate on demand and capacity and do not think about the flow of patients through the system to identify potential bottlenecks
- You assume demand and capacity issues only impacted on your service and do not consider constraints imposed by other services or involve them in identifying solutions
- You only think about one aspect of demand, for example, number of referrals, or one element of capacity, for example, number of staff rather than the broad spectrum of issues related to demand, capacity and flow
- Analysis of demand and capacity is based on poor quality information
- The analysis is focussed on process – clinical outcomes and quality standards are not included
- Unmet demand is not taken into account – service re-design can have an unexpected impact on demand which needs to be accounted for

---

Demand, capacity and patient flow

Understanding demand, capacity and patient flow is fundamental to improving the way every aspect of the service is delivered and should be central to all re-design projects.

Demand

> Demand = all the requests and/or referrals coming in to the service from all sources and the resources required to meet the needs of these.

Demand is inextricably linked with service provision it is not necessarily constant – it can vary from one time to another depending on the nature of the service. Much of the variation – and the approaches used to control it – will depend on where the service fits in care pathways, at what point patients are referred and who is referring. Demand is not uncontrollable or unmanageable – there are many things that can be done to more effectively manage and control it. This can be through initiatives, such as waiting list validation, improving communication or changing the way referrals are made.

Box 19.4 Useful information for demand management.

- Who – the range of individuals and organisations referring patients
- How many – the number of referrals received and how many are accepted
- Variation and trends – referral fluctuation, such as, day of week, time of year
- What is missing – what do you know about unmet demand
- What is changing – this can be about changes in referral practice

---

If demand is increasing and capacity is not aligned with this, then waiting lists may grow leading to referrer, patient and staff dissatisfaction.

Capacity

> Capacity = resources available to meet demand. Resources include financial, human, physical space, equipment and information, all of which are interdependent.

Capacity may not be constant over time. There are numerous reasons why services experience capacity gaps leading to problems in meeting demand for services. This may be due to shortfalls in resources but may also be caused by available capacity not being maximised.

Box 19.5 What limits capacity?

- DNAs and cancellations
- Inappropriate referrals
- Unnecessary follow-up appointments or delayed discharges
- Unnecessarily long appointments
- Patients not being discharged appropriately
- Inappropriate skill mix
- Insufficient staff
- Poor scheduling and appointments management
- Under-scheduling of clinic sessions
- Poor use of staff time

- Insufficient administrative support – wasting clinical time
- Missing or unavailable equipment or information
- Lack of clinic space or access to consulting rooms
- Delayed starts or early finishes in clinic sessions
- Duplication of effort collecting data
- Patients allocated to wrong members of staff

Patient flow

Patient flow = the movement of patients, information or equipment between departments, staff groups or organisations as part of their care pathway.

To improve patient flow, services need to address the systems and processes which create interruptions or delays.

In order to improve patient flows, it is necessary to process map, identifying 'bottlenecks' and their causes. It is important to ensure that any changes to the patient journey do not have a detrimental impact on quality of care or outcomes.

Box 19.6 What causes delay?

Process mapping will highlight many reasons for interruptions and delay to patient flow.
- Referrals waiting too long before being processed.
- Complex patient pathways which require movement of patients and staff between locations.
- Cancelled or rearranged appointments; waiting for equipment, drugs or specialist staff.
- Poor scheduling of appointments.

Mapping the whole 'pathway' will help identify opportunities for improvement; highlighting points of inefficiency, waste and variation. This generates ideas and helps teams to know where to start making improvements. There are a variety of approaches to process mapping. Which one is selected depends on:

- the detail of what you need to know
- resources and timescales
- engagement of staff.

When process mapping, look at the number of steps in each component to help streamline the pathway. Analysis often shows that a proportion of the process gives no added value; by identifying these elements the process can be shortened. The new pathway should be reviewed on an agreed timescale. It is important to include user views.

Box 19.7 Tips for pathway mapping for service improvement.

- Look at the journey from different perspectives – think about how patients move between staff and locations and how staff move between patients

- Use reliable data – the case for change must be robust
- Understand the expectations of service users
- Identify resources, including staff, finance, time, facilities
- Scrutinise possible causes of delay
- Keeping things simple – process mapping should be about simplifying patient journeys not making them more complicated

There are other 'tools' such as spaghetti diagrams – a method whereby a continuous line is used to represent the patient travelling through various services. It helps to identify inefficient process layouts and unnecessary travel distance between stages.

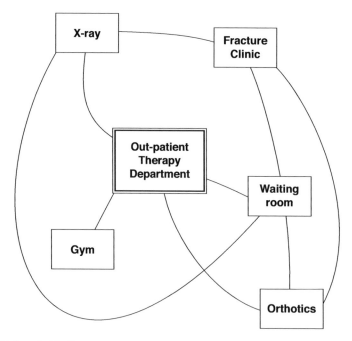

Figure 19.2 Spaghetti diagram.

Lean

Removing waste from the system is an important way of ensuring that effectiveness and efficiency are maximised. 'Lean' is the process of identifying and eliminating waste, and 'value' is determined by the customer.[6] The principles of 'Lean' are used widely in manufacturing industry[7, 8] and are equally applicable to healthcare.[9] Figure 19.3 shows five key principles of 'lean' methodology.

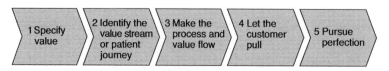

Figure 19.3 Lean methodology: five key principles.

> **Box 19.8 A checklist for process re-design.**
>
> 1   Understand key strengths and weaknesses
> 2   Understand the patient flow through our services
> 3   Understand what each step in the process is designed to achieve
> 4   Identify steps in the pathway that do not add value
> 5   Considered the pathway from patients' perspective
> 6   Involve relevant staff in the process
> 7   Identify improvements based on the patient flow analysis
> 8   Quantify patient flow

Examine referral processes

Service providers need to be clear about sources and volumes of referrals. Services operate a variety of referral mechanisms, including self-referral,[10] GP referral and consultant referral. Services need to define clear referral criteria. Lack of criteria may lead to unnecessary and inappropriate demand in turn leading to long waits.

Some commissioners and providers, in their quest to ensure that waiting time targets are met and resources used efficiently, have moved away from a system where referrals are received by individual services, to one where a centralised referral management centre receives all referrals. This system may be clinically inappropriate causing unnecessary waiting and delay.

> **Box 19.9 A checklist for referrals.**
>
> 1   Understand referral rates
> 2   Map the referral pathways
> 3   Identified areas for improvement
> 4   Make referral criteria clear evidence-based
> 5   Issue guidance on referral criteria
> 6   Communicated any changes to all stakeholders
> 7   Ensure training needs are met
> 8   Put in place monitoring and evaluation

Interview stakeholders

It is worthwhile undertaking discussions with stakeholders to identify:

• their perceptions of the service
• key issues
• ideas for change and development.

This interaction is best undertaken in the early stages of the review process as it provides focus and clarification of some of the issues. Information gathered must be carefully collated and used to provide feedback to the service. The process needs to be managed carefully to provide fair and accurate feedback.

> **Box 19.10 Opening questions for stakeholders.**
>
> 1 What is your role and how do you relate to the service?
> 2 What do you believe the service does best/worst and why?
> 3 If you have a question about the service where do you go to find the answer?
> 4 Do you know the current waiting times for the service?
> 5 What improvements do you feel need to be made and why?
> 6 Have you directly experienced receiving the service?
> 7 What were your impressions?
> 8 What interests you most about the service?
> 9 Would you recommend the service to others?

This is a powerful method for obtaining valuable, largely qualitative, information as well as inviting those closest to the service who may want to input. The whole process can be beneficial to inform future developments.

Experience from stakeholder interviews shows:

- a few minutes introductory explanation is time well spent
- stakeholders are usually keen to be involved and appreciate being included
- plan the questions carefully, ensuring relevance to stakeholder groups
- be prepared to adopt a flexible approach to the interview
- take note of qualitative comments or quotes which will help to bring home key messages
- quotes from patients are particularly powerful
- value contributors' time.

Principles of re-design

The adoption of a set of re-design principles will help provide a logical framework. Principles can be used to support planning and development and also to guide work streams which may have been established. Some examples are provided below but will need to be developed using local priorities.

- Service objectives:
  - clear service purpose and objectives to be in place.
- Improve access and reduce unnecessary waits:
  - services to be provided without delay
  - eliminate or reduce areas of waste
  - streamline pathways.
- Sustainable change informed by evidence:
  - good quality and safe services
  - clear entry and exit criteria
  - clear evidence-based assessment processes.
- Sustainable change informed by stakeholder views:
  - information availability to support users navigating the service.

It is often assumed that reducing delays and increasing access will increase cost. The opposite is often true: delays and restricted access are associated with poorly

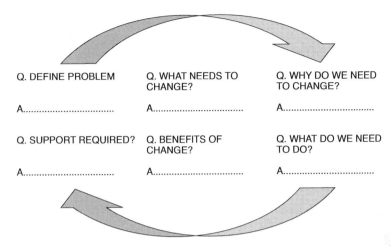

Figure 19.4 Framework for prioritisation.

designed, costly systems. The same changes that reduce delays can also reduce costs.

Each emerging priority needs to be examined. Teams can be established to work through specific issues for discussion, prior to decision-making on possible implementation or testing. A simple framework to assist teams may be helpful.

Instructive information

Set up comprehensive processes to collect, analyse and interpret relevant information and ensure it is processed into useful information, which can be used to support work on demand and capacity management.

- Identify and be clear about information needs and how the data is going to be collected.
- Agree definitions and standards for all data collected and ensure these are communicated to all staff.
- Check regularly that the standards are being maintained, by ongoing monitoring.
- Good data quality needs to be the responsibility of all members of staff.
- Information is needed on a wide range of aspects including for example, clinical outcomes, efficacy of service provision, throughputs, time use.
- Good quality data is comprehensive, timely, complete, consistent, accurate and meaningful.
- Work to reduce duplication of effort – ensure data is collected only once.
- Meet the information needs of service users, and stakeholders.

Objective outcomes

At the heart of service re-design projects, objectives should be related to improving clinical outcomes. Ensure the proposed changes impact positively on the health and experience of patients. Design pathways around outcomes and quality standards rather than these being secondary objectives.

Reasonable referrals

AHP services need to take a proactive approach to the way referrals are received and processed by their service to minimise the impact of unnecessary or incomplete referrals on patients and service delivery. These referrals could be:

1 patients referred inappropriately still need to be processed, however, the patient may never be seen and the referral is sent back to the referrer
2 patients referred with incomplete details about the reason for the referral may waste time when further information is required
3 patients referred with incorrect information may be allocated to an inappropriate clinician.

Scheduling

Investigate service scheduling to maximise capacity. Sessions which start late, finish early or have long periods without patients are wasteful. If this pattern is repeated on a regular basis, waiting lists will increase and patient satisfaction will fall. Every session needs to be scheduled to maximise the number of patients who can be seen and minimise the amount of time that is lost.

Making it happen

Clear action plans need to be put in place to guide implementation of the service re-design. There is a variety of ways in which this can be accomplished.

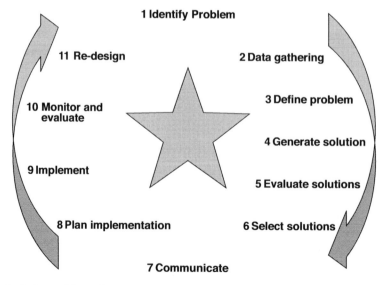

Figure 19.5 Control-loop for monitoring.

Table 19.1 Re-design simple action plan.

Lead:

Objective:
to streamline the pathway for paediatric services ensuring
clear and consistent processes across localities

Tasks:	Due date:	Completed:
Complete re-design of patient pathway identifying each element of service and identify actions	April	April
Identify administrative support required, time and skill mix	April – May	June
Complete validation of existing waiting list	On-going	On-going
Examine need for closure of cases to release clinical capacity and identify procedures to ensure appropriate discharge	Monthly	Monthly
Calculate the demand and capacity required	April – June	July
Review referral and discharge procedures	May	May
Identify training requirements	On-going	On-going

Outcomes:
Clear and streamlined processes in place
Release of clinical time for patient related activities
Clear relationship between demand and capacity required

Implementation plans can be developed simply and quickly, an example is
included in Table 19.1.

The implementation plan must be monitored carefully and adjusted in light of
evaluation. Plans need to be 'owned' and implemented by teams otherwise the
benefits of change may not be fully realised.

Monitor and evaluate

There is a danger that once implementation has started, monitoring takes a lower
priority. Regular monitoring of changes is essential to ensure that any problems
are recognised and rectified quickly. Test progress against the implementation
plan and desired outcomes. This 'control-loop' is a framework for monitoring.

References

1 NHS Modernisation Agency. *Improvement Leaders Guides*: www.institute.nhs.uk/
building_capability.
2 NHS Institute for Innovation and Improvement: www.nodelaysachiever.nhs.uk/
ServiceImprovement.
3 DH 18 weeks: www.18weeks.nhs.uk.
4 The Access Partnership. *5 Steps to successful re-design*: www.accesspartnership.co.uk.
5 Jones R, Jenkins F. *Key Topics in Healthcare Management – understanding the big picture*.
Oxford: Radcliffe Publishing; 2007.

6 Womak J, Jones D, Roos D. *The Machine That Changed the World*. New York: Rawson Associates; 1990.
7 Liker J. *The Toyota Way: 14 management principles from the world's greatest manufacturer*. New York: McGraw-Hill; 2004.
8 http://leanmanufacturingmadeeasy.com.
9 NHS Institute for Improvement and Innovation: www.institute.nhs.uk/building_capability/general/lean_thinking.html.
10 DH. *Self-referral Pilots to Musculoskeletal Physiotherapy and the Implications for Improving Access to Other AHP Services*: www.dh.gov.uk/en/Publicationsandstatistics/Publications/PublicationsPolicyAndGuidance/DH_089516.

Further reading

- AHP Services Information Handbook: www.18weeks.nhs.uk/Content.aspx?path=/achieve-and-sustain/AHP-services/information-management-handbook.
- AHP Services Pathway Improvement Tool: www.18weeks.nhs.uk/Content.aspx?path=/achieve-and-sustain/AHP-services/physiotherapy-tool.

Index